KINETICS
OF EXPERIMENTAL
TUMOUR PROCESSES

KINETICS
OF EXPERIMENTAL
TUMOUR PROCESSES

by

N. M. EMANUEL

Institute of Chemical Physics, Academy of Sciences of the USSR, Vorobyevskoye Chaussee 2B
Moscow V-334, USSR

PERGAMON PRESS

OXFORD · NEW YORK · TORONTO · SYDNEY · PARIS · FRANKFURT

U.K.	Pergamon Press Ltd., Headington Hill Hall, Oxford OX3 0BW, England
U.S.A.	Pergamon Press Inc., Maxwell House, Fairview Park, Elmsford, New York 10523, U.S.A.
CANADA	Pergamon Press Canada Ltd., Suite 104, 150 Consumers Rd., Willowdale, Ontario M2J 1P9, Canada
AUSTRALIA	Pergamon Press (Aust.) Pty. Ltd., P.O. Box 544, Potts Point, N.S.W. 2011, Australia
FRANCE	Pergamon Press SARL, 24 rue des Ecoles, 75240 Paris, Cedex 05, France
FEDERAL REPUBLIC OF GERMANY	Pergamon Press GmbH, 6242 Kronberg-Taunus, Hammerweg 6, Federal Republic of Germany

First English edition 1982

Library of Congress Cataloging in Publication Data

Emanuel, N. M. (Nikolai Markovich), 1915-
Kinetics of experimental tumour processes.
Translation of Kinetika eksperimental'nykh opukholev-ykh protsessov.
Includes index (es)
1. Oncology, Experimental. 2. Cancer cells—Growth.
3. Antineoplastic agents. 4. Dynamics.
RC267.E413   1982   616.99'407   81-17753
AACR2

British Library Cataloguing in Publication Data

Emanuel, N. M.
Kinetics of experimental tumour processes.
1. Tumours—Chemotherapy
2. Pharmacokinetics 3. Cytokinesis 4. Cancer cells
I. Title II. Kinetika eksperimental'nykh opukhlevylch protsessov. *English*
616.99'4061   RC270.8

ISBN 0-08-024909-4

This translation is based on the first Russian edition of *Kinetika eksperimental'nykh opukhlevylch protsessov* published by Isdatel' stvo 'Nauka'©1977.

In order to make this volume available as economically and as rapidly as possible the author's typescript has been reproduced in its original form. This method unfortunately has its typographical limitations but it is hoped that they in no way distract the reader.

Printed in Great Britain by A. Wheaton & Co. Ltd., Exeter

CONTENTS

FOREWORD TO THE ENGLISH EDITION

Cancer research has for a long time, and for various reasons, attracted the attention of chemists, physicians and mathematicians, but the greatest contributions have come from physicians and biologists.

In-depth studies of oncological problems in various scientific disciplines have acquired international importance.

In the USSR, investigations of kinetics and physico-chemical (especially free radical) mechanisms of carcinogenesis, tumour growth, and the molecular biology of chemotherapy, are very well developed. Advances have been made in techniques for objectively assessing cancer treatment statistically with the aid of computers. This research parallels that of the Chester Beatty Research Institute in London, the Paterson Research Laboratory at the Christie Hospital in Manchester and in many similar institutions.

This monograph was published in the USSR in 1977. In the following three years, Soviet research paid great attention to the fundamental principles of creating new effective antitumour drugs. The basic laws of pharmacokinetics, the mathematical investigations of the quantum kinetics of antitumour activity and drug structures, and the results of biochemical and biophysical investigations underlie these principles.

A survey of these investigations was presented in the author's lecture 'Physical, Biochemical and Biophysical Bases for Creation of New Effective Anticancer Agents' at the 28th Congress of the International Union of Pure and Applied Chemistry (IUPAC) in Helsinki in August 1979. The lecture was published in the journal *Pure and Applied Chemistry* and constitutes an addition to this monograph.

I hope that the publication of the English edition of the monograph will be welcomed by our colleagues and will assist our mutual efforts for the solution of the most important current problems in oncology.

Professor N. M. Emanuel
Member of the Academy of Science

FOREWORD

Clinical reactions are subject to the laws of kinetics and thus kinetic studies are of great importance in many fields of natural science. While physical kinetics and chemical kinetics have already become independent scientific fields, the kinetics of biological processes are less well understood. However, knowledge of molecular mechanisms and of the general quantitative principles of the development of biological processes with time is essential for further progress of biology and medicine.

In the past two decades this has become so obvious that mathematicians, physicists, chemists, biologists and physicians from many countries have joined forces to solve biological and medical problems.

Cancer is one of the most formidable problems of humanity; any advance here is of extreme importance. Systematic studies of the kinetic principles and molecular (mostly free radical) mechanisms of malignant growth, as well as the search for rational principles of approach to the creation of efficient anticancer drugs were started at the Institute of Chemical Physics in the USSR in 1957.

These problems are investigated now by a team of researchers at the Department of Kinetics of Chemical and Biological Processes in the Institute of Chemical Physics in the USSR.

Numerous studies on the kinetics and mechanisms of tumour growth have yielded results of theoretical and practical value. Several chemotherapeutic drugs proposed by this Department have been clinically effective.

This monograph develops the principles of the kinetics of experimental malignant growth. The molecular mechanisms of chemotherapy and certain problems of carcinogenesis and biochemistry are discussed.

The first chapter is theoretical. It introduces the notion of a true average kinetic curve for tumour growth and discusses the principles for obtaining experimental kinetic curves. Various analytical functions for the approximation of experimental kinetic curves are given. These functions are obtained by integration of the population growth equation under certain simple assumptions about the time dependence of the specific rate of growth. Attention is given to a large set of exponential and power functions, and Gompertz, Bertalanffy and logistic functions, the dependences for curves with an extremum (polynomial exponents), etc.

These dependences are widely used in describing kinetic curves that have to be
applied in experiments. Simple equations for the kinetic survival curves are also
given. The procedures of analytical functions by means of their linearization are
described. This section is included for convenience of readers in order to save
them from the need to resort to special handbooks on regression analysis.

A whole section is devoted to quantitative criteria used in estimating the effectiveness of antitumour drugs. Many are proposed for the first time. It is
expected that the use of these criteria in specific experimental research will
show the expediency and advantages of their application, in particular in standard-
izing the experiments conducted in different laboratories.

The second chapter contains experimental data on tumour growth from the USSR and
elsewhere. The general treatment of the experimental results and plots, using the
analytical functions given in the first chapter, is described. This seems to be
the first systematic survey of data on the kinetics of tumour growth. This chapter
contains valuable reference material on over 40 tumour models.

The third chapter deals with kinetic analysis of the results obtained by various
treatments of tumours (chemotherapy, surgery and combined treatment). Drug effectiveness is estimated with the same kinetic criterion — the effectiveness coefficient.

The fourth chapter is a survey of pharmacokinetic methods of major regularities
connected with general problems of cancer chemotherapy, in particular with kinetic
analysis of the behaviour of certain antitumour drugs in the body.

The molecular mechanisms of chemotherapy discussed in the fifth chapter are considered only from the standpoint of the biological action of the new antitumour
drugs developed at the Department of the Kinetics of Chemical and Biological
Processes of the Institute of Chemical Physics. These are inhibitors-antioxidants
(phenol compounds), alkylnitrosoureas and diazoketones. The alkylnitrosoureas are
of particular interest because of their interaction with nucleic acids. In studying the mechanism of the action of diazoketones, attention was paid to their
effect on biosynthesis. The inhibitors-antioxidants were considered in terms of
the free-radical mechanisms of their action.

In the last fifteen years the role of free radicals in the mechanisms of carcinogenesis and tumour growth have become one of the most important developing trends
in the biophysics of cancer; this field is still at the stage of phenomenological
description. The kinetic approach allowed the solution of many problems and
enabled the finding of certain general patterns (e.g. the change in content of
free radical species during the initial period of tumour growth, the step-wise
nature of changes in the free radical content during chemical carcinogenesis, etc.).
The limiting factor for the development of these studies is the absence of methods
for identification of the individual nature of paramagnetic species exhibiting EPR
signals. These problems are discussed in the sixth chapter.

The seventh chapter deals with the kinetic analysis of biochemical shifts occurring
in tumour tissues. It is suggested that knowledge of the quantitative kinetic
parameters characteristic of these shifts and of various therapeutic treatment
effects can help in developing methods of strictly controlled therapy.

The last chapter contains a survey of the present data on disturbance of structure
and biosynthesis of informational macromolecules occurring in tumour growth.
These are new fields for effective application of kinetic methods; their discussion in the monograph seems to be expedient.

The author wishes to thank his colleagues of the Department of Kinetics of Chemical and Biological Processes for their participation in the development of this new field of oncology — the physico-chemical study of cancer. The author also expresses his thanks to V.M. Andreev, G.N. Bogdanov, V.A. Gor'kov, N.P. Konovalova, V.I. Naidich, V.V. Suchchenko, L.S. Ter-Vartanyan, I.N. Todorov, O.K. Shiyataya for help in writing this monograph and also to V.N. Varfolomeev and L.P. Zaikova for preparation of the figures.

CHAPTER 1

THE KINETICS OF TUMOUR GROWTH

Theoretical and experimental studies of tumour growth and of the accompanying biochemical and biophysical changes are concerned with general patterns, the nature and mechanism of a process, the setting up of criteria for evaluation of the effectiveness of therapeutic drugs, and with a rational search for new principles in the prophylaxis, diagnosis, and medical treatment of cancer.

Kinetics, as a science, deals with the development of various (physical, chemical and biological) processes in time: it is of particular value for investigating these problems. Tumour growth progresses regularly in time; kinetic studies have become important in experimental and clinical oncology. A formal mathematical approach, the creation of tumour growth models and kinetic analysis of these results concerning the rules for development of malignant processes and the mechanisms of drug action are required. Mathematical description of the kinetic regularities yields numerous parameters that can be used to model these processes and computer techniques can be used to evaluate the vast amount of data generated.

1.   KINETIC CURVES

Kinetic curves are the most usual means of representing the results of kinetic studies. Besides the two definitions: 'kinetics' and 'kinetic curve', a general one, namely 'dynamics', is often used in biology and medicine.

A kinetic curve is a graphical representation of changes in a certain value, F, characteristic of the process development in time. This value denotes any measurable property of the system studied and the result of measurements is given as a numerical value corresponding to each fixed moment of time.

Values of a different mathematical nature are used in plotting kinetic curves. Certain values continuously change with time (are continuous time functions), others can change only discretely (discrete time functions). The volume, diameter, area or weight of a solid tumour can serve as an example of continuous time functions of tumour development. A discrete function is, for instance, the change in number, N, of tumour cells. It will obviously be represented by integer numbers only. Naturally, the discrete number of changes in N will be important only for low N values.

Kinetic studies of tumour growth and the effect of various drugs reveal a great diversity of kinetic functions (exponentially decreasing or increasing curves, curves which pass through a minimum or maximum, and curves going from minimum to maximum extremes). These graphs reflect the phenomena of tumour growth inhibition, regressions, recurrences, etc. Figure 1 presents kinetic curves obtained in the study of experimental tumour processes. The common S-shaped kinetic curve is taken as a standard and treatments giving different results are considered.

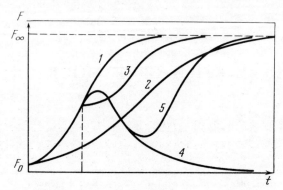

Fig. 1 Types of kinetic curves for tumour growth. 1 — Control; 2 — Inhibition after early therapy; 3-5 — Treatment of a developed process with inhibition effects (3), with complete (4) and partial (5) regressions; F — Tumour size (F_0 — initial, F_∞ — attainable limit).

Experimentally, kinetic curves are obtained by means of many data from a large number of animals. However, kinetic curves can be plotted for individual animals as well: the shape will then be prone to individual fluctuations during the experiment. Tumour growth in another animal will not give exactly the same kinetic curve, even if the experimental conditions are exactly the same. This lack of reproducibility cannot be helped; it is due to the variable proliferation of tumour cells: different animals are not genetically identical and their individual physiology can differ widely, resulting in large deviations from mean values.

Figure 2 presents kinetic curves for individual animals. These curves show the random nature of tumour growth. Each point in an individual kinetic curve is defined by its time coordinate, t, and a relevant value, F, characteristic of tumour growth. All kinetic curves have a natural original point (0, F_0) corresponding to an initial F value at the time of tumour transplantation when $t = 0$. Each individual curve also has its final point (τ, F_τ) at the death of the animal. Death can be caused by the tumour, as a result of toxic therapy, or old age in cases of successful chemotherapy. Therefore a group of animals must be used for the study of tumour growth. Tumour models are amenable techniques for use in large groups of animals; the results are reproducible and are suitable for statistical analysis. Mathematical models help in planning experiments and analyzing the data obtained (Kramer, 1948; Nalimov, 1971; Malenvo, 1975).

The theory of random processes helps to construct the model (Prokhorov and Rozanov, 1973; Feller, 1967; Grenander, 1961). We may imagine an infinite number of all potentially possible kinetic curves for tumour growth. Each of these curves is denoted by ω so that the functions $F(t)$ and the set Ω of all ω have the same value. Each curve originates at a point (0, $F_{0\omega}$) and ends at a point (τ_ω, $F_{\tau\omega}$). Let the subset B in set Ω be probability $P\{B\}$.

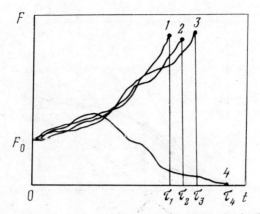

Fig. 2 Examples of kinetic curves for tumour growth in individual animals. 1-3 — Control; 4 — Regression as a result of treatment; τ_i ($i = 1, 2, 3, 4$) — time of death.

Denote by Ω_t the set of all ω that correspond to curve F_ω still present to the time t, i.e. those for which $\tau_\omega \geq t$. It will be seen that $P\{\Omega_t\}$ is the probability of survival at time t. This probability $v(t)$ is:

$$v(t) = P\{\Omega_t\} \tag{1}$$

The curve $v(t)$ is the true survival curve. Obviously $v(0) = 1$, and $v(\infty) = 0$. Consider two procedures of averaging the individual kinetic curves.

1. Introduce the notion 'true average kinetic curve' $\mu(t)$. Define $\mu(t)$ for each moment of time as the mathematical expectation of the value F_ω

$$\mu(t) = MF_\omega(t) = \int_{\Omega_t} F_\omega(t) \frac{P\{d\omega\}}{P\{\Omega_t\}} = \int_{\Omega_t} F_\omega(t) \frac{P\{d\omega\}}{v(t)}, \tag{2}$$

where M is the mathematical expectation symbol, and integration is made over set Ω_t.

Another equivalent expresssion can also be given for curve $\mu(t)$. Estimate for any t the distribution function of the random value F as the probability that $F_\omega(t) \leq F$. Then

$$P_t(F) = P\{F_\omega(t) \leq F\} = \int \frac{P\{d\omega\}}{P\{\Omega_t\}}, \tag{3}$$

with integration over the set of all $\omega \in \Omega_t$ such that $F_\omega(t) \leq F$. The equation

$$\mu(t) = \int_{-\infty}^{+\infty} F dP_t(F) \tag{4}$$

is then valid. The true dispersion of F is defined as

$$\sigma_t^2 = M[F - \mu(t)]^2 = \int_{-\infty}^{+\infty} [F - \mu(t)]^2 dP_t(F).$$

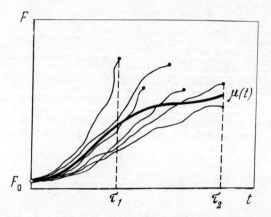

Fig. 3 Plotting of kinetic curves for $\mu(t)$ from the mean
arithmetic values of F.

Figure 3 shows the position of curve $\mu(t)$ in the set of individual curves $F_\omega(t)$.

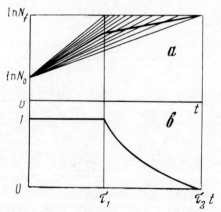

Fig. 4 Averaging of kinetic curves for exponentially growing
tumours (a) and the relevant survival curve (b).

Take a simple example of the definitions (1-4) (Fig. 4a). Assume an entity of
animals each having a number of tumour cells increasing strictly exponentially,
$N = N_0 \exp(\phi t)$. The same number of tumour cells, N_0, has been transplanted to all
animals at $t = 0$. Let the exponential factor differ for different animals, the
possible values ϕ being distributed uniformly in the order $\phi_1 \leq \phi \leq \phi_2$.

Assume that the death of animals occurs at a certain value $N = N_f$, independently of
ϕ. For this case index ω can be identified with the value ϕ. F_ϕ will be chosen as

$$F_\phi = \ln N = \ln [N_0 \exp(\phi t)] = \phi t + \ln N_0.$$

Every individual curve is plotted only up to time

$$\tau_\phi = \frac{1}{\phi} \ln (N_f/N_0).$$

The probability that ϕ will fall within the range $(\phi, \phi + d\phi)$ is:

(1) at $\phi < \phi_1$ $P\{d\phi\} = 0;$

(2) at $\phi_1 < \phi < \phi_2$ $P\{d\phi\} = \dfrac{d\phi}{(\phi_2 - \phi_1)}$;

(3) at $\phi > \phi_2$ $P\{d\phi\} = 0.$

Over the time range

$$0 \le t \le \tau_1 = \frac{1}{\phi_2} \ln \frac{N_f}{N_0}$$

all F_ϕ curves are defined. Consequently Ω_t coincides here with the whole range $\phi_1 \le \phi \le \phi_2$, and thus $P\{\Omega_t\} = 1$. Over the time range

$$\tau_1 \le t \le \tau_2 = \frac{1}{\phi_1} \ln \frac{N_f}{N_0}$$

only a part of the curves is defined. Here Ω_t coincides with the range

$$\phi_1 \le \phi \le \frac{1}{t} \ln \frac{N_f}{N_0}$$

and therefore

$$P\{\Omega_t\} = \frac{1}{\phi_2 - \phi_1} \left(\frac{1}{t} \ln \frac{N_f}{N_0} - \phi_1 \right).$$

The kinetic curves are not defined for $t > \tau_2$, and here $P\{\Omega_t\} = 0$.

Thus the survival curve $v(t)$ plotted using Eq. (1) consists of three segments of different analytical shapes (see Fig. 4b). Its descent represents an hyperbola.

Calculate (t) by Eq. (2). At $0 \le t \le \tau_1$,

$$\mu(t) = \int_{\phi_1}^{\phi_2} (\phi t + \ln N_0) \frac{d\phi}{\phi_2 - \phi_1} = \frac{\phi_1 + \phi_2}{2} t + \ln N_0$$

At $\tau_1 \le t \le \tau_2$,

$$\mu(t) = \int_{\phi_1}^{\frac{1}{t} \ln (N_f/N_0)} (\phi t + \ln N_0) - \frac{d\phi}{\phi_2 - \phi_1} \cdot \frac{\phi_2 - \phi_1}{\frac{1}{t} \ln \frac{N_f}{N_0} - \phi_1}$$

$$= \frac{1}{2} \left(\phi_1 t + \ln \frac{N_f}{N_0} \right) + \ln N_0.$$

At $t > \tau_2$, $\mu(t)$ is not evaluated.

Thus $\mu(t)$ represents a broken line consisting of two straight segments, though all individual $F_\phi(t)$ represent straight lines. This example suggests that generally the shape of the curve $\mu(t)$ will probably be very different from the shapes of individual curves $F_\omega(t)$ over the time range corresponding to the death of the animals. The curves for $\mu(t)$ and individual $F_\omega(t)$ certainly can differ not only in the death section, but also throughout the range of tumour growth. An example of this can be found in Comfort (1965).

Now calculate $P_t(F)$, using the definitions

$$F_1(t) = \phi_1 t + \ln N_0,$$
$$F_2(t) = \phi_2 t + \ln N_0.$$

Eq. (3) yields the expressions for $0 \le t \le \tau_1$

$$P_t(F) = \begin{cases} 0 \\ \dfrac{F - F_1(t)}{F_2(t) - F_2(t)} \\ 1 \end{cases} \quad \begin{array}{l} \text{for } F \le F_1(t) \\ \text{for } F_1(t) \le F \le F_2(t) \\ \text{for } F \ge F_2(t) \end{array}$$

and at $\tau_1 \le t \le \tau_2$

$$P_t(F) = \begin{cases} 0 \\ \dfrac{F - F_1(t)}{\ln N_f - F_1(t)} \\ 1 \end{cases} \quad \begin{array}{l} \text{for } F \le F_1(t) \\ \text{for } F_1(t) \le F \le \ln N_f \\ \text{for } F \ge \ln N_f \end{array}$$

The function $P_t(F)$ is not determined for $t > \tau_2$.

The $P_t(F)$ probability distributions enable calculation of $\mu(t)$ using Eq. (4). The function obtained coincides with $\mu(t)$ calculated by Eq. (2).

A more satisfactory model of tumour cell population growth is the 'branching process', or the process of 'birth-death', It starts with a number, $N = N_0$, of tumour cells and is characterized by parameters representing the probabilities of division and decay of a cell in unit time. Such a model can provide a precise solution (Prokhorov and Rozanov, 1973; Feller, 1967; Beili, 1970; Bartlett, 1958; Karlin, 1971; Harris, T.E., 1963). At high N values, N can be considered as continuously changing with time. The process 'birth-death' then becomes a 'diffusion process' (Venttsel, 1975). The theory of diffusion processes is well developed (Ito and McKean, 1965).

The 'birth-death' models are representative of the kinetic patterns of population growth of pathogenic micro-organisms in animals where growth begins with a small number of cells (Shortley and Wilkins, 1965). In certain cases these models might also be used to represent tumour growth kinetics. The practical value of these and other detailed mathematical models in experimental oncology depends on how well they represent the factors controlling tumour growth. The most important of these factors are:

(a) The heterogeneity of the tumour cell population which is more like a series of interacting subpopulations with different biological properties. This hetero-geneity can increase with tumour growth due to the appearance of mutant cells, metastases, etc.

(b) The lack of synchrony of internal physiology of different cells, even in a uniform subpopulation.

(c) The necessity of allowing for the time-dependent interaction of tumour cells with host systems responsible for feeding the tumour, systems creating anti-tumour immunity (specific and nonspecific), and systems controlling the prolif-eration of normal cells.

Examples of mathematical population growth models allowing for such factors can be found in ecology, demography, and the theory of evolution (Moran, 1962; Eigen, 1973; Crow and Kimura, 1970). However, the creation of mathematical models for tumour growth that would find wide application and would adequately reflect the proliferation mechanisms of tumour cells needs further investigation.

2. Take a group of individual kinetic curves (Figure 5b) that were presented earlier in Figure 3. Every curve terminates at a time τ_ω corresponding to the death of the animal. However, these curves can be rearranged in such a way that a fraction of an individual animal life-span after tumour transplantation $\theta = t/\tau_\omega$ would be chosen as an independent dimensionless variable. Then all kinetic curves will originate at $\theta = 0$ and terminate at $0 - 1$. As a result of this procedure the curves will transform as shown in Figure 5a. We can now define the true average kinetic curve for the set of curves in Figure 5a as the curve for mathematical expectation of F for each θ:

$$\mu(\theta) = M(F) = \int_\Omega F_\omega(\theta) P(d\omega)$$

To define the true average life-span of animals as the mathematical expectation of individual life-span τ_ω:

$$\tau = \int_\Omega \tau_\omega P(d\omega)$$

Let function $\mu(\theta)$ correspond to the time $t = \theta\tau$. Thus the true average kinetic curve will be defined as the function $\mu = \mu(t/\tau)$ that terminates at $t = \tau$ (Fig. 5b).

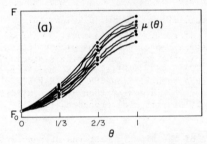 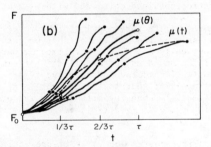

Fig. 5 Plotting the mean kinetic curve for time
relative to the animal's life-span

Consider the example of a family of semilogarithmic anamorphoses of the exponential kinetic curves in Figure 4. The curve for mathematical expectation (the semi-logarithmic anamorphosis of the true average kinetic curve) will then be a straight line instead of a broken line within the range $t = 0$ to $t = \tau$, i.e. to the mean lifespan of tumour-bearing animals (compare the straight line 2 with the broken line 1 in Figure 6a). Passing from semilogarithmic anamorphoses to kinetic curves we obtain accordingly two types (3 and 4) of mathematical expectation curves (Figure 6b). With both averaging procedures the kinetic curves virtually coincide up to time $t = \tau_1$ (time of death of the first animal) and then the curves diverge. This divergence might appear to be immaterial, if the time interval between τ_1 and τ_2 (death time of the last animal) is small.

At the same time it will be noted that curve 4 belongs to the same family of curves as do the individual kinetic curves, and in this sense it describes better than curve 3 the tumour growth kinetics, just as does the curve $\mu(\theta)$ in Fig. 5b.

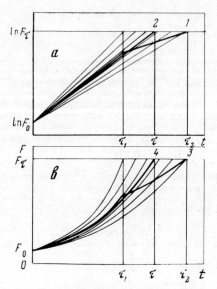

Fig. 6   Comparison of two averaging procedures
for exponential kinetic curves

2.   EXPERIMENTAL POINT AND THE EXPERIMENTAL
KINETIC CURVE

In practice the individual kinetic curve $F_j(t)$ referring to an animal with index
j is recorded not in full, but only for a finite number of points or only for one
point if measurement necessitates slaughter of the animal.   Thus the experimental
data obtained for a group of Q animals represent a set of n separate measurements
of F made at various m times.   These measurements are represented in Table 1.

TABLE 1   Sample of Experimental Data

Time of measurement	Index j					Number of measurement
	1	2 ...	j	...	Q	
t_1	F_{11}	F_{12} ...	F_{1j}	...	F_{1Q}	n_1
t_2	F_{21}	F_{22} ...	F_{2j}	...	F_{2Q}	n_2
...	...	... ...	...	... ...		...
t_i	F_{i1}	F_{i2} ...	F_{ij}	...	F_{iQ}	n_i
...	...	... ...	...	... ...		...
t_m	F_{m1}	F_{m2} ...	F_{mj}	...	F_{mQ}	n_m
Number of measurement	ν_1	ν_2 ...	ν_j	...	ν_Q	n

Certain F_{ij} values may be absent if relevant measurements were not made.   The
number of all measurements is

$$n = \sum_{j=1}^{Q} \nu_j = \sum_{i=1}^{m} n_i .$$

The pairs of numbers (t_i, F_{ij}) that can be plotted in co-ordinates (t,F) are referred to as experimental points. The times t_i must not be considered as random, since they are usually fixed by the investigators, whereas F_{ij} represent random values.

Generally, the values F_{ij} representing measurements for the same animal j made at various times t_i are stochastically dependent. The value F_{ij} for the same time t_i can be considered as stochastically independent, as measurements refer to different animals.

As stated before, the probability distribution for the random value F_{t_i} is $P_{t_i}(F)$. The distribution $P_{t_i}(F)$ is characterized first of all by its mathematical expectation $\mu(t_i)$ and by dispersion δ_i^2. The following sample characteristics are calculated to estimate these values:

1) Sample means

$$\overline{F}_i = \frac{1}{n_i} \sum_{j=1}^{n_i} F_{ij}$$

that can serve as estimates for $\mu(t_i)$, since $M F_i = \mu(t_i)$;

2) Sample dispersions

$$S_i^2 = \frac{1}{n_i - 1} \sum_{j=1}^{n_i} (F_{ij} - \overline{F}_i)^2$$

and the corresponding root-mean-square deviation $S_i = \sqrt{S_i^2}$. The values S_i can serve as estimates for δ_i^2, since $M S_i^2 = \delta_i^2$.

3) Root-mean-square deviations of the sample means $S_{\overline{F}_2} = S_i / (n_i)^{\frac{1}{2}}$. The mean experimental points (t_i, F_i) together with the intervals $\pm S_{\overline{F}_i}$ can be plotted (Figure 7a). These intervals determine the scope of deviations of the sample means $\overline{F}_i$ from the true averages $\mu(t_i)$.

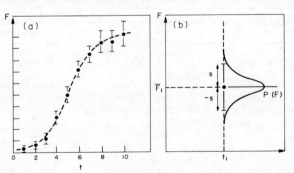

Fig. 7 Experimental kinetic curve (a) and the mean experimental point (b). S — mean quadratic equation; $P(F)$ — distribution density of experimental points.

It can often be considered that the distribution of values $\overline{F}_i$ is normal and in this case the probabilistic deviations of $\overline{F}_i$ from $\mu(t_i)$ can be estimated by plotting a reliable interval using the Student's t-distribution (Beili, 1970; Khald, 1956; Bolshev and Smirnov, 1965). In practice the Student distribution can be used in two cases:

1)   at high n_i (it is virtually sufficient in practice that $n_i \geq 30$) the distribution of $\overline{F}_i$ will be approximately normal, with mathematical expectation $\mu(t_i)$ and dispersion $\delta_i{}^2/n_i$, whatever the F_{t_i} distribution;

2)   if the F_{t_i} distribution can be assumed to be normal, then the distribution of $\overline{F}_i$ will also be normal.

A certain hypothesis must be chosen in studying the type of distribution $P_t(f)$. The distribution can be assumed to be normal, log-normal, or some other type. The consistency can be checked by comparing the obtained results with those expected from the hypothesis. Use can be made of χ^2, Kolmogorov-Smirnov, Reigni, or other criteria (Khald, 1956; Bolshev and Smirnov, 1965; Owen, 1962). The hypothesis of normal distribution can be checked using the criterion of absolute mean deviation (d), the asymmetry coefficient criterion (g_1) (Bolshev and Smirnov, 1965), as well as the graphical, but purely qualitative probit analysis which entails discovering whether the sample distribution plot on 'probabilistic paper' straightens (Khald, 1956; Meinell and Meinell, 1967).

The experimental kinetic curve is often drawn by hand from plotted points of the experimental data, but this graph is not totally objective. A more scientifically satisfying result is obtained by first deciding the shape of the curve and then plotting the time function afterwards. This would involve finding the function $F(t)$ — the best approximation to the true mean kinetic curve $\mu(t)$ — and evaluating the probable deviation of $F(t)$ from $\mu(t)$. The curve $F(t)$ represents the mean experimental kinetic curve: this is plotted by regression analysis; the curve $F(t)$ is referred to as the curve for regression of the random value F relative to t.

Regression analysis is conducted using a standard program. Choice is made of a family of functions:

$$F = F(t; a_1, a_2, \ldots a_g)$$

of a certain analytical shape and depending on parameters a_1, a_2, ..., a_g that can have various numerical values. A hypothesis that the true average kinetic curve $\mu(t)$ is among the function of the chosen family is accepted. In this case there must exist true, though unknown, parameters $a_1 = \alpha_1$, $a_2 = \alpha_2$, ..., $a_g = \alpha_g$ for which the equation

$$\mu(t) = F(t; \alpha_1, \alpha_2, \ldots, \alpha_g)$$

holds. Then a function showing the best fit with the sample is chosen from the family $F(t; a_1, \ldots, a_g)$. As a rule, the least squares procedure is used for optimization, i.e. one finds parameters $\hat{a}_1$, $\hat{a}_2$, ..., $\hat{a}_g$ to give the smallest sum of weighted deviations squares

$$S(a_1, a_2, \ldots, a_g) = \sum_{i=1}^{m} w_i [\overline{F}_i - F(t_i; a_1, a_2, \ldots, a_g)]^2$$

The weights w_i depend on dispersions $\delta_i{}^2$ and on numbers n_i. The estimates of $\hat{a}_1$, ..., $\hat{a}_g$ are assumed to be the best approximations to the true parameter a_1, ..., a_g. The regression curve

$$F = F(t; \hat{a}_1, \hat{a}_2, \ldots, \hat{a}_g)$$

is considered as the best approximation to the true average kinetic curve $\mu(t)$.

Such an estimation is reliable only if all random F_{ij} are stochastically independent. This is only true when one animal represents one point in the sample. If several sample points refer to the same tumour at different times, certain F_{ij} might appear to be stochastically dependent. If there is stochastic dependence, the calculation of estimates becomes more complicated. Regression procedures that can be used in such cases have been described (Malenvo, 1975, 1976;   Khennan, 1964, 1974;   Box and Jenkins, 1970;   Plackett, 1960). They will not be considered here and we will assume that all F_{ij} are stochastically independent.

The last stage of regression analysis is the evaluation of the fit of the regression curve and the sample. Now, if the original hypothesis about the analytical shape of $\mu(t)$ is rejected, some other hypothesis about it has to be made.

If the original hypothesis is not rejected, probable deviations of the estimating values $\hat{a}_1$, $\hat{a}_2$, ..., $\hat{a}_g$ from the true values α_1, α_2, ..., α_g have to be calculated and the reliable zone for the true curve $\mu(t)$ must be found.

3.   FUNCTIONS USED IN THE DESCRIPTION OF TUMOUR GROWTH

The deterministic population growth models of cells and living bodies (Williamson, 1975; Watt, 1968; Romanovskii *et al.*, 1975; Pechurkin and Terskov, 1975; Bertalanffi, 1960) are commonly used to determine the shape of the analytical kinetic curve: the regression curve $F = F(t; a_1, a_2, ..., a_g)$. The differential equation for population growth can be written as

$$\frac{1}{F} \frac{dF}{dt} = \phi(t), \tag{5}$$

where $\phi(t) = \phi_1(t) - \phi_2(t)$.

The value

$$\frac{1}{F} \frac{dF}{dt}$$

is known as the specific rate of growth. Function $\phi_1(t) \geq 0$ characterizes the overall rate of cell proliferation; function $\phi_2(t) \geq 0$ the overall rate of their decay. These values allow also for tumour cell transport factors. The function $\phi(t)$ may be both positive and negative.

The differential equation is

$$F = F_0 \exp \left[\int \phi(t) \, dt \right].$$

We require deterministic models of tumour growth to give the appropriate functions $\phi(t)$. The most commonly used models are:

1. An exponential dependence is obtained when ϕ = const. Integration of Eq. (5) then gives

$$F = F_0 \exp (\phi t). \tag{6}$$

2. An exponential function with a constant additive term

$$F = F_0 \exp (at) + F_1 \tag{7}$$

will be a solution to Eq. (5) when $\phi = 1/[1/a + c \exp(-at)]$.

The exponential law with $\phi = \text{const}$ usually holds at the first stage of growth of the transplanted tumour: this stage may be more or less prolonged. In later stages of tumour development the growth rate usually becomes less and various decreasing functions $\phi(t)$ will also be considered hereafter.

3. A power function is obtained when $\phi(t) = b/(t + a)$. In this case integration of Eq. (5) gives

$$F = F_0(1 + t/a)^b. \tag{8}$$

When $t \ll a$, $F = F_0 \exp(t/a)$, i.e. the growth can be considered to be exponential. At $t \gg a$ $F \simeq F_0(t/a)^b$, i.e. this will be maximum growth.

It will be noted that the specific growth rate can be expressed not only as $\phi(t)$. but also as $f(F)$, in a manner conventional for kinetic equations used in ecology or in chemical kinetics. For instance, in the case considered, function (8) satisfies also the equation

$$\frac{1}{F}\frac{dF}{dt} = \left(\frac{b}{a}F_0^{1/b}\right)F^{-1/b} .$$

4. When $\phi(t) = b/(t + a) - c$, solution of the differential equation (5) gives

$$F = F_0(1 + t/a)^b \exp(-ct). \tag{9}$$

This function describes curves with an origin at zero. It is seen that as $t \to \infty$, the value $F \to 0$. This function is valid for description of tumour regression processes. Transformation of the differential equation (5) to the form

$$\frac{1}{F}\frac{dF}{dt} = f(F)$$

in elementary functions is impossible here.

5. The Gompertz function is obtained by integration of Eq. (5) at $\phi(t) = ab \exp(-bt)$

$$F = F_0 \exp[a(1 - e^{-bt})] = F_\infty \exp(-ae^{-bt}), \tag{10}$$

where $F_\infty = F_0 \exp(a)$.

When $a > 0$, $b > 0$, the function $F(t)$ is a monotonically ascending S-shaped curve. At low $t(bt \ll 1)$, $F \simeq F \exp(abt)$, i.e. the function is near-exponential. At $t \to \infty$ the value $F \to F_\infty$. When $a < 0$, $b < 0$, the function $F(t)$ decreases monotonically, fairly approximating, for instance, the distribution of human population lifespans. Such a mortality law was first found by Gompertz in 1825 (Streler, 1964; Gompertz, 1825) and the dependence (10) is referred to accordingly as the Gompertz function at any a,b parameters.

A logistic function is obtained when $\phi(t) = b/[1 + \exp(bt)/a]$, $(a > 0, b > 0)$. The solution of Eq. (5) yields in this case

$$F = F_0\frac{1 + a}{1 + a \exp(-bt)} = \frac{F_\infty}{1 + a \exp(-bt)} \tag{11}$$

where $F_\infty = F_0(1 + a)$. This is an S-shaped curve with an asymptote $F = F_\infty$.

The differential equation for $F(t)$ can be transformed as

$$\frac{dF}{dt} = \frac{b}{F_0} (F_\infty - F) = \phi (F_\infty - F) F, \tag{12}$$

where $\phi = b/F_0$.

The expression (12) is used in chemical kinetics for analysis of autocatalytic processes.

7. When $\phi(t) = b \exp(-bt)/[1/a - \exp(-bt)]$, integration of Eq. (5) yields the Bertalanffi function (Bertalanffi, 1960)

$$F = F_\infty [1 - a \exp(-bt)]. \tag{13}$$

8. For a general case, over a restricted time range, function $\phi(t)$ can be considered to be a polynomial:

$$\phi(t) = \phi_0 + \phi_1 t + \ldots + \phi_s t^s. \tag{14}$$

The solution of the differential tumour growth equation takes then the form of a polynomial exponent:

$$F = F_0 \exp \left\{ \phi_0 t + \tfrac{1}{2}\phi_1 t^2 + \ldots + \frac{1}{s+1} \phi_s t^{s+1} \right\}. \tag{15}$$

A function of this form is applicable to kinetic curves characterized by the presence of one or several points at zero. For instance, when $a_1 < 0$, a function of the form

$$F = F_0 \exp(a_0 t + a_1 t^2) \tag{16}$$

can describe the kinetic tumour regression curves, and the function of the form

$$F = F_0 \exp(a_0 t + a_1 t^2 + a_2 t^3) \tag{17}$$

is valid for approximation of the kinetic curves for recurring tumours.

The axial symmetry of the quadratic parabola function (16) will describe only kinetic curves with an appropriate symmetry, and this is only rarely found. The expression of asymmetric kinetic curves would require polynomials of a higher power, i.e. a larger number of parameters would be required.

9. The asymmetric polynomial exponent with

$$\phi(t) = (a_0 + a_1 t + a_2 t^2 + \ldots + a_s t^s) \exp(-bt)$$

can be used for description of asymmetric kinetic curves. Sometimes this permits using a smaller number of parameters. Integration of Eq. (5) with the function $\phi(t)$ of this form yields the expression

$$F = a \exp \left\{ [c_0 + c_1 t + \ldots + c_s t^s] \exp(-bt) \right\}. \tag{18}$$

Introduction of the factor $\exp(-bt)$ into the index produces an absolute rate of function variation in regions to the left of extreme points and is higher than the rates in the next curve sections. Such a picture is observed for fast partial regression of the tumour with subsequent gradual recurrence of its growth. Parameter b can be used here as a measure of the difference between the average rate of tumour size reduction and that of its subsequent growth. The Gompertz function and the polynomial exponent are particular cases of an asymmetric polynomial exponent. Indeed, assuming a parameter $b = 0$ in function (18), we obtain a polynomial exponent. When $b \neq 0$ and $c_i = 0$, we obtain the Gompertz function for all i, except $i = 0$ (i.e. for $c_0 \neq 0$), whereas assuming parameter $b = 0$ and all $c_i = 0$, except $c_1 \neq 0$, we obtain the usual exponential dependence.

Thus the asymmetric polynomial exponent (18) can be used for description of kinetic curves of different types.

The types of kinetic curves corresponding to the functions discussed here are shown in Figure 8. The exponential function (curve 1) is seen to ascent faster than the power curve (curve 2). The same figure presents the S-shaped autocatalysis curve and the logistic function (curve 4), and the Gompertz function (curve 3): all these functions are monotonic. To describe kinetic curves with zero points use can be made of the polynomial exponent (curves 5 and 6). The kinetic curves 7 to 9 are described by the symmetric polynomial exponent (18).

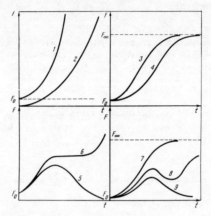

Fig. 8   Plots of functions used for description of
tumour growth kinetics

The functions considered in this section can be used also for descriptions of the survival curves, provided the parameters are taken with the corresponding signs. The most often encountered types of such curves are presented in Figure 9.

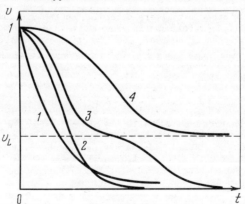

Fig. 9   Plots of analytical functions used for
description of survival curves

Survival curves are described by an averaged exponential function:

$$v = \exp(-\alpha t) \tag{19}$$

where α is a constant value (curve 1') and is frequently encountered. Use can also be made of function

$$v = \exp(-\alpha t^k) \tag{20}$$

where α and k are constant parameters (curve 2).

Complicated survival curves with several inflexion points (curve 3) can be represented by the polynomial exponent (15) with appropriate parameter a_i.

When there is a certain fraction v_L of surviving animals (curve 4) the function

$$v = (1 - v_L) \exp(-\alpha t^k) + v_L \tag{21}$$

can be used. If the survival curve has both several inflexion points and a non-zero asymptote (curve 5) use can be made of the asymmetric polynomial exponent (18) at appropriate parameters of a_i and b.

4. ESTIMATION OF KINETIC PARAMETERS

After choice of a certain family of functions

$$F = F(t; a_1, a_2, \ldots a_8),$$

assumed to involve the true mean kinetic curve $\mu(t)$, regression analysis can be made.

Transformation of the Co-ordinate System

As a rule, function F is nonlinear relative to parameters $a_1, a_2, \ldots a_8$. It is expedient to transform it in a way such that the function obtained, $y = y(F)$, be of the form

$$y(F) = c_1 x_1(t) + c_2 x_2(t) + \ldots + c_8 x_8(t),$$

where $c_1, \ldots, c_8$ are other parameters depending on the previous ones only, and the functions $x_1(t), \ldots, x_8(t)$ must in general be independent of the parameters, the real values of which are unknown. Thus function y will become linear in all its unknown $c_1 \ldots c_8$ parameters. The sample transformed in the same way, i.e. $y_{ij} = y(F_{ij})$ has to be calculated.

Linearization of parameters is not essential for regression analysis, but, when possible, it substantially simplifies the estimating of parameters. If linearization is not carried out (it is often impossible), the calculation of parameter estimates becomes very time-consuming and a computer is needed. The relevant methods have been described (Malenvo, 1975; Klepikov and Sokolov, 1964).

Some examples of the linearization of model functions enumerated in the previous section follow.

1. The exponential dependence (6)

$$F = F_0 \exp(\phi t)$$

where $a_1 = F_0$, $a_2 = \phi$ is transformed by simply using a logarithmic scale

$$\ln F = \ln F_0 + \phi t$$

In this case $y = \ln F$, $c_1 = \ln F_0$, $c_2 = \phi$, $x = t$.

2. The exponential function with a constant additive term (7) can be linearized over two parameters only, assuming that the true value F_i is known. Then

$$y = \ln(F - F_1) = \ln F_0 + bt$$

Here $c_1 = \ln F_0$, $c_2 = b$, $x = t$.

3. The power function $F = at^b$. The corresponding transformation will be

$$y = \ln F = \ln a + b \ln t$$

The regression analysis is made in co-ordinates $\{y = \ln F, \ x = \ln t\}$; here $c_1 = \ln a$, $c_2 = b$.

4. Function (9) cannot be linearized relative to the parameters.

5. The Gompertz function (10) can be linearized in co-ordinates $\{\ln(\ln F_\infty - \ln F), t\}$, i.e.

$$y = \ln(\ln F_\infty - \ln F) = \ln a - bt; \quad c_1 = \ln a, \ c_2 = -b; \ x = t.$$

The true value F_∞ is assumed to be known.

6. The logistic function (11) linearizes as a result of transformation

$$y = \ln(F_\infty/F - 1) = \ln a - bt; \quad \text{here } c_1 = \ln a, \ c_2 = -b, \ x = t.$$

The true value of F_∞ is again assumed to be known.

7. The Bertalanffi function (13) is linearized in the same way as the function of type (7), i.e.

$$y = \ln(1 - F/F_\infty) = \ln a - bt.$$

When the true value of F_∞ is unknown, graphical and analytical methods are used for calculation of the parameters a, b, F_∞. A procedure for estimating the initial values of the parameters of three-parametric functional dependences is reduced to the general form

$$y = \alpha + \beta \gamma^t$$

(Gorkov, 1977). For instance, the Gompertz, Verhulst, and Bertalanffi functions are reduced to this form by the change of parameters (Table 2).

This method assumes that m values are obtained after equal periods of time, since otherwise interpolation of the initial data would have to be made. Under this assumption the equation for neighbouring y values yields the relationship

TABLE 2 Parameters for reducing Gompertz (1825) (1), Verhulst (2) and Bertalanffi (1960) (3) equations to a general form

Initial equation	y	α	β	γ
1. $F = F_\infty e^{-ae-bt}$	$\ln F$	$\ln F_\infty$	$-a$	e^{-b}
2. $F = F_\infty / (1 + ae^{-bt})$	$1/F$	$1/F_\infty$	a/F_∞	e^{-b}
3. $F = F_\infty (1 - ae^{-bt})$	F	F_∞	$-aF_\infty$	e^{-b}

$$y_{k+1} = \gamma y_k + \alpha(1-\gamma), \quad k = 0, 1, \ldots, m-1$$

Using the least squares procedure, we obtain for the parameters α and γ

$$\alpha = A/(B-A); \quad \gamma = C/B$$

where
$$A = \Sigma y_{k+1}\, \Sigma y_k^2 - \Sigma y_k\, \Sigma y_k y_{k+1} ;$$

$$B = m\Sigma y_k^2 - \left(\Sigma y_k\right)^2;$$

$$C = m\Sigma y_k y_{k+1} - \Sigma y_k\, \Sigma y_{k+1}$$

(summation is made everywhere over index k from 0 to $m-1$).

Substituting the obtained values   and   into the initial equation and using the least squares procedure, we obtain an estimate of parameter

$$\beta = \frac{\sum_{k=0}^{m} y_k \gamma^k - \alpha \sum_{k=0}^{m} \gamma^k}{\sum_{k=0}^{m} \gamma^{2k}}$$

Using a back change of parameters α, β and γ we obtain the first approximation to parameters a, b, and F_∞ for the original kinetic curve equation.

8. For the polynomial exponent (1) the linearizing transformation is obtained by using the logarithmic scale

$$y = \ln F = \ln F_0 + \phi_0 t + \tfrac{1}{2}\phi_1 t^2 + \ldots + \frac{1}{s+1}\phi_s t^{s+1}$$

The co-ordinate sysem for regression analysis is $y = \ln F$, $x = t$.

Thus, after linearization, in all virtually important cases, the function

$$y(F) = \sum_{i=1}^{s} c_i x_i(t)$$

acquires the form of a polynomial

$$y = \sum_{k=0}^{r} c_k x^k$$

where x is a certain time function ($x = t$ or $x = \ln t$). The regression analysis has been described in detail (Malenvo, 1975; Wilks, 1962; Klepikov and Sokolov, 1964; Mitropolskii, 1971) for the cases in which $r > 1$, or function y is not reduced to a polynomial. Only the simplest case of a linear dependence between y and x, i.e. $y + ax + b$, will be considered hereafter. This type of the regression curve is most often used in the statistical treatment of biological and medical data.

Choice of Statistical Weights

By definition, the weights are calculated using the expression

$$w_i = \frac{\dfrac{n_i}{\sigma_i^2}}{\displaystyle\sum_{k=0}^{m} \dfrac{n_k}{\sigma_k^2}}$$

However, this expression involves the true values of dispersion σ_i^2: as a rule these are unknown. Consequently, one of the following procedures has to be chosen in calculations:

1. All dispersions σ_i^2 are assumed to be equal. Then $w_i = n_i/n$. If the distribution of values y_{ij} is normal for all x_i, the suggestion about the possible equality of all σ_i^2 can be checked by means of Barlett's or Cochran's criteria, or better, by Fisher's criterion v^2 which is unaffected by small deviations from normal distributions (Nalimov, 1971; Malenvo, 1975; Bolshev and Smirnov, 1965).

2. It is assumed that $\sigma_i^2 = \sigma^2 h^2(x_i)$ where $\sigma^2 = \text{const}$, and $h(x)$ is a known function.

3. The true dispersions σ_i^2 are replaced by their estimates

$$S_i^2 = \frac{1}{n_i - 1} \sum_{j=1}^{n_i} (y_{ij} - \overline{y}_i)^2$$

Calculation of Estimates

In the case of a simple linear regression the expression for S becomes

$$S(a,b) = \sum_{i=1}^{m} w_i \left[\overline{y}_i - (a + bx_i) \right]^2$$

The parameters a and b corresponding to minimal S are found from equations $\partial S/\partial a = 0$, $\partial S/\partial b = 0$. This yields the expressions for the estimates

$$\hat{a} = \frac{(\Sigma w_i \overline{y}_i)(\Sigma w_i x_i^2) - (\Sigma w_i x_i)(\Sigma w_i x_i \overline{y}_i)}{\Sigma w_i x_i^2 - (\Sigma w_i x_i)^2},$$

$$\hat{b} = \frac{\Sigma w_i x_i \bar{y}_i - (\Sigma w_i x_i)(\Sigma w_i \bar{y}_i)}{\Sigma w_i x_i^2 - (\Sigma w_i x_i)^2}$$

Allowing that the distributions of y_{ij} are normal, and their dispersions are equal to σ_i^2, the estimates $\hat{a}$ and $\hat{b}$ will also be distributed normally with the following dispersions

$$D\{\hat{a}\} = \sigma^2 \frac{\Sigma w_i x_i^2}{\Sigma w_i x_i^2 - (\Sigma w_i x_i)^2},$$

$$D\{\hat{b}\} = \frac{\sigma^2}{\Sigma w_i x_i^2 - (\Sigma w_i x_i)^2}$$

where

$$\sigma^2 = \left(\sum_{i=1}^m \frac{n_i}{\sigma_i^2} \right)^{-1}.$$

The estimates $\hat{a}$ and $\hat{b}$ are stochastically dependent.

Analysis of the Fit of the Regression Curve and Experimental Sample

When the kinetic curve for the true average values are approximated by the polynomial

$$y = \sum_{k=0}^r c_k x^k$$

it has to be established whether the polynomial power r is adequate. Consider the procedure of selecting the optimal r value, which will be valid if the random values y_{ij} are distributed normally at any value of x_i. For details see, for instance, Bolshev and Smirnov, 1965; Klepikov and Sokolov, 1964. These calculations are very time-consuming; a computer is needed.

It is convenient to write down the function y in the form of an expansion over orthonormed polynomials

$$L_k(x) = \sum_{\lambda=0}^k L_{\lambda k} x^\lambda$$

rather than over power series of x.

The polynomial $L_k(x)$ has the power k. The coefficients $L_{\lambda k}$ are found from the orthonormation condition

$$\sum_{i=1}^m w_i L_k(x_i) L_{k^1}(x_i) = \begin{cases} 1, & \text{if } k = k^1; \\ 0, & \text{if } k \neq k^1. \end{cases}$$

In these definitions the regression curve obtained by the least squares procedure will have the form

$$y = \sum_{k=0}^r g_k L_k(x).$$

After the estimates g_0, ..., g_r are found, the values s_1^2 and s_2^2 are calculated. The value s_1^2 depends on the scatter of individual y_{ij} values around the mean y_i

$$s_1^2 = \frac{1}{n-m} \sum_{i=1}^{m} \frac{w_i}{n_i} \sum_{j=1}^{n_i} (y_{ij} - \overline{y}_i)^2$$

The value $s_2^2(r)$ is controlled by the scatter of mean $\overline{y}_i$ around the regression line y:

$$s_2^2(r) = \frac{1}{m-r-1} \sum_{i=1}^{m} w_i \left[\overline{y}_i - \sum_{k=0}^{r} g_k L_k(x_i) \right]^2 = \frac{1}{m-r-1} \left(\sum_{i=1}^{m} w_i \overline{y}_i^2 - \sum_{k=0}^{r} g_k^2 \right)$$

The regression line can be considered to be adequate if the following three conditions are fulfilled:

1. The coefficient g_r has to be significantly greater than zero. This is checked using Fisher's v^2 criterion (Bolshev and Smirnov, 1965). The inequality

$$g_r^2 / s_2^2(r) > v_p^2(1, m-r-1)$$

has to hold (p is the significance level). If the reverse inequality is fulfilled, a lower order polynomial is chosen as the regression curve.

2. The coefficient g_{r+1} will not significantly differ from zero. In calculating g_{r+1} the regression curve is assumed to be a polynomial of power $r+1$, and the coefficient for $L_{r+1}(x)$ is calculated. Checking of the significance is done in the same way as for g_r.

3. Finally, the inequality $v_1^2 - p(f_1, f_2) < s_2^2(r)/s^2 < v_p^2(f_1, f_2)$ has to hold,

where $f_1 = m-r-1$, $f_2 = \sum_{i=1}^{m} \frac{w_i^2}{n_i-1}$.

It will be borne in mind that the same experimental data can be satisfactorily approximated by several regression curves of a different analytical form (Khald, 1956; Steel and Lamerton, 1966).

5.   QUANTITATIVE EFFICIENCY CRITERIA FOR TUMOUR GROWTH TREATMENT

Treatments of the tumour growth process induce changes in the kinetic curves for tumour growth and subsequent survival of the experimental animals. Objective criteria for determination of the effectiveness of chemotherapy have to be found. These criteria can be based on comparison of the tumour growth and of the survival curves.

Accurate kinetic curves for tumour growth can be obtained experimentally. Large-scale screening of new chemotherapeutic compounds requires techniques involving as little labour as possible. This imposes constraints on the number of experimental animals used and on the amount of data obtained in each experiment. Screening regimens used in Russia and America require that the experiment must involve six to ten animals, each animal giving only one or two points (Larionov, 1962). Thus screening gives no possibility of obtaining kinetic curves for tumour growth. One experiment is just the measurement of a small number of values.

Clinical investigations meet with other difficulties as well. As a rule, the value F characterizing the tumour size (except for leukaemia and pulmonary metastases) is difficult to measure and thus the plotting of kinetic curves for tumour growth is possible only in rare cases. The lifespans and survival of patients usually are the values observed. Taking into account the characteristic features found in some other studies, a number of criteria for the efficiency of tumour treatment can be proposed.

Parametric Criteria

If the experimental kinetic curve belongs to the same family of functions $F(t; a_1, a_2, \ldots a_s)$ as the control curve, the comparison of curves can be restricted to comparison of the relevant parameters for these curves. As stated earlier, within a limited time interval any kinetic curve can be approximated by function (15), or in a reduced form (after linearization) it will be

$$y = a_0 + a_1 t + \ldots + a_m t^m$$

Since the task is to compare the control and experimental curves, the time of starting therapeutic treatment can be chosen as the reference point in time. The control and experimental curves are polynomials of finite power:

$$\text{control curve:} \qquad y_c = \ln F_c = a_0 + a_1 t + \ldots + a_m t^m$$
$$\text{experimental curve:} \qquad y_e = \ln F_e = a' + a' t + \ldots + a'_{m'} t^{m'}.$$

The powers of these polynomials m and m' may appear to be different.

The procedure of choosing the polynomial power was described above. However, the same curves can formally be represented as polynomials of the same power n equal to the value of m or m' whichever appears to be higher. It will appear then that certain parameters of one of the curves will not differ significantly from zero. Consequently, it can be accepted formally that the experimental and control curves belong to the same family of functions. To compare the parameters of these curves it is necessary to check whether the differences in parameters a_i and a_i' are significant at corresponding polynomial powers for the control and experimental curves. If the differences are not significant in all $a_i - a_i'$ pairs, it will be concluded that the curves do not differ. If the differences are significant at least in one pair, the curves have to be considered as dissimilar. This will mean that therapeutic treatment results in varying shapes of the kinetic curve. Some function $\chi = f(a_0, a_1, \ldots, a_n; a_0', a_1', \ldots, a_n')$ equal to zero or unity at $a_0 = a_0'$, $a_1 = a_1'$, $\ldots$, $a_n = a_n'$, or a certain set of such functions can be taken as a measure of the effect obtained. In case of a set of functions the effect will be characterized not by one number, but by a set of numbers. The effectiveness criteria of this type can be called 'parametric', since they are expressed via parameters of kinetic curves. Many similar functions can be found. For instance one can choose as a measure of the effect a set of differences

$$\varkappa_0 = a_0 - a_0'; \quad \varkappa_1 = a_1 - a_1'; \quad \ldots; \quad \varkappa_n = a_n - a_n'$$

a function of the type

$$\varkappa = \left[\sum_{i=0}^{n} (a_i - a_i')^2 \right]^{\frac{1}{2}}$$

or a set of ratios of relevant parameters

$$\varkappa_0 = \frac{a_0}{a_0'}; \quad \varkappa_1 = \frac{a_1}{a_1'}; \quad \dots; \quad \varkappa_n = \frac{a_n}{a_n'}.$$

In the simplest case, when the tumour grows exponentially both in control

$$F_c = F_0 \exp(\phi_c t)$$

and in experiment

$$F_e = F_0 \exp(\phi_e t),$$

the set of parameters reduces to two pairs: $(\ln F_0, \phi_c)$ and $(\ln F_0, \phi_e)$. Then the measure of the effect will be the relation

$$\varkappa = \frac{\phi_e}{\phi_c} \tag{22}$$

showing how many times the experimental process is slower than the control process.

With efficient drugs $(\phi_e < \phi_c)$ comparison of the control and the experimental curves in any points where $F_e = F_c$ gives

$$\phi_c t_c = \phi_e t_e \quad \text{or} \quad \phi_c / \phi_e = t_e / t_c.$$

This equality represents similarity in the experimental and control kinetic curves and it implies that the efficiency criterion (22) can be represented also as

$$\varkappa = \frac{t_e}{t_c} \tag{23}$$

Such a form of representation permits calculating $\varkappa$ from the shift of the experimental relative to the control curves.

The inhibition coefficient $\varkappa$ is determined by Eq. (23) for the case when therapeutic treatment is started soon after tumour transplantation. Whereas if treatment is started at t_1, $\varkappa$ is obtained by expression

$$\varkappa = \phi_c / \phi_e = (t_e - t_1) / (t_c - t_1).$$

Nonparametric Criteria

These criteria are valid whatever the type of kinetic tumour growth curves for controls and for experimental data.

Criteria for estimating the effectiveness from the survival curves are:

1. Criteria using the fractions of animals surviving in the experiment (v_e) and in the controls (v_c) in the time t. The time t is chosen by the experimentalist. The value

$$\varkappa_1 = v_e(t)$$

or the difference

$$\varkappa_2 = v_e(t) - v_c(t)$$

can be used as the measure of effectiveness.

With screening, t can always be chosen so high that v_c will be zero (rejecting from the control group the animals that survived because transplantation failed). Criterion $\varkappa_1$ is commonly used in clinical treatment in estimating the effectiveness of treating people (Emanuel and Evseenko, 1970).

2. Criteria using animal life-spans as controls and experiments. The effectiveness measure will be

$$\varkappa_3 = \frac{\tau_e}{\tau_c}$$

where τ_e is the mean life-span in experiment, τ_c that in controls. Another criterion is the relation

$$\varkappa_4 = \frac{(\tau_{1/2})_e}{(\tau_{1/2})_c} \, ,$$

where $\tau_{1/2}$ is the time of death of 50% of animals (median of life-span distribution). Both criteria are basic in the system of screening adopted in America.

Criteria Requiring Measurement of the Value F

1. Criteria using comparison of times needed for the value F to attain a certain value F^*. Though in principle this level can be chosen arbitrarily, there are several obvious ways of choosing F^*.

(i) Treatment results in remission, i.e. the tumour diminishes and becomes so small that it cannot be observed within time T_R (remission time). Then the minimally detectable value $F^* = F_{min}$ can be taken as the level F^*. The duration of remission

$$\varkappa_5 = T_R$$

i.e. the time interval over which $F < F_{min}$ can be adopted as the effectiveness measure. This criterion is used in clinical oncology, mainly in treating leukaemia (see, for instance, Weissand and Zelan, 1963).

(ii) Treatment results in temporary reduction of the tumour (regression). It is natural to adopt as the effectiveness measure the time interval T_r (regression time) over which $F < F_1$, where F_1 is the tumour size at the start of treatment

$$\varkappa_6 = T_r$$

A somewhat modified criterion is sometimes more convenient

$$\varkappa_7 = T_r/T_2$$

where T_2 is the doubling time of F to the start of treatment $t = t_1$, i.e.

$$T_2 = \frac{\ln 2}{\phi(t_1)} = \ln 2 \Big/ \left(\frac{1}{F} \frac{dF}{dt} \right)_{t = t_1}$$

Criterion $\varkappa_7$ permits comparing the effects obtained by treatment of tumours exhibiting different specific growth rates. The criteria $\varkappa_6$ and $\varkappa_7$ are used in investigating tumour radiotherapy.

(iii) After the treatment is terminated, the tumour growth recommences and the value F reaches a certain level F^*. The efficiency measure will then be the relation

$$\varkappa_8 = (t^*_e - t_1)/(t^*_c - t_1),$$

where t_1 is the time of starting treatment, t^*_e is the time of reaching level F^* in experiment or in clinic, t^*_c is the time of reaching F^* in controls (control group).

The criteria $\varkappa_5$ to $\varkappa_8$ based on determining the time of reaching level F^* or F_1 require plotting of the kinetic curves, and thus they are somewhat inconvenient in mass screening.

2. Criteria using F values in controls and in experiment at time t. The efficiency measure here is usually the relation

$$\varkappa_9 = \frac{\overline{F}_{te}}{\overline{F}_{tc}}$$

where $\overline{F}_{te}$ is the mean value of F in experiment, $\overline{F}_{tc}$ is the mean value in controls (in the American system of screening), or else the value

$$\varkappa_9{}' = (1 - \varkappa_9) \cdot 100 \ = (1 - \overline{F}_{te}/\overline{F}_{tc}) \cdot 100,$$

which is referred to as the inhibition percent (in the Russian system of screening: Anon, 1958; Larionov, 1962). The time t is chosen to a certain extent arbitrarily and thus it is a parameter of the criterion. In practice the choice of t is very restricted. The treatment usually takes a certain time. It starts at the time t_1 and ends at $t_1 + T$, where T is the treatment duration. Consequently conditions $t > t_1 + T$ and $t > t^*_{fc}$ have to be fulfilled (t^*_{fc} is the time at which control animals start dying). The value $t - t_1 + T$ is often chosen. If treatment is continued beyond the time by which most control animals have died (in screening this takes place, for instance, for L-1210 ascites leukaemia) these inequalities are incompatible and the criteria $\varkappa_9$ and $\varkappa_9{}'$ cannot be used.

It will be noted that the kinetic criterion $\varkappa$ (22) characterized exponentially-growing tumours better than does the inhibition percent criterion, since its value is independent of the time the experiment ends. The relation between these two criteria is

$$\varkappa_9{}' = \left\{1 - \exp\ [(1 - \varkappa)\phi_{et}]\right\} \cdot 100$$

An advantage of the kinetic criterion is its high 'sensitivity' in the evaluation of effective drugs. It will be seen from Figure 10 that $\varkappa$ is approximately directly proportional to $\varkappa_9{}'$ and this persists up to $\varkappa_9{}'$ values of 50-60%. In terms of the $\varkappa$ criterion this means that the drugs used are not very effective and can inhibit tumour growth only 1.3 - 1.5 fold. With very effective drugs, when $\varkappa_9{}'$ reaches 80-100%, the $\varkappa$ criterion values increase very markedly. Because of the inevitable scatter present in experimental data, the experimentalist most often notices only a drug which gives a high percentage of inhibition (for instance, 80-100%). A finer differentiation of drugs with respect to their activity is very difficult in this field, whereas the kinetic criterion is very convenient for finding the solution to one of the main problems of chemotherapy, namely the establishing of the relation between the chemical structure and the anticancer activity of the most effective drugs.

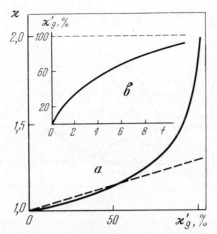

Fig. 10 Relation between criteria $\varkappa$ and $\varkappa_9'$ (a) and
dependence of $\varkappa_9'$ on the time of measurement (b) for
exponentially growing tumours

Complex Kinetic Effectiveness Criteria Method of Equivalent Exponents

The specific growth rate $\phi(t)$ is an important characteristic of the tumour state at
a given time. To calculate the mean specific growth rate for the time interval
(t_1, t_2)

$$\overline{\phi}(t_1, t_2) = \frac{1}{t_2 - t_1} \int_{t_1}^{t_2} \phi(t) \, dt$$

Since $\qquad \phi(t) = \frac{1}{F} \frac{dF}{dt} = \frac{d \ln F}{dt}$

the equation

$$\overline{\phi}(t_1, t_2) = \frac{1}{t_2 - t_1} \int_{t_1}^{t_2} \frac{d \ln F}{dt} \, dt = \frac{\ln F(t_2) - \ln F(t_1)}{t_2 - t_1}$$

holds. Thus, the specific growth rate averaged over the whole time interval
(t_1, t_2) depends only on the F values at the end points of this interval. The value
$\overline{\phi}(t_1, t_2)$ is equal to the power of the 'equivalent exponent' which passes through
the ends of the kinetic curve $F(t)$ within the time interval investigated (Figure 11).

Take as the efficiency measure the ratio of the mean specific tumour growth rates
of controls to experiment

$$\overline{\varkappa} = \frac{\overline{\phi}_C(t_{1C}, t_{2C})}{\overline{\phi}_e(t_{1e}, t_{2e})} = \frac{t_{2e} - t_{1e}}{t_{2C} - t_{1C}} \cdot \frac{\ln F_C(t_{2C}) - \ln F_C(t_{1C})}{\ln F_e(t_{2e}) - \ln F_e(t_{1e})} \tag{24}$$

Generally the value $\overline{\varkappa}$ depends on the choice of both mean time intervals (t_{1C}, t_{2C})
and (t_{2e}, t_{2e}). The common start of these intervals will obviously be at the time
t_1, at which the effect of treatment begins. The choice of the ends of the time
intervals can be made in different ways:

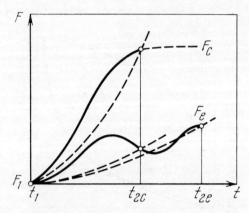

Fig. 11 Plotting of equivalent curves

1. The ends of the mean kinetic curves for tumour growth are taken as the end of the mean time intervals. Then

$$\varkappa_{10} = \frac{\overline{\varphi}_c(t_1, t_{fc})}{\overline{\varphi}_e(t_1, t_{fe})} = \frac{t_{fe} - t_1}{t_{fc} - t_1} \cdot \frac{\ln F_c(t_{fc}) - \ln F_c(t_1)}{\ln F_e(t_{fe}) - \ln F_e(t_1)}$$

2. Any time t_2 for which the compared kinetic curves are valid can be chosen as the common end of the time intervals

$$\varkappa_{11} = \frac{\overline{\varphi}_c(t_1, t_2)}{\overline{\varphi}_e(t_1, t_2)} = \frac{\ln F_c(t_2) - \ln F_c(t_1)}{\ln F_e(t_2) - \ln F_e(t_1)}$$

When the tumour development processes are exponential both in experiment and controls

$$\overline{\varphi}_c(t_1, t_{2c}) = \varphi_c; \quad \overline{\varphi}_e(t_1, t_{2e}) = \varphi_e \quad \text{and} \quad \overline{\varkappa}_{10} = \overline{\varkappa}_{11} = \varphi_c/\varphi_e = \varkappa$$

i.e. the criterion obtained is the same as that derived earlier.

Returning to Figure 11 presenting experimental and control kinetic curves and the equivalent exponents (dotted), we shall show for this hypothetic example the procedure of calculating case (1) by the method of equivalent exponents. In arbitrary units:

$$t_1 = 0; \quad t_{fc} = 7; \quad t_{fe} = 11; \quad F_c(t_1) = 1; \quad F_c(t_{fc}) = 9,2;$$

$$F_e(t_1) = 1; \quad F_e(t_{fc}) = 5,2 .$$

Substituting these values into the equation for $\varkappa_{10}$, we have

$$\varkappa_{10} = 2, 12$$

Thus, the observed inhibition effect is equivalent to a double decrease in tumour growth relative to the control.

Let (22) be written as

$$\overline{\varkappa} = 1 \Big/ \frac{\overline{\phi_e}}{\phi_e}$$

Then the plot of this dependence in co-ordinates $\{\overline{\varkappa}, \overline{\phi_e}\}$ will represent a hyperbola (Figure 12a). Since for any particular model $\phi_c = \text{const}$, this function will depend on the specific rate $\overline{\phi_e}$ of tumour growth in experiment.

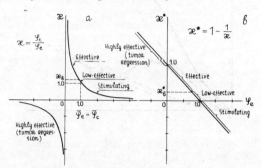

Fig. 12   Regions of therapeutic treatment effectiveness
$\varkappa_b = 1.25$ and $\varkappa_b^* = 0.2$ conditional values separating the
low-effective and effective treatments

Effective therapeutic action is seen as a decreasing value of ϕ_e. The value $\varkappa = 1$ corresponds to no effect ($\phi_e = \phi_c$). All values $\varkappa > 1$ are characteristic of effective treatment — from immaterial inhibition to complete termination of the tumour growth ($\phi_e = 0$). The treatments for which $1.0 < \varkappa < 1.25$ are low-effective. The choice of such limits is based on the screening rules for antileukaemic drugs in America, where only the drugs that ensure no less than 1.25 times prolongation of the life-spans of mice with L-1210 leukaemia are accepted for further investigation.

Accordingly, the effective actions of drugs are those for which $\varkappa > 1.25$. A stimulating action is characterized by $\phi_e > \phi_c$ and $0 \leqslant \varkappa \leqslant 1$. Negative ϕ_e values, as well as negative $\varkappa = \phi_c/(-\phi_e)$, correspond to tumour regression. With increasing rate of regression, i.e. with increase in effectiveness, the absolute $\varkappa$ value decreases, since $|\varkappa| = \phi_c/|\phi_e|$.

A disadvantage is that the values $\varkappa_{10}$ and $\varkappa_{11}$ tend to infinity with complete inhibition of growth ($\overline{\phi} = 0$). Consequently, it is more convenient to use modified $\varkappa_{10}^*$ and $\varkappa_{11}^*$ criteria, that have no such disadvantage:

$$\varkappa_{10}^* = 1 - 1/\varkappa_{10}$$
$$\varkappa_{11}^* = 1 - 1/\varkappa_{11}$$

Since both modified criteria are in this case linear functions of the mean specific growth rate in experiments, i.e.

$$\varkappa_{10\,(11)}^* = 1 - (1/\phi_c)\phi_e$$

the value $\varkappa_{10}^* = \varkappa_{11}^* = 0$ corresponds to no effect, the positive values of $\varkappa_{10}$ and $\varkappa_{11}$ refer to effective treatment (inhibition of tumour growth, and the negative values to an action stimulating the tumour growth (Figure 12b).

It will be noted that calculation of $\varkappa_{10}$ and $\varkappa_{11}$ uses the F values taken from the mean kinetic curves for tumour growth in experiment and controls. Since the plotting of these curves is rather tedious, the criteria $\varkappa_{10}$ and $\varkappa_{11}$ can be replaced by $\varkappa_{10}'$ and $\varkappa_{11}'$, that can be readily calculated from experimental data

$$\varkappa_{10}' = \frac{\tau_e - t_1}{\tau_c - t_1} \cdot \frac{<\ln F_c> - <\ln F(t_1)>}{<\ln F_e> - <\ln F(t_1)>}$$

$$\varkappa_{11}' = \frac{<\ln F_c(t)> - <\ln F(t_1)>}{<\ln F_e(t)> - <\ln F(t_1)>}$$

Here τ_c and τ_e are the median lifespan of animals in the control and experimental groups, $<\ln F_c>$ is the mean value of $\ln F$ for the moments of death of control animals, $<\ln F_e>$ the same for the experimental group, $<\ln F_c(t)>$ and $<\ln F_e(t)>$ are the corresponding mean values for the time t.

The criteria $\varkappa_{10}$, $\varkappa_{11}$, $\varkappa_{10}^*$, $\varkappa_{11}^*$ possess a very important feature — their values are only slightly dependent on choice of F — the characteristic of the tumour process development (the diameter, area, volume, mass of the tumour, the number of malignant cells). Any two of the cited characteristics are approximately connected by the power dependence $F_1 = aF_2^b$: the coefficients a and b can change but slightly in the course of the process. The expression (24) is invariant relative to replacement of F_1 by F_2 (the coefficients a and b reduce here, if assumed as constant in time). The criteria $\varkappa_9$ and the 'inhibition percent' $\varkappa_9'$ often used in screening, as stated above, possess no such lack of variance.

Integral Effectiveness Criterion

This criterion accounts simultaneously for the tumour growth kinetics and for the survival curve. The most important factor representing an integral characteristic of the tumour process in each animal is its life-span τ. The second important characteristic is the kinetic curve for tumour growth in the animal studied

$$F = F_0 \exp(\phi t) \quad \text{where} \quad \phi = \phi(t).$$

The value $\quad x = \overline{\phi}/\tau$

where

$$\overline{\phi} = \frac{1}{\tau} \int_0^{\tau} \phi \, dt \tag{26}$$

can be taken as a characteristic of the tumour process involving both factors for an individual animal.

Using the survival function $v(\tau)$ or the death function $u = 1 - v$ average the value χ over a group of animals

$$\psi = \int_{t_0}^{\infty} \chi u' d\tau \tag{27}$$

where t_0 is the moment of starting treatment, u' is a derivative over τ. This integral converts, since $u' = 0$ when $\tau > \tau_{max}$, where τ_{max} is the maximal life-span of the animal.

The efficiency criterion can be expressed by the relation

$$\varkappa_{12} = (\psi_c - \psi_e)/\psi_c, \tag{28}$$

where ψ_e and ψ_c are ψ values for the experimental and control groups of animals.

With such a definition of effectiveness we have

at $\psi_e = \psi_c$ — no effect ($\varkappa_{12} = 0$)

at $\psi_e > \psi_c$ — stimulation of growth ($\varkappa_{12} < 0$)

at $\psi_e < \psi_c$ — positive effect ($\varkappa_{12} > 0$).

When $\psi_e < 0$ regression takes place ($\varkappa_{12} > 1$).

Making use of expressions (25) to (28) we obtained for the integral effectiveness criterion

$$\varkappa_{12} = 1 - \frac{\displaystyle\int_{t_0}^{\infty} \frac{u'_e}{\tau^2} \int_0^{\tau} \phi_e \, dt \, d\tau}{\displaystyle\int_{t_0}^{\infty} \frac{u'_e}{\tau^2} \int_0^{\tau} \phi_c \, dt \, d\tau}$$

It will be noted, however, that in order to calculate this criterion the individual curve for tumour growth in each animal up to its death and its survival curve must be known.

Thus, there are many possibilities for quantitatively expressing the effectiveness of various therapeutic actions on experimental tumour growth processes. Many of the criteria cited in this chapter can be used also in clinical studies into the various methods of treating cancer. The choice of the criterion depends on the task envisaged by the researcher. However, certain criteria are already used more often then the others. It has to be expected that further selection of the criteria most convenient for various aims will be made, especially of those opening up the best possibilities for evaluation of experimental and clinical data by computer.

CHAPTER 2

KINETICS OF EXPERIMENTAL TUMOUR GROWTH

Experimental tumour models were predominant in the earliest biological studies searching for an effective antitumour treatment. Much information on the biology of transplanted, induced and spontaneous malignant tumours in animals is now available. Statistical evaluation of data obtained in experimental oncology, setting up guidelines for the development of experimental malignant processes and finding quantitative criteria of tumour growth are particularly important. Since any malignant process develops regularly with time, a concept based on kinetic analysis of the data would obviously be the most satisfactory. This chapter attempts to discuss the data available for most of the experimental tumour models from a kinetic standpoint.

Experimental oncology has leaned heavily towards kinetics in the USSR for twenty years. Recently, kinetics have been studied in other countries. The results obtained are given in this chapter, expressed mathematically by the statistical techniques used by the Soviet kinetic school. This allows discussion of all the data reported and unifies the kinetic parameters to give a mathematical comparison.

Knowing the kinetic rules and numerical parameters of tumour growth makes it possible to propose general criteria by which to measure the therapeutic treatment of tumour growth and forms a basis for standardized screening of chemotherapeutic compounds.

1. SOLID TUMOURS AND THEIR ASCITES FORMS

The largest number of studies is concerned with transplanted, induced, and spontaneous solid tumours. These tumours are closest to cancer in humans, though most solid tumours lose their tissue and organ specificities in the course of repeated transplantation.

Solid tumours are very convenient for experimental kinetic studies. The models permit measurement of tumour size in a living body, both in control and treated animals. Solid tumours often give metastases and there have been recent studies on metastasization; the study of Walker sarcoma, Lewis carcinoma, certain melanomas, etc., are of great interest in this respect. Solid tumours also make suitable models for surgical treatment and for study of relapses when surgery was not sufficiently radical.

31

With few exceptions, kinetic curves in this section have in common either the
experimental data obtained by the authors cited or the ways of analyzing these
data.

Walker Sarcoma

This carcinoma was first produced in 1928 from a spontaneous carcinoma of the
mammary gland. It takes in rats of various lines, but mostly in non-inbred animals.
It has complete transplantability and is accompanied by infiltration and movement
out to lymph nodes and lungs (Larionov, 1962).

Schreck (1935) gave a linear description of the growth of this tumour:

$$D = b(t - t_0)$$

where D is the mean tumour diameter (mm), b is the growth rate (in mm/day), t_0 is
the crossing point of the straight line with the time axis (latent period). The
value b depends only slightly on the inoculum value, whereas the latent period
increases with decreasing inoculum size. The mean values of b (~ 1.25 mm/day) and
of t_0 for various inocula and the plots of typical deviations from the linear
dependence are given.

The Gompertz equation

$$v = 3.9 \ 10^{-6} \exp\{17.1[1 - \exp(-0.21t)]\} \ cm^3$$

is used by McCredie $et \ al.$, 1965, for description of the tumour growth kinetics
(Figure 13A). It will be seen from the numerical parameters that the tumour size
approaches asymptotically the value $V_\infty = 3.9 \cdot 10^{-6} \exp(17.1) = 104 \ cm^3$. The
initial size obtained by extrapolation to the transplantation time is $3.9 \cdot 10^{-6} \ cm^3$,
which is considerably smaller than the inoculum size ($1.8 \cdot 10^{-2} \ cm^3$) and the volume
of the viable cells it contains ($\sim 5.7 \cdot 10^{-5} \ cm^3$).

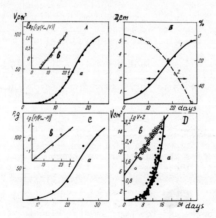

Fig. 13 Kinetics of Walker carcinosarcoma growth.
A — data from McCredie $et \ al.$, 1965; B — (1) tumour
growth, (2) mortality — Schmid $et \ al.$, 1966; C —
from Harding $et \ al.$, 1964

A kinetic curve for changes in the tumour diameter (Figure 13B, curve 1) described by the autocatalytic expression

$$D = \frac{5.5}{1 + 18.22 \exp(-0.18t)} \text{ cm}$$

is plotted using data from Schmid *et al.*, 1966. The limiting tumour volume calculated from the value $D_\infty = 5.5$ cm is 87 cm^3. More than 50% of the animals die by the end of the experiment (Figure 13B, curve 2).

According to Harding *et al.* (1964) the kinetics of changes in tumour weight can be described by equation

$$P = \frac{123.2}{1 + 513 \exp(-0.27t)} \text{ g}$$

with a limiting tumour size close to the values obtained previously (Figure 13C). Indeed, it has been found (McCredie *et al.*, 1965) that the limiting value of the tumour size was 104 cm^3. When calculated using data from Schmid *et al.* (1964) this value appeared to be 87 cm^3, and Harding *et al.* (1964) report the highest weight was 123 g.

In all cases studied the tumours were transplanted subcutaneously into the animal's flank. If the transplantation site is changed, the kinetic regularities appear to be different. For instance, the kinetics of changes in the size of a tumour transplanted subcutaneously into the animal's tail is exponential (Figure 13D). The mean exponential index was $\phi = 0.30 \pm 0.06$ day^{-1}. The close ϕ parameter values in Harding *et al.* (1964) seem to be due to the fact that the exponential growth corresponds to the initial section of the autocatalytic curve before the point of inflection. The mean kinetic curve equation (Figure 13D) is

$$V = 0.12 \exp(0.3t) \text{ cm}^3.$$

Here, as well, tumour size calculated by extrapolation to the time of transplantation (0.12 cm^3) is lower than the inoculum size (0.3 cm^3).

Guérin Carcinoma

This strain was produced in 1934 from a spontaneous adenocarcinoma of rat uterus; it takes to non-inbred animals. Transplantability varies from 50% to 90%; spontaneous regression is rare and it sometimes moves out to regional and distant lymph nodes (Guérin and Guérin, 1934).

The change in tumour diameter may be described by an autocatalysis equation

$$D = \frac{3.9}{1 + 48 \exp(-0.3t)} \text{ cm}$$

(Figure 14A). The average size of tumours V was calculated from the same experimental data. Its changes are described by a power expression $V = 2.3 \cdot 10^{-6} t^{5.3}$ cm^3 (Figure 14B, curve 1). At a half size of the inoculum the curve for diameter changes and that for relevant volumes (Figure 14B, curve 2) are described by power equations

$$D = 6.2 \cdot 10^{-3} t^2 \text{ cm}$$

$$V = 1.3 \cdot 10^{-7} t^6 \text{ cm}^3.$$

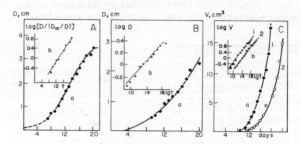

Fig. 14   Changes in mean diameters and Guérin carcinoma
volumes after transplantation of 50% malignant cell suspensions of various volumes. A, B (1) — transplantation of
0.30 ml;   B, C (2) transplantation of 0.15 ml.

In part of the kinetic curve experimental results can be satisfactorily approximated by various functions (Evseenko *et al.*, 1971). Here, the change in kinetics
on passing from tumour diameters to relevant volumes is interpreted as follows:
if the S-shaped function $D(t)$ has an inflection point at the time t^*_d found from
the condition $d^2D/dt^2 = D''(t^*_D) = 0$, the inflection point t^*_v for the function
$V(t) = \pi/6 \ D^3(t)$ will shift to the right along the time axis. In this case the
value $V'' = \pi/D(D')^2 + 2D^2D''$ in point t^*_D is known to be higher than zero. In
particular, for the autocatalysis equation the values t^*_D and t^*_v are related as

$$t^*_v = t^*_D + \frac{1.1}{\phi D}$$

In Figure 14A, $t^*_v = 17$ days, and this corresponds to the end section of the curve,
and consequently the S-shaped form of the curve $V(t)$ is not attained.

The absence of the S-shaped form in Figure 14B (for a smaller inoculum) becomes
clear if one takes into account that the time corresponding to the point of
inflection is related to the initial tumour size by the autocatalysis equation:

$$t^*_D \sim \log \frac{D_\infty}{D_0}$$

Thus D_0 decreases with inoculum size, and t^*_D shifts towards higher time values.
This conclusion is supported by the fact that the maximal tumour diameter in
Figure 14B approximately coincides with the diameter value at the inflection point
in Figure 14A. The same rate of tumour growth in the two cases follows from the
parellelism of linear anamorphoses (Figure 14B).

The rate of Guérin carcinoma growth depends on the site of transplantation. When
the tumour is transplanted in the kidneys or in the epididymis the rate of tumour
growth is higher, and when it is in the liver or spleen, it is lower.

Sarcoma 45

This was produced in 1949 from a tumour induced by dimethylbenzoanthracene in
subcutaneous tissue. It has the structure of a fascicular sarcoma with central
necrosis; it is encapsulated, it does not metastasize, and the strain is sustained
in non-inbred rats (Larionov, 1962; Konoplev, 1960).

The kinetics of tumour growth were first studied by Kiseleva *et al.* (1969). The mean diameter change is described by the autocatalysis equation

$$D = \frac{3.6}{1 + 21.3 \exp (-0.31t)} \text{ cm}$$

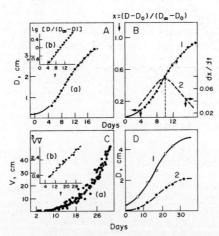

Fig. 15 Kinetic curves for sarcoma 45 growth.
A — change in tumour diameter; B — (1) generalized curve,
(2) change in the growth rate (Kiseleva *et al.*, 1969);
D — sarcolysine-susceptible (1) and sarcolysine-resistant
(2) strains (Larionov, 1962).

The data in Figure 15A are reconstructed so that the tumour size is expressed in dimensionless units

$$x = (D - D_0)/(D_\infty - D_0)$$

(Figure 15B). Such a transformation can be used for comparison of the tumour growth rates at various values of D_∞. The same figure shows the time dependence of the growth rate dx/dt with a maximum corresponding to the inflection curve in the initial kinetic curve (approximately to the 10th day).

The kinetics of changes in tumour volume (Figure 15B) have a cube root dependence

$$(v)^{1/3} = -0.23 + 0.13t \text{ cm}$$

The cube root equation is equivalent to linearity of increase in tumour size, since the mean values of volume and diameter are connected by the relationship $D = 1.24(V)^{1/3}$. Thus tumour diameter increases at a rate of 0.17 cm/day, whereas according to Kiseleva *et al.* (1969) the rate on the linear part of the S-shaped curve is 0.27 cm/day (Figure 15A). These differences might be due to biological peculiarities of the transplanted cells and of the host body.

Indeed, Larionov (1962) reports results on the growth kinetics of sarcolysine-sensitive and sarcolysine-resistant strains of sarcoma 45. The kinetic curves are S-shaped in both cases (Figure 15D). Comparison of the numerical values of the autocatalysis equation parameters obtained by computerizing Larionov's results reveals substantial differences in the values D_0, D_∞ and V_{max}:

	Sensitive	Resistant
D_0, cm	0.32	0.06
D_∞, cm	4.94	2.20
ϕ, day^{-1}	0.16	0.19
V_{max}, cm/day	0.21	0.11

In the autocatalysis equation the maximal rate at the inflection point
($V_{max} \cong \frac{1}{4} \phi D_\infty$) will have the same value as that obtained from the slope of the
linear part of the S-shaped curve. In this example the ratio of D_∞ values is
almost the same as that of V_{max} values, and the latter (0.11 and 0.21 cm/day) are
close to those calculated from the data from Kiseleva $et\ al.$ (1969) (0.17 and 0.27
cm/day).

This kinetic evaluation supports the observed fact that the growth-rates of
experimental tumour strains responsive to chemotherapeutic treatment are higher
than those for resistant strains.

The results obtained by analysis of the statistical distribution of individual
tumour sizes at any point of the curve (Figure 15A) are presented in Figure 16,
where z is the cumulated probability for each individual value D, D^{-1}, log D, or V
observed experimentally. The values $\psi(z)$ (probit values) are taken from the table
in the monograph by Urbakh (1964).

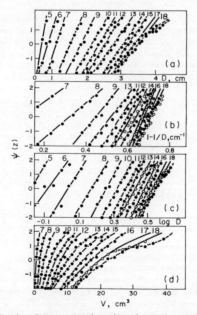

Fig. 16 Check of normal distribution of tumour sizes on
various points of the sarcoma 45 growth curve (according to
Fig. 15A): (a) diameters; (b) reciprocals; (c) diameter
logarithms; (d) volumes. z — cumulative frequency;
$\psi(z)$ — probits. The numbers over curves denote measurement
times in days.

The linear nature of dependences (Figure 16A) shows that at any point in time the distribution of D values is approximately normal. The parallelism of straight lines is evidence of the constancy of statistical scatter (dispersion) at any point of the kinetic curve. The fulfilment of these conditions permits estimation by the least squares procedure of the parameters of approximated expressions from the experimental results (Urbakh, 1964). The dispersion at the start of the experiment is caused by measuring difficulties due to the small size of lymph nodes. The deviation from normality at its end is probably due to the death of the animals with the largest tumours. In order to obtain a better pattern of growth and fairer estimates of the kinetic function parameters, it would be advisable to reject the early and late end points.

A normal distribution was found also for the logarithms and reciprocals of diameters (Figure 16B,C) and this permits evaluating the parameters for kinetic equations also from the values $\log D$ or $1/D$.

The distribution of the volume values (Figure 16D) differs from normal and the scatter substantially increases in the course of the experiment. Consequently, when the analytical function parameters are evaluated from values V, there will be a shift towards higher V values, for which dispersion often exceeds the absolute values of the initial section of the curve. Since $\log V = \log (\pi/6) + 31 gD$, the $\log V$ values are distributed following the same law as the $\log D$ values, i.e. the distribution is approximately normal.

Besides revealing the most reliable section of the kinetic curve for determination of the parameters, such an analysis permits important conclusions on the nature of the effect of various factors, including chemotherapy, on tumour growth (Pelevina et al., 1968).

Sarcoma SSK

This was produced in 1954; it has the structure of a fibrosarcoma. It takes subcutaneously in about 90% of cases. Spontaneous resolution is observed in about 20% of cases (Larionov, 1962). It has not been used frequently in experimental work. The changes in tumour size over the whole range of measurements are exponential. The rate constants of tumour growth in individual animals are approximately the same $(0.38 \pm 0.05$ days). The kinetic curves differ mostly in the pre-exponential factor values. Figure 17A shows kinetic curves for tumour growth in 12 animals (in certain cases the curves coincide). The other experimental points corresponding to the other 50 animals fall between curves 1 and 6.

The averaged kinetic curve (Figure 17B) obtained by the normalization method of combining individual dependences (shift along the time axis) is described by equation

$$V = 0.02 \exp (0.38t) \quad \text{cm}^3$$

It will be noted that as a rule the exponential dependence described the growth of solid tumours only up to the point of inflection of the S-shaped curve. In this research the measurements were terminated when ulceration of the tumour began and consequently the further trend of the curve could not be observed.

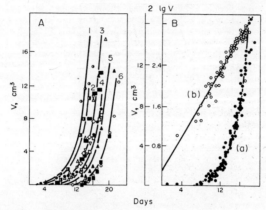

Fig. 17 Kinetics of sarcoma SSK growth.
A — individual curves; B — generalized curve (a) and
its semi-logarithmic anamorphosis (b).

Radiation-induced Skin Tumours

The pecularities of growth and morphology of 740 skin tumours induced in rats by single high doses of α- and β-radiation were studied by Albert *et al.* (1969). The morphological characteristics of tumours fall to three major categories: cornified, non-differentiated, and glandular (i.e. arising from the sebaceous glands). The duration of the induction period and the growth rates are very different, irrespective of the histological type. The authors divide the tumours into six groups with respect to the growth rates from the time of appearance of palpable nodules (D = 1-2 mm). The progression kinetics of the most rapidly growing tumours are described by the exponential functions given in Table 3.

TABLE 3   Kinetic parameters of growth of radiation-induced
skin tumours in rats (Moran, 1962)

Group of tumours	D_0, mm	ϕ, week^{-1}	$T_2 = \ln \frac{2}{\phi}$, weeks
1	0.39	0.063	11.00
2	0.60	0.053	13.10
3	0.63	0.065	10.65
4	$2.6 \cdot 10^{-5}$	0.295	2.35

It will be seen from Table 3 and Figure 18a that the tumour of the first to third group (curves 1, 2, 3) grow at approximately the same rate, but the rate of the fourth group growth (curve 4) is much higher. The lowest D_0 value corresponds to the latter group.

Statistical analysis of the size distribution of 488 tumours measured 20 weeks after each tumour attained the diameter of 1-2 mm was made by Bagg and Jackson (1937). The distributions of diameters of all tumours, divided into groups both with respect to histological type (Figure 18b) and to the extent of radiation-induced skin damage (Figure 19c) are logarithmically normal. This permits

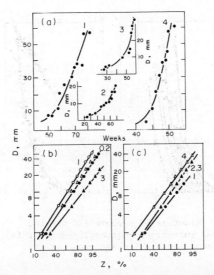

Fig. 18 Radiation-induced skin tumours (Albert *et al.*, 1969).
(a) Kinetic curves of growth;   (b) statistical distribution
of tumour sizes in relation to their morphological types:
0 — all tumours, 1 — keratinous, 2 — non-differentiated,
3 — glandular tumours;   (c) tumour size distribution depending on the extent of irradiation: 1 — weak, 2 and 3 —
moderate, 4 — strong.

characterization of the difference between groups by differences in the normal
log distributions. For instance, the mean diameter of the 488 tumours is
$D = 4.8 \pm 3.2$ mm. The rate of tumour growth in individual groups decreases in the
order: cornified ($D = 6.6$ mm), non-differentiated ($D = 4.8$ mm), and glandular
($D = 3.2$ mm). More rapid growth corresponds to more serious radiation-induced
damage. The frequency of tumour appearance in time is of a polymodal nature.

Adenocarcinoma 755

This strain was produced from a spontaneous tumour in the mouse from a low-cancer
C57 line. The tumour has the structure of an alveolar adenocarcinoma and in
certain cases metastasizes to the lungs (Bagg and Jackson, 1937).

The kinetic regularities of changes in tumour weight in mice of the BDF_1 line have
been studied by Wilcox *et al.* (1965), Laster *et al.* (1969) and Adams and Bowman
(1963). The experimental results of Wilcox *et al.* (1965) and Laster *et al.* (1965)
(Figure 19A,B) are described by the autocatalysis equations as listed in Table 4.

When the tumours are inoculated as a 0.2 ml suspension (Figure 19A,B, curve 2) the
kinetic parameters of changes in tumour weight are close. When transplanted as
25 mg fragments (Figure 19B, curve 1) the initial (P_0) and the limiting (P_∞)
values of the tumour weight are substantially lower and the growth rate constant ϕ
increases somewhat (0.44 compared to 0.31 and 0.36 day^{-1}).

According to Adams and Bowman (1963), tumour growth is exponential (Figure 19B)
over the whole time of observation (20 days):

TABLE 4   Parameters of autocatalysis equations for
adenocarcinoma 755 growth curves (Crow and Kimura, 1970;   Khald, 1956)

P_0 , r	P_∞ , r	ϕ, day^{-1}	References
0.04	14.0	0.36	Crow and Kimura, 1970
0.06	18.0	0.31	Khald, 1956
0.01	6.5	0.44	Khald, 1956

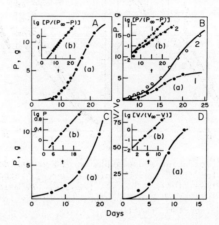

Fig. 19   Adenocarcinoma 755 growth in accordance with the
results reported by various authors. A — Wilcox *et al.*
(1965); B — (1) transplantation by 25 mg fragments, (2)
inoculation with 0.2 ml suspension (Laster *et al.*, 1969);
C — Adams and Bowman (1963); D — Summers (1966).

$$P = 0.39 \exp (0.17t) \text{ g}$$

At the end of this time the tumour weight attained 10 g. The substantially lower
ϕ value compared to those in Table 4 should be noted.

The adenocarcinoma 755 growth in C57Bl mice is described by the relation

$$V_r = 2^{t(K-K_1 V_r)}$$

where $K = 0.27$ day^{-1} and $K_1 = 0.0014$ day^{-1}, $V_r = V_t/V_0$; V_0 is the inoculum volume
(Summers, 1966). A disadvantage of this equation is the impossibility for its
explicit solution relative to V, and also the incorrect identification of inoculum
size with the initial tumour volume. Moreover, the limiting relative tumour size
calculated from the parameters given by Summers ($V_\infty/V_0 = K/K_1 = 200$) is more than
three times that observed experimentally (approximately 70). The treating of
Summers' results by the autocatalysis equation

$$V_r = \frac{75.5}{1 + 74.5 \exp (-0.53t)}$$

gives a more real value of $V_\infty/V_0 — 75.5$ (Figure 19D). In this case the exponential
index $\phi = 0.53$ day^{-1} is higher than the values in Table 4 (0.31 - 0.44 day^{-1}). This

might be due to the use of animals of another line.

It was found later than the tumour growth rate constants differ depending on the animal's sex (Figure 20A) and on the inoculum 'age' (Figure 20B) (D'iachkovskaia and Konovalova, 1973). The relevant parameters of the autocatalysis equation are given in Table 5.

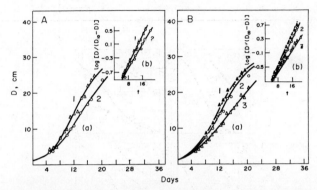

Fig. 20 Kinetics of adenocarcinoma 755 growth depending upon inoculum 'age' and the animal's sex (D'iachovskaia and Konovalova, 1973). A — (1) females, (2) males, 12-day inoculum; B — (1) 9-day inoculum, (2) 12-day inoculum, (3) 15-day inoculum, females.

TABLE 5 Effect of inoculum 'age' and animal sex on adenocarcinoma 755 growth kinetics in C57Bl mice (Owen, 1962)

Inoculum 'age', days	Animal sex	D_0, cm	D_∞, cm	ϕ, day^{-1}
9	female	0.12	3.0	0.27
12	female	0.12	3.0	0.26
12	male	0.12	3.0	0.21
15	female	0.12	3.0	0.21

The values $V_\infty/V_0 = 90$ ($V_0 = 0.15$ ml) and $\phi_V = 3\phi_D = 0.6$–0.8 day^{-1} corresponding to the results of D'iachkovskaia and Konovalova are sufficiently close to the values $V_\infty/V_0 = 75.5$ and $\phi = 0.5$ day^{-1} calculated using the data from Summers (1966).

The differences in growth kinetics of adenocarcinoma 755 reported by various authors may be due to the influence of the kind, size and age of the inoculum, the procedure and site of transplanting, the animal's sex and line, to accuracy in estimating parameters, and to the choice of approximating expresssions.

Hepatomas

Hepatomas were first induced in mice by inoculation of 2-aminoazotoluene; other azodyes representing hepatocarcinogenic agents were used later (Morris, 1966). Hepatomas in mice may arise from spontaneous tumours; these have fast invasive growth and 100% transplantability.

This group of tumours are characterized by different amounts of deviation from normal liver tissue, by the differentiation level and by growth rates. The transplanted hepatomas (from the slow-growing 'minimally deviated' hepatomas to rapidly growing tumours with distinct loss of tissue specificity) represent various stages of tumour progression and are convenient for the study of malignant growth pecularities at cellular and subcellular levels.

Morris studied hepatoma 5123 in greatest detail. This arose in 1956 from a tumour in a Buffalo line rat which received N-(2-fluorenide phthalamic acid in food (Weber, 1961). It showed slow growth and was highly differentiated biochemically and morphologically.

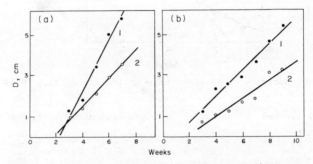

Fig. 21   Hepatoma 5123 growth in animals of different sex and age.   (a) 1 — males, 2 — females;   (b) 1 — 1.1-month age, 2 — 8.9-months age to the time of transplantation.

The effects of the age and sex of recipient animals on the growth of hepatoma 5123 have been studied. Kinetic treatment of these data (Figure 21) revealed that tumour growth was characterized by a linear function. Below are the data on the growth of hepatoma 5123 in relation to the recipient's sex and age.

Sex	Age, months	Growth rate, cm per week
Male	—	1.22
Female	—	0.67
Female	1.1	0.63
Female	8.9	0.44

The average diameter of hepatoma 3924A (Figure 22) calculated from the table in Lo *et al.* (1973) increases in the same way and with a close rate constant (1.01 cm per week). In this case a prolonged linear phase is preceded by an initial exponential period with an exponent $\phi = 0.077$ day^{-1}, which differs only slightly from the value $\phi = 0.069$ day^{-1} obtained earlier (Knox *et al.*, 1970; Tsou *et al.*, 1974; Looney *et al.*, 1973). A mathematical model of solid tumour development involving continuous transition from exponential to linear growth will be considered in the next section.

Comparison of the indices of hepatoma 5123's exponential growth with another strain of Morris hepatoma was made using the data from Knox *et al.* (1970), Tsou *et al.* (1974) and Looney *et al.* (1973).

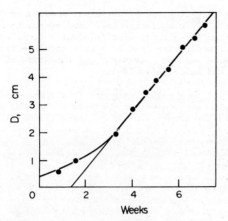

Fig. 22   Kinetics of hepatoma 3924A growth (Lo *et al.*, 1973)

Tumour strains	ϕ, day^{-1}	Tumour strains	ϕ, day^{-1}
7800	0.025	7777	0.045
7793	0.031	3924A	0.069
5123^{tc}	0.043	3683F	0.105

The growth kinetics of three transplanted hepatomas with different growth rates and extents of differentiation induced in C3HA mice under the action of o-amino-azotoluene described by Gelshtein (1966) have been further studied (Bogdanov *et al.*, 1973). These were: hepatoma 22a (anaplastic, glycogen absent, time between generations 15 days), hepatoma 60 (trabecular, abundance of glandular side struc-tures and glycogen present in certain cell groups, time between generations 1.4 months) and hepatoma 46 (trabecular, of an ultrastructure resembling that of normal hepatocytes, non-uniform glycogen distribution, time between generations 3 months).

The curves for tumour size changes are S-shaped and are well described by auto-catalysis equations (Figure 23, A-C). The kinetic parameters are listed in Table 6.

Fig. 23   Mouse hepatomas
         (Bogdanov *et al.*, 1973)

A — Hepatoma 22a;   B — Hepatoma 60;
     C — Hepatoma 46;
D — Relation between volume and
     weight of hepatoma 22a.

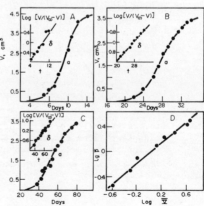

TABLE 6   Kinetic parameters of transplanted hepatoma growth (Williamson, 1975)

Hepatoma strain	V_∞, cm^3	ϕ, day^{-1}	(dx/dt) max, day^{-1}	Induction time, days	Inflection point, days
22a	4.7	0.63	0.17	4	10
60	3.8	0.47	0.12	23	28
46	3.9	0.10	0.03	39	58

The relation between tumour volume and weight of hepatoma 22a was estimated as: log P = $-0.26 + 0.82 \log V$ (Figure 23D). These parameters are connected by the relation $P = \delta V$, where δ is the density of the tumour tissue. Then $\log P = \log \delta + \log V$, and thus the coefficient of log V would be 1, instead of the experimental value 0.82. This difference is probably due to insufficient accuracy in evaluating the tumour volume, and also to a possible change in its density in the process of growth. Lo *et al.* (1973) found a positive relationship between weight and volume for rat hepatoma 3924A.

Taper *et al.* (1966) investigated the growth kinetics of transplanted spontaneous mouse hepatoma characterized by rapid growth. Figure 24, A–C, gives data on time-dependent changes in tumour size with various transplantation procedures. After intramuscular transplantation (Figure 24A) the tumour weight grows exponentially

$$P = 0.06 \exp(0.42t) \text{ g.}$$

The change in diameter of a tumour transplanted subcutaneously (Figure 24B) obeys the linear function

$$D = 0.09 + 0.14t \text{ cm.}$$

With intraperitoneal transplantation the change in the number of tumour cells in the ascitic fluid is described by a function with a maximum on the 13th day (Figure 24C). The doubling time of tumour cells in the exponential phase of growth (up to 9 days) is about 21 hours, i.e. almost half the time of weight doubling after intramuscular transplantation (~39.3 hours).

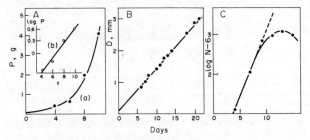

Fig. 24   Kinetics of mouse hepatoma growth for various transplantations (Taper *et al.*, 1966): A — intramuscular; B — subcutaneous; C — intraperitoneal.

Melanomas

Transplanted melanomas differ in the extent of pigment content, histological characteristics, capacity for metastasization, etc.

Melanoma Harding-Passey

Harding and Passey (1930) reported that this melanoma had been produced in 1925 from a spontaneous tumour in a brown mouse. It is strongly pigmented, takes to mice of any line with almost 100% transplantability. It consists of melanoblasts and macrophages containing melanin granules of identical structure and is considered to be close to a melanoma in humans (Shanin, 1959).

The increase in mean tumour diameter in C3HA mice over the time span of 14 to 32 days after subcutaneous transplantation of a tumour cell suspension (Figure 25A) is described by an autocatalysis equation of the form

$$D = \frac{2}{1 + 36 \exp{(-0.22t)}}$$

with computed parameters (Vasileva *et al.*, 1969). The measurements were not made at earlier times: the tumour sizes were too small. The growth rate at the point of inflection of the kinetic curve (17th day) was 0.11 cm/day.

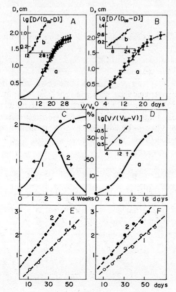

Fig. 25 Transplanted melanomas.
A — Harding-Passey melanoma (Vasileva *et al.*, 1969); B — melanoma B-16 (Vasileva *et al.*, 1974); C — melanoma B-16: (1) tumour growth, (2) death of animal (Schmid *et al.*, 1966); D — Cloudman melanoma (Summers, 1966); E, F — Cloudman melanoma, growth in DBA/1 (E) and BDF₁ (F) mice on subcutaneous transplantation in the mouse tail (1) or in axillary space (2) (Vedrich *et al.*, 1961).

Melanoma B-16

This melanoma arose from a spontaneous tumour of C57Bl mice. It takes to mice of
the same line: transplantability is up to 100% and in a number of cases it
metastasizes to the lungs, liver and spleen. It is characterized by the heterogeneity of its cell population involving both strongly pigmented zones, and
fragments with an inappreciable content or complete absence of melanin.

The kinetic characteristics of tumour growth given by Vasileva *et al.*. (1974) and
those calculated from Schmid *et al.*'s (1966) results virtually coincide (Figure 25,
B,C), though the transplantation procedure were different. Schmid *et al.* transplanted the tumour in fragments, whilst Vasileva's team inoculated it as a cell
suspension. The kinetic parameters of melanoma B-16 growth (Schmid *et al.*, 1966;
Vasileva *et al.*, 1974) are

	Vasileva	Schmid
D_0, cm	0.17	0.14
D_∞, cm	2.15	2.28
ϕ, day^{-1}	0.18	0.21
V_{max}, cm/day	0.10	0.13

The kinetic parameters of tumour growth in male and female C57Bl mice or F_1
hybrids do not differ statistically. A summary curve is given in Figure 25B.
Between the 10th and 14th days tumour growth results in progressive death of the
animals (Figure 25C, curve 2).

Cloudman melanoma S-91

This melanoma was produced from a spontaneous tumour from a DBA mouse. It is
slightly pigmented, takes to animals of the same line with 100% transplantability,
has a high frequency of pulmonary metastasization, and has a well-developed
vascular metwork and poor connective tissue.

Processing the experimental kinetic data obtained by Summers (1966) using the autocatalysis equation yielded the parameters ϕ = 0.3 day^{-1} and V_∞/V_0 = 37 (Figure 25D).
The V_0 value was not reported, so that the absolute growth rate at the point of
inflection could not be calculated.

Analysis of the data from Vedrich *et al.* (1961) on the growth kinetics of tumours
transplanted in the axillary space or subcutaneously in DBA/1 and BDF$_1$ mice shows
that in all cases the change in tumour diameter follows a linear dependence (Figure
25E,F). The growth kinetics of melanoma S-91 as a function of the animal line and
transplantation site are given in Vedrich *et al.* (1961).

Animal line	Axillary space	Tail
DBA/1	$D = 4.0 + 0.65t$	$dD = -1.9 + 0.50t$
BDF$_1$	$D = 1.9 + 0.56t$	$D = -0.3 + 0.41t$

(D measured in mm, t in days after transplantation).

The difference in growth rates Δb of a tumour transplanted at various sites
(0.15 mm/day) is seen to be independent of the animal line; the value Δb for the
same transplantation sites in various animals (0.09 mm/day) also is constant.

A functional expression for linear tumour growth rate was reported by Gorkov and
Vasileva (1973):

$$b = (\phi/3)D_{tr}$$

where ϕ is the index of exponential growth at the initial stage and D_{tr} is the diameter after which growth becomes linear. Assuming that ϕ remains constant, the observed differences in the values of b will be due to D_{tr} only and the latter depends also on the blood supply. Δb values are constant and the various mice lines are characterized by different intensities of blood supply generally, but the ratio of rates for various body organs keeps approximately constant.

Comparison of the kinetic characteristics of various melanomas shows that those for Harding-Passey and B-16 growth are only slightly different. According to Summers (1966) the Cloudman melanoma attained the same size relative to the inoculum size in shorter periods of time (Figure 25A,D), but according to Vedrich et al. (1961) it takes approximately twice the time taken by the first two melanomas. In the latter case the linear growth constants are also approximately half those for the first two strains (0.41 - 0.65 and 1.05 - 1.30 mm/day). Comparison of the exponential factor ϕ in the autocatalysis equation recalculated in terms of diameters ($\phi_D = \phi_V/3$) shows that the Cloudman melanoma growth was slower also in Summers' work in 1966 ($\phi_D = 0.10$ compared to $\phi_D = 0.18 - 0.21$ day^{-1}). Achieving the same size in a shorter time could be the result of a larger inoculum: its size is not reported.

Sarcoma 180

This was produced in 1914 from a spontaneous gland carcinoma (Larionov, 1962). The tumour is non-differentiated and has 100% transplantability. As a rule there are no spontaneous regressions. It can be used in the solid form and in ascites forms.

Kinetic studies of the solid tumour form were conducted over the period 1963 to 1970 using diverse experimental methods recording many characteristics (weight, volume, etc.) of tumour growth (Wilcox et al., 1965; Adams and Bowman, 1963; Summers, 1966; Minenkova et al., 1968; Humphrey, 1963). This has resulted in differences in the types of kinetic regularities and in the relevant parameters used for description of experimental results (Figure 26).

Tumour growth in mice of the Swiss line over the time span 4 to 12 days is described by the exponential function

$$P = 0.06 \exp(0.37t) \text{ g}$$

(Wilcox et al., 1965)(Figure 26A), but the pre-exponential factor (60 mg) at the time of transplantation, obtained by extrapolation, is higher than the true inoculum value (15 mg). This paper gives a plot on a modified scale: tumour growth is exponential only at the initial phase (4 to 8 days) with an exponential index $\phi = 0.62$ day^{-1}.

According to Minenkova et al. (1968) the exponential phase of tumour growth in non-inbred mice is longer (up to 16 days), and the exponent is lower (0.19 day^{-1}). Over the whole time span (up to 22 days) the change in tumour volume is approximated by a power dependence (Figure 26B)

$$V = 0.026t^{2.11} \text{ cm}^3$$

The change in the value R^3 (Humphrey, 1963) proportional to the volume (R is the mean radius) also follows a power dependence with the index close to that of Minenkova et al. (1968):

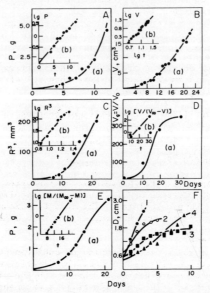

Fig. 26 Kinetics of solid sarcoma 180 growth from reported
data. A — Wilcox *et al.* (1965); B — Minenkova *et al.* (1968);
C — Humphrey (1963); D — Summers (1966); E — Adams and
Bowman (1963); F — complete diet and thymectomy (1), as
above with pseudo-operation (2), B_6 deficiency and thymectomy
(3), as above with pseudo-operation (4).

$$R^3 = 0.035t^{2 \cdot 85} \text{ mm}^3.$$

The time span of changes also coincides (22 days), but the maximum volume attained
at the end of the experiment is considerably shorter (Figure 26B). This seems to
be connected with experimental conditions, as in Humphrey (1963) the tumour was
transplanted to mice that were given potassium-deficient food. Processing the
results of Adams and Bowman (1963) and Summers (1966) by the autocatalysis
equation, we have (Figure 26D,E)

$$V_r = \frac{345}{1 + 344 \exp(-0.36t)}$$

$$P = \frac{3.7}{1 + 37 \exp(-0.26t)} \text{ g.}$$

However, the parameters of these equations are difficult to compare, since, in the
former, the tumour growth is characterized by a dimensionless value $V_r = V/V_0$, and
the inoculum size V_0 is not shown. Assuming in the second equation that $t = 0$, we
get $P_0 = 0.1$ g, whence $P_\infty/P_0 = 37$. This is considerably lower than the value
$V_\infty/V_0 = 345$ in the first equation.

Ferrer and Mihich (1967) report experimental kinetic results using an autocatalysis
equation suggesting that thymectomy seems to favour tumour growth, whereas a
vitamin B_6 deficient diet somewhat retards tumour growth (Figure 26F, Table 7).

TABLE 7   Dependence of solid sarcoma 180 growth kinetics on diet and
immunological factors (Steel and Lemerton, 1966)

Curve no. in Fig. 26B	Diet	Surgical treatment	D_0 (cm)	D_∞ (cm)	ϕ (day^{-1})
1	Full diet	Thymectomy	0.7	3.0	0.14
2	Full diet	'Control' surgery	0.5	2.1	0.17
3	Vitamin B_6 deficient	Thymectomy	0.4	1.6	0.10
4	Vitamin B_6 deficient	'Control' surgery	0.4	3.0	0.02

The kinetic regularities of the development of the ascites sarcoma 180 in mice of
different lines were studied by Ostrovskaia (1968). The surves for increase in
the ascitic fluid volume always were S-shaped (Figure 27a-d, curves 1). The change
in the number of cells is extreme (Figure 27a-d, curves 2) and up to the maximum
point it is well approximated by the cubic root equation. The numerical equations
describing both types of curves are given in Table 8.

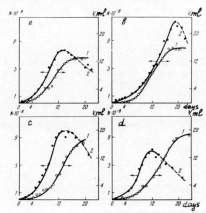

Fig. 27   Ascites sarcoma 180 in mice of various lines
(Ostrovskaia, 1968): (a) non-inbred; (b) BALB/C; (c)
C3HA; (d) C57Bl. Curves 1 — volume of ascitic fluid;
2 — number of cells.

TABLE 8   Kinetic equations for changes in ascitic fluid and tumour cell number
for sarcoma 180 in animals of different lines   (Anon, 1958).

Characteristic of tumour growth		Non-inbred	BalB/C	C3HA	C57Bl
V, ml	=	$\dfrac{13.2}{1+100e^{-0.45t}}$	$\dfrac{15.8}{1+333e^{-0.50t}}$	$\dfrac{18.0}{1+143e^{-0.42t}}$	$\dfrac{19.0}{1+333e^{-0.43t}}$
$10^{-2}(N)^{1/3}$	=	$2.08 + 0.61t$	$2.38 + 0.46t$	$1.63 + 0.73t$	$1.29 + 0.74t$

Comparison of the curves in Figure 27 and of the relevant parameters (see Table 8) shows that the kinetics of tumour growth in C3HA, C57B1 mice and in non-inbred mice is similar, whereas in BALB/C mice the ascitic fluid accumulates somewhat faster, and the increase in the number of cells is slower. The maximum point is characterized by a higher value and is reached at a later time. The lifespan of the BALB/C line mice is also longer.

Sarcoma 37
===

This is a non-differentiated, polymorphocellular tumour produced in 1906 from a transplanted carcinoma from a mouse mammary gland (Larionov, 1962). It sometimes metastasizes to lymph nodes and the lungs; when transplanted intravascularly it may invade the ovaries and the adrenal gland. Peripheral necrosis is inherent in the solid form. It shows 100% transplantability, but transplantation as an acellular filtrate fails. It can be passed in linear and non-inbred animals.

The solid tumour form takes a long time to develop (up to 80 days) with a substantial induction period (5-22 days) (Minenkova *et al.*, 1968). Changes in tumour size in mice of different lines is described by a power dependence within a considerable time span (up to 40-45 days) by an exponential equation (Figure 28A-E). The kinetics of tumour growth in animals of certain lines differs in one or both parameters of these dependences (Table 9).

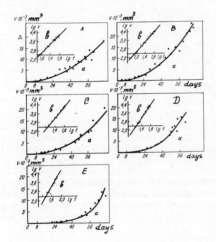

Fig. 28. Solid sarcoma 37 in mice of various lines (Minenkova *et al.*, 1968). (A) C57B1; (B) non-inbred; (C) C3HA; (D) BALB/C; (E) C3H/He.

TABLE 9 Kinetic parameters of development of solid sarcoma 37 in mice of different lines and non-inbred (Wilks, 1962)

| Line of mice | Kinetic function and parameters | | | | Induction time, days | Mean lifespan, days |
| | exponential | | power | | | |
	V_o, mm^3	ϕ, day^{-1}	a, mm^3	b		
C57B1	356	0.07	4.95	1.93	6	60
Non-inbred	111	0.11	2.36	2.18	8	76
C3HA	161	0.08	0.80	2.35	10	69
BALB/C	76	0.10	0.10	2.92	13	46
C3H/He	51	0.08	0.005	3.44	22	49

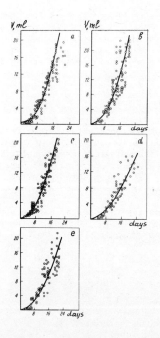

Fig. 29   Change in the ascitic fluid
volume after transplantation of
sarcoma 37 to mice of various lines
(Minenkova *et al.*, 1967).
(a) C57Bl;   (b) non-inbred;   (c) C3HA;
(d) BALB/C;   (e) C3H/He.

The growth of ascites tumours is faster. Mice live for 16 to 29 days, depending on
the animal's line (Minenkova *et al.*, 1967). The change in the volume of the
ascite tumour (Figure 29A-E) is described by a power function over the whole
experimental range and by an exponential function at the initial time (up to 14
days). The change in the number of tumour cells is finite, as for sarcoma 180,
and up to the maximum point it can also be described by a power dependence (Figure
30, A-E); in the latter case the exponential period is shorter (5-8 days). The
kinetic parameters for changes in the number of tumour cells show no significant
differences in most animal lines. The kinetics of ascitic fluid accumulation
depend to a greater extent on the animal line (Table 10). The accumulation of
tumour cells is slower than the increase in the ascitic fluid volume (Figure 31).
The concentration of tumour cells (N/V) continuously decreases with tumour growth,
and this seems to be the cause of the finite nature of the cell accumulation
curves. Perhaps, before the maximum value $N(t)$ is reached, the concentration of
nutritional compounds in the ascites becomes insufficient, and as a result the
cells either cease to divide or perish (Erokhin, 1968).

A mathematical description of the diffusion of nutritional compounds into ascitic
fluid implies an exponential decrease in the number of cells in the fall-off phase
and an exponential increase in their doubling time at the terminal stages of tumour
growth.

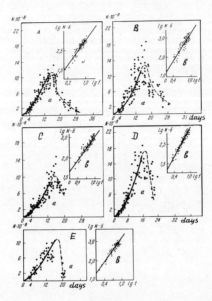

Fig. 30   Change in cell number of ascites sarcoma 37 in
mice of various lines (Minenkova *et al.*, 1967).
(A) C57Bl;   (B) non-inbred;   (C) C3HA;   (D) BALB/C;
(E) C3H/He.

TABLE 10   Kinetic parameters of sarcoma 37 ascitic form in mice
of different lines and non-inbred   (Larionov, 1962)

Characteristic of growth	Parameters	C57Bl	Non-inbred	C3HA	BALB/C	C3H/He
	$a \cdot 10^{-1}$	2.57	1.47	2.55	1.55	1.99
	b	1.32	1.60	1.40	1.60	1.44
N						
	$N_0 \cdot 10^{-7}$	3.52	2.62	2.10	1.75	1.26
	ϕ, day^{-1}	0.35	0.39	0.51	0.49	0.60
	a, ml	0.05	0.03	0.04	0.06	0.05
	b	1.97	2.23	2.12	1.79	2.03
V						
	V_0, ml	0.15	0.22	0.36	0.19	0.31
	ϕ, day^{-1}	0.33	0.30	0.25	0.27	0.28

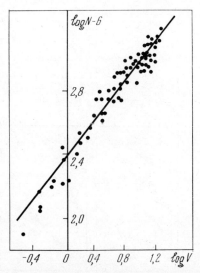

Fig. 31 Dependence between ascitic fluid volume and number
of sarcoma 37 malignant cells in C3HA mice (Erokhin, 1968)

Ehrlich Ascites Cancer

This was produced in 1906 by transplantation of a spontaneous cancer from a mouse
mammary gland (Larionov, 1962; Ehrlich, 1907). The tumour is non-differentiated
and takes to all mouse lines with 100% transplantability. The solid form is used
infrequently and has been little studied from the kinetic standpoint.

A detailed kinetic study of the Ehrlich ascites carcinoma was first conducted in
1953 by Klein and Revesz. The kinetics of change in the number of cells in the
ascitic fluid was described by equation

$$(N)^{1/3} = (N_0)^{1/3} + b(t - t_0)$$

where N_0 is the number of inoculated cells, b is a constant coefficient and t_0 is
the moment of time when $(N)^{1/3} = (N_0)^{1/3}$. With an increase in the inoculum size
from $7.3 \cdot 10^5$ to $1.75 \cdot 10^7$ the coefficient b increased from 3.8 to 4.8, and with a
further increase in N_0 to $4.0 \cdot 10^7$ it fell to 3.0. The b value is independent of
the inoculum 'age'. A proportional dependence between the ascites fluid volume
and the number of tumour cells it contains was noted (Figure 32D). This is
evidence of a constant specific content of cells in this case, and seems to explain
the absence of the fall-off phase from the curve for the cell number change
characteristic of the ascites form of sarcoma 37, for which the specific cell
content decreases monotonically with time (Minenkova, 1967).

The changes in values of N reported by Klein and Revesz (Figure 32, A-D) can also
be described by autocatalysis equations:

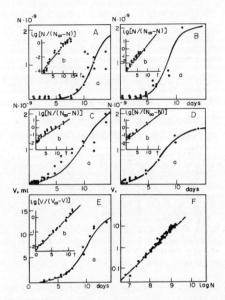

Fig. 32   Ehrlich ascites carcinoma (Klein and Revesz, 1953).
A-D — Change in the number of malignant cells per inoculum:
7×10^5 (A), 1.8×10^6 (B), 4.0×10^7 (D). E — Ascitic fluid
volume; F — relationship between the ascitic fluid volume
and the number of cells in the ascites.

$$N_A = \frac{1.9 \cdot 10^9}{1 + 11900 \exp(-0.81t)} \qquad N_B = \frac{2.0 \cdot 10^9}{1 + 935 \exp(-0.81t)}$$

$$N_C = \frac{2.3 \cdot 10^9}{1 + 63.5 \exp(-0.42t)} \qquad N_D = \frac{1.6 \cdot 10^9}{1 + 38.0 \exp(-0.5t)}$$

The change in the ascitic fluid volume (Figure 32E) is satisfactorily described
by an autocatalysis equation

$$V = \frac{15}{1 + 234 \exp(0.55t)} \quad \text{ml.}$$

The Gompertz equations (Laird, 1964) and a function of the form

$$V_r = 2^{(K - K_1 V_r)^t}$$

proposed by Summers (1966) were also used in analyzing the above data.

Computer processing of the results of Baserga (1963) and Tannock and Steel (1970)
using the autocatalysis equation yields parameters close to those for the equations
given earlier: $N_0 = 4.9 \cdot 10^6$ and $3.8 \cdot 10^6$ cells; $N_\infty = 1.9 \cdot 10^9$ and $1.4 \cdot 10^9$,
$\phi = 0.66$ and 0.70 day^{-1} (Figure 33, A and B). The hypotetraploid tumour was studied
by Baserga and the hyperploid tumour by Tannock and Steel. The close parameter
values seem to show that the ploidy of tumour cells has no great effect on the
kinetics of tumour growth. The kinetics of change in the number of cells of the
near-diploid (N_2) and near-tetraploid (N_1) variants is finite and up to the

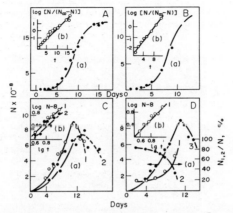

Fig. 33   Change in number of malignant cells in Ehrlich
ascites carcinoma sublines.   A — Hypertetraploid subline
(Baserga, 1963);   B — hyperdiploid subline (Tannock and
Steel, 1970);   C — near-diploid (1) and near-tetraploid (2)
strains;   D — relative cell content for various lines (1,2)
and their total number (3) after transplantation of the
conventional strain.

maximum is described by power functions with close parameter values (Figure 33B)

$$N_1 = 1.8 \cdot 10^7 t^{1.61}; \qquad N_2 = 1.5 \cdot 10^7 t^{1.56}.$$

Two cell lines have also been found in the heterogeneous strain of Ehrlich ascites
cancer: one with 44 chromosomes and a set of markers A_1-B-2C (line 1), and the
other with 45 chromosomes and a set of markers A-B-2C (line 2).   As the malignant
process develops, there occurs a change in these stem cells: an equilibrium in
their relative content sets in about two days before the start of fall-off (Figure
33D).

Qualitative and quantitative differences in the kinetics of tumour growth in
animals of different lines were reported by Ostrovskaia in 1968.   The kinetic
surves for accumulation of ascitic fluid in the BALB/C line and in non-inbred mice
were S-shaped.   For C3HA and C57Bl mice these lines were exponential over the whole
experimental range (Figure 34a-d, curves 1).   The number of tumour cells in the
BALB/C and C57Bl mice reached a maximum and then decreased, whereas for C3HA and
non-inbred mice the fall-off phase was absent (Figure 34a-d, curves 2).   Just as
for sarcomas 37 and 180 the changes in the cell number of the whole range
(Figure 34a,c) or up to the maximum point (Figure 34b,d) was approximated by the
cube root equation, and the S-shaped increase in the ascitic fluid volume — by the
autocatalysis equation.   The mean life-span of hosts differed only slightly.   The
numerical equations are:

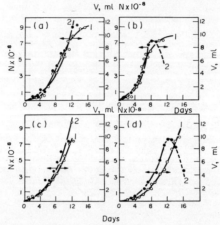

Fig. 34   Development of Ehrlich ascites carcinoma in mice
of various lines (Ostrovskaia, 1968):   (a) non-inbred;
(b) BALB/C;   (c) C3HA;   (d) C57Bl (1 — ascites volume,
2 — number of cells).

	Ascitic fluid volume	Number of cells
Non-inbred	$V = \dfrac{11.3}{1 + 35.8 \exp{(-0.64t)}}$	$\sqrt[3]{N} = 10^2(1.89+0.63t)$
BALB/C	$V = \dfrac{9.4}{1 + 22.2 \exp{(-0.83t)}}$	$\sqrt[3]{N} = 10^2(1.18+0.99t)$
C3HA	$V = 0.28 \exp{(0.31t)}$	$\sqrt[3]{N} = 10^2(1.90+0.70t)$
C57Bl	$V = 0.15 \exp{(0.31t)}$	$\sqrt[3]{N} = 10^2(1.12+0.68t)$

Ilina and Merkle (1973) proposed one might describe the kinetics of change in the
number of Ehrlich ascites cancer cells by the equation

$$N(t) = \frac{a}{b} \frac{1}{1 + \left(\dfrac{a}{bN_0} - 1\right) \exp{[-a(t-t_0)]}}$$

where a, b, and N_0 are constant parameters, $(t - t_0)$ is the time elapsed after
transplantation. By substituting the variables

$$\frac{a}{b} = N_\infty; \quad a^* = \left(\frac{a}{bN_0} - 1\right); \quad b = a; \quad t_0 = 0$$

this equation reduces to a first order autocatalysis equation or to an equivalent
logistic function

$$N = N_\infty/[1 + a^* \exp{(-bt)}]$$

and substituting the reported numerical coefficients a, b and N_0 to yield
parameter estimates $N_\infty = 0.06 \cdot 10^9$ and $\phi = b = 0.65$ day^{-1}, close to those obtained by
processing the results given in other papers.

Thus this equation is another form of the equations widely used in experimental
oncology, but it is less convenient for practical use. The original equation used
by Ilina and Merkle is known to have been first proposed for population growth by
Verhülst in 1837 (see Chapter 1):

$$\frac{dN}{dt} = aN - bN^2.$$

It will be noted that the biological sense of the quadratic form of the negative-
additive term is not discussed by Ilina and Merkle. The identification of the N_0
value with inoculum size and the semi-qualitative evaluation of two other parameters from the approximate position of the asymptote and of the point of inflection
also are unjustified.

Other Experimental Models

The adenocarcinoma EO771, sarcoma T241, the osteogenic Ridgway sarcoma (ROS) and
carcinoma C1025 transplanted to mice of various lines have been proposed for
screening of antitumour drugs in 1966 (Schmid et al.). Kinetic treatment of the
experimental data obtained by Schmid et al. shows that the growth of these four
tumour types is satisfactorily approximated by the autocatalysis equation with the
parameters in Table 11.

TABLE 11 Kinetic growth parameters of adenocarcinoma EO771, sarcoma T241,
osteogenic Ridgeway sarcoma and carcinoma C1025 (Schmid et al., 1966).

Type of tumour	D_0, cm	D_∞, cm	ϕ, day^{-1}	V_{max}, cm/day
EO771	0.08	3.1	0.22	0.18
C1025	0.28	3.0	0.11	0.09
POC	0.23	2.8	0.14	0.10
T241	0.27	3.0	0.16	0.13

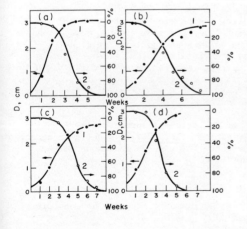

Fig. 35 Solid mouse tumours
(Schmid et al., 1966)
(a) Adenocarcinoma EO771;
(b) Carcinoma C1025;
(c) Ridgway osteogenic sarcoma;
(d) Sarcoma T241 (1 — tumour growth,
2 — death of animals).

Figure 35a-d shows the kinetic curves (curves 1) plotted from these parameters and their experimental points, together with the animal mortality curves (curves 2).

The tumour transplanted to CBA mice from spontaneous sarcomas have also been studied (Hewitt and Blake, 1966). The tumours are known to be both fast and slow-growing. In both cases the tumour diameter increases linearly at a rate of 1.2 mm/day for a fast-growing tumour and 0.27 mm/day for a slow-growing tumour (Figure 36a). The kinetics of tumour growth are independent of the animal's age (Figure 36b) and the inoculum size (Figure 36c). A decrease in the inoculum size causes a parallel shift of the curves. Pre-irradiation of the transplantation site with a 2000 r dose causes a similar decrease in the growth rate in all cases (Figure 36, a-d). The minimal effective dose inducing a decrease in the growth rate lies within 500 - 1000 r. Over the 1000 - 4000 r dose range the linear growth rate decreases by 30-50%. Gorkov and Vasileva (1973) state that the linear growth constant b is expressed by the parameters of the exponential (ϕ) and transition (D_{tr}) phases

$$b = (\phi/3)D_{tr}.$$

The pre-irradiation effect is thought to change the D_{tr} value corresponding to a transition from exponential to linear growth. A decrease in ϕ would be expected to prolong the latent period and this was not observed in practice (Figure 36c,d).

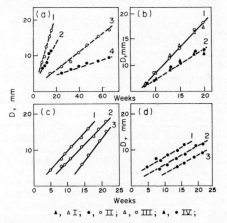

▲, ▵ I; •, ○ II; ▵, ○ III; ▲, • IV;

Fig. 36 Sarcoma growth kinetics in CBA mice (Hewitt and Blake, 1968). (a) Fast-growing (1,2) and slow-growing (3,4) variants; (b) growth in young animals and adults; (c,d) transplantation with inocula of decreasing volume (I — young animals, II — adults, III — without irradiation, IV — with pre-irradiation of the transplantation site at a dose of 2000 rad).

Subcutaneous inoculation of a suspension of the original tumour cells grown in culture produced a mouse fibrosarcoma (Frindel et al., 1967). Kinetic treatment of their experimental results shows that the curve for changes in tumour volume (Figure 37A) is described by a power equation

$$V = 2.5 + 0.21t^{3 \cdot 1} \quad \text{mm}^3.$$

Since the exponent is negligibly higher than 3, tumour growth can be considered as

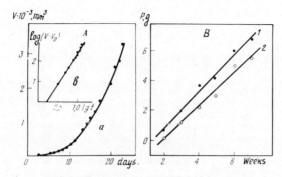

Fig. 37 Growth of solid tumours.
A — Fibrosarcoma transplanted with culture cells (Frindel
et al., 1967); B — alveolar cell carcinoma in intact (I)
and pre-irradiated (II) BALB/C mice (Yuhas and Pazmino,
1974).

linear in co-ordinates D vs t (D is the diameter), if the small (2.5 mm^3) additive
term is disregarded. It was suggested by Frindel *et al.* that the change in tumour
volume could be described by the Gompertz equation, though no numerical parameters
were given.

The growth of the alveolar cell carcinoma in BALB/C mice is unusual: the
increase in tumour weight is linear (Figure 37B) (Yuhas and Pazmino, 1974). Pre-
irradiation of the tumour cells with a 500 r dose two hours before subcutaneous
transplantation slightly retards the tumour growth, as expressed quantitatively by
equations

$$P_1 = -1.81 + 1.25t; \qquad P_2 = 2.23 + 1.11t.$$

Here P_1 and P_2 are the tumour weight values (in g) for non-irradiated and
irradiated mice, and t is the time (in weeks) elapsed after transplantation.

Experimental Leukaemias

Transplanted mouse and rat leukaemias are widely used in experimental oncology as
models of human leukaemias. These strains are very convenient for haematological
studies because the development of the malignant process is readily seen from
quantitative and qualitative shifts of the cellular forms.

Intraperitoneal and intravascular transplantation usually results in generalization
of the process. Leukaemia develops as a systemic disease with characteristic
changes in the peripheral blood (high leucocytosis, the appearance and progressive
increase of leukaemic cells, a decrease in the number of erythrocytes), with
infiltration of the bone marrow, spleen, liver, lymph nodes by leukaemic cells.
With subcutaneous transplantation of leukaemia a tumour arises at the inoculation
site, and it becomes the active centre responsible for subsequent development of
generalized leukaemia. A number of transplanted leukaemias of an ascitic form are
known. These are accompanied by the appearance of leukaemic cells in blood and in
haemopoietic organs (bone marrow, spleen and lymph nodes).

Leukaemia La

This leukaemia was developed in 1955 in C57Bl mice by transplantation of leukaemic organs of a mouse irradiated with high doses. Acute haemocytoblastosis developed as a generalized process with distinct infiltration of leukaemic cells into various organs, mostly spleen, bone marrow, liver and lymph nodes.

The kinetic regularities in leukaemia development were first studied in 1962 by Emanuel *et al*. The changes in spleen weight (S), in the number of leucocytes (L) and in malignant cells (haemocytoblasts) in peripheral blood (H) and in bone marrow (M) are described by exponential functions (Figure 38):

$$S = 110 + 20 \exp{(0.67t)}, \text{ mg}$$

$$L = 12000 + 3.7 \exp{(1.64t)}, \text{ } 1/\text{mm}^3$$

$$H = 0.01 \exp{(2.36t)}, \text{ } 1/\text{mm}^3$$

$$M = 1.85 + 0.24 \exp{(0.66t)}, \text{ %.}$$

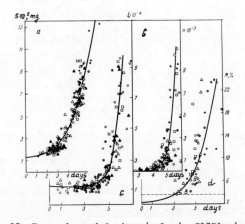

Fig. 38   Transplanted leukaemia La in C57Bl mice.
(a) Spleen weight;   (b) leucocytes in peripheral blood;
(c) haemocytoblasts in blood;   (d) haemocytoblasts in bone
marrow.

An accurate assessment of the parameters characteristic of increase in spleen weight was obtained by Bogdanov *et al*. (1971):

$$S = 110 + 23 \exp{(0.58t)}, \text{ mg,}$$

an expression for the relative content of haemocytoblasts in spleen having been first found:

$$H_S = 1.11 \exp{(0.54t)}, \text{ %.}$$

The doubling time of the total number of leukaemic cells in an animal's body was calculated by Gorkov and Ostrovskaia (1977). Assuming that the animal dies after the malignant cell population has reached the threshold value N_i, an equation was proposed for host life-span as a function of the number of transplanted cells

$$t_i = t_{max} - 3.32\ T_d \log N_i$$

where t_{max} is the expected life-span upon transplantation of one cell, N_i is the number of cells in the inoculum, T_d is the population doubling time. Experimental study of t_i as a function of inoculum N_i (Figure 39) yielded the expression

$$t_i = 22.8 - 2.2 \log N_i, \quad \text{days}$$

thus the doubling time is $T_d = 2.2/3.32 = 0.66$ days $= 15.9$ hours. The average spleen weight of dead mice (S = 890 ± 66 mg) was independent of the inoculum size, and this is an indirect support of the assumption that N_i is constant and independent of N_i.

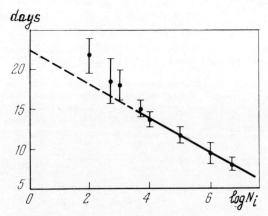

Fig. 39 Life-span of mice with leukaemia La as a function of amount of transplanted cells (Bogdanov *et al.*, 1971).

Over the range of N_i changes from $1.5 \cdot 10^4$ to $4.0 \cdot 10^7$ cells the kinetic parameters ϕ_S, ϕ_L, ϕ_H, ϕ_M remain unchanged and the mean shift Δt_i of experimental curves for changes in S, L, H, M indices for any N_i value is independent of the nature of the parameter studied (Emanuel *et al.*, 1964). It follows from the preceding equation that

$$\Delta t_i = 3.32\ T_d \log (N_i^*/N_i), \quad \text{days}$$

where N_i^* is the inoculum size corresponding to the standard curve. Processing the data obtained in 1964 by Emanuel *et al.* making use of this expression yielded a doubling time of 20 hours. This is higher by about 25% than the T_d value obtained in 1974. But during the past 10 years the maximal spleen weight decreased approximately from 1300 to 1000 mg, the life-span at $N_i = 10^8$ cells decreased from 7-8 to 5-6 days, the critical inoculum value fell from 10^4 to 10^2 cells. Thus, leukaemia development was accelerated.

At the same time the strain is characterized by high stability of the kinetic parameters for serial transplantations and is consequently very convenient for chemotherapeutic experiments.

Leukaemia L-1210

Law *et al*. reported in 1949 a subcutaneous tumour in a DBA mouse after painting the skin with methylcholanthrene. The strain is transplantable intravenously, intraperitoneally, subcutaneously or intracerebrally. All transplantation methods give 100% transplantability. DBA/2, C57B1, BALB mice and the BDF$_1$ hybrid mice are used.

Leukaemia L-1210 is widely used as a model in the selection of antitumour drugs. It gives the best correlation with human leukaemias with respect to drug action. There are strain sublines resistant to certain compounds, such as amethopterin, 6-mercaptopurine, azoguanine, etc. These sub-strains are used in the selection of drugs that could be effective in treating human leukaemias resistant to the above compounds. Leukaemia L-1210 is also used as a model for studying combined therapy.

The ascites leukaemia form is accompanied by generalization of the process: the number of leucocytes in the peripheral blood increases, leukaemic cells appear in increasing numbers. Sometimes leukaemic cells are found in the brain of the animal.

Transplantation of leukaemic cells into the brain results in a meningeal form. Generalization of the process starts 3-4 days after transplantation.

A quantitative study of the ascites form of leukaemia L-1210 was first conducted in 1958 by Shelton and Rice. Curves for the change in total number of cells and for the relative content of malignant cells in the ascitic fluid of DBA/2 mice were given for two generations. The curves are S-shaped (Figure 40) and can be described by autocatalysis equations

$$N = \frac{8 \cdot 10^8}{1 + 124 \exp(-1.5t)} \qquad \eta = \frac{100}{1 + 1.78 \exp(-1.67t)}$$

where N is the total number of cells in the ascitic fluid, and η is the percentage of malignant cells.

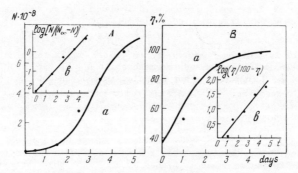

Fig. 40   Leukaemia L-1210 in DBA/2 mice (Shelton and Rice, 1958). (A) Total number; (B) relative number of leukaemic cells in ascitic fluid.

The development of ascitic and meningeal forms of leukaemic L-1210 was studied by Skipper *et al*. (1964). With intraperitoneal transplantation $10^5 - 10^6$ malignant cells appeared in the brain on the fourth day after transplantation: curves for the increase in number of leukaemic cells were obtained. One of these can be described by an exponential function

$N = 0.775 \exp(1.6t)$.

When leukaemic cells were transplanted into the brain, it did not seem possible to find the regularity of changes in the number of malignant cells owing to the great scatter of experimental points. Within four to seven days after intracerebral transplantation malignant cells also appeared in other organs and tissues.

Leukaemia development in hybrid mice has been studied with respect to changes in the number of leucocytes (L) and leukaemic cells (C) in peripheral blood (Figure 41). The kinetic curves for changes in L and C are described by exponential functions

$$L = 12000 + 580 \exp(0.63t), \text{ mm}^{-3};$$

$$C = 0.007 \exp(0.94t), \%.$$

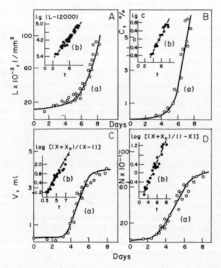

Fig. 41   Leukaemia L-1210 in hybrid C57Bl — DBA/2 mice.
(A) Leucocytes;   (B) leukaemic cells in peripheral blood;
(C) ascitic fluid volume;   (D) number of leukaemic cells
in ascitic fluid.

The increases in ascitic volume and in the number of malignant cells in the ascitic fluid are described by S-shaped curves

$$V = \frac{4}{1 + 11.5 \exp(-1.7t)}, \text{ ml}; \qquad N = \frac{7.4 \cdot 10^8}{1 + 36 \exp(-1.08t)}$$

The time of attaining the maximum accumulation rate of ascitic fluid and malignant cells in the fluid was 4.9 days.

The developmental kinetics of leukaemia L-1210 sublines resistant to cyclophosphamide (Johnson *et al.*, 1965) and to methotrexate (Johnson *et al.*, 1966) in DBA/2 mice and in CDF$_1$ hybrids was studied. The kinetic curves for increase in the number of ascites cells in both sublines (Figure 42a,b) are approximated by the

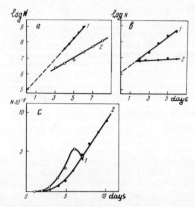

Fig. 42 Changes in total number of cells in ascitic fluid
for leukaemia L-1210 and P-388. (a) 1 — original line L-1210,
2 — subline resistant to cyclophosphamide (Johnson *et al.*, 1965);
(b) 1 — original line L-1210, 2 — subline resistant to
methotrexate (Johnson *et al.*, 1966); (c) leukaemia P-388
in DBA/2 (1) and BDF₁ (2) mice (Harris *et al.*, 1973).

exponential functions

$$a: \quad N_1 = 10^5 \exp(1.5t), \quad N_2 = 2.2 \cdot 10^5 \exp(0.8t)$$

$$b: \quad N_1 = 1.3 \cdot 10^6 \exp(1.0t); \quad N_2 = 5.5 \cdot 10^6 \exp(0.075t).$$

It is characteristic that the change in the main sign of leukaemia L-1210 development — in the number of cells in the ascitic fluid — is described, as a rule, by
first order autocatalysis equations with parameters close in magnitude. An
exception was observed for the results in Johnson *et al.* (1965, 1966). In this
case the exponential nature of the process seems to be due to use of CDF₁ hybrid
mice with different genotypical characteristics.

Leukaemia P-388

This was produced in 1955 by transplantation of lymphatic leukaemia induced by
methylcholanthrene in DBA/2 mice. It has been used as a model for the choice of
antitumour drugs only recently, mostly when investigating drugs of natural origin.
It is applied at present in the ascites form in BDF₁ hybrid mice. The cell cycle
duràtion in the course of tumour development increases from 8.5 hours after
transplantation to 22 hours at the terminal stages (Harris *et al.*, 1973). Figure
42c shows the kinetic results for changes in the number of cells in the ascitic
fluid after intraperitoneal transplantation of 10⁶ P-388 cells to DBA/2 and BDF₁
mice. The changes in cell numbers in mice DBA/2 are of an extreme nature and
reach a maximum (about 5·10⁸ cells) on the sixth day; 90% of animals die within
7 days after transplantation (Harris *et al.*, 1973). Characteristically from the
fifth day the increase in the number of cells in BDF₁ mice becomes linear and its
mean rate is 1.54·10⁷ cells a day. It attains twice the values for the DBA/2
mice (Konovalova, 1975). Most animals die around the fifth day, but more prolonged
life-spans were reported (more than 12 days). Such differences in the kinetics of
growth and the duration of life-spans might be due to further progression of the
strain, the properties of which did not reach stabilization.

Reticulum Cell Sarcomatosis

This strain was produced in 1968 in mice after inoculation of a spleen cell suspension passaged in tissue culture. Cells from the brain of a human who died from acute haemocytoblastosis produced the same condition. It is transplantable intraperitoneally in C57Bl mice. The development of reticulum cell sarcomatosis is characterized by lesions of the lymph system and internal organs, by enlarged liver and spleen, and by spread of tumour nodes in the intestine. Microscopically the metaplastic organs revealed large young cell forms belonging to reticular cells of the haemopoietic system.

The kinetics of changes in weight of liver, kidneys, spleen, mesenteric lymph nodes, the leucocyte concentration in blood and chemical changes have been studied. The total number of cells and the number of leukaemic cells in the liver and spleen were also counted. The original segments of kinetic curves for weight changes of individual organs and in their summary weight are described by exponential functions (Figure 43):

Index	Equation
Weight of liver, mg	$P = 1220 + 54.5 \exp (0.13t)$
Weight of kidneys, mg	$P = 290 + 1.3 \exp (0.26t)$
Weight of mesenteric nodes, mg	$P = 404 + 79.5 \exp (0.14t)$
Weight of spleen, mg	$P = 140 + 0.28 \exp (0.29t)$
Number of leukaemic cells in liver, $\times 10^6$	$N = 0.28 \exp (0.29t)$
Summary weight of: liver, kidney, spleen, mesenteric lymph nodes, mg	$P = 2050 + 94.5 \exp (0.17t)$

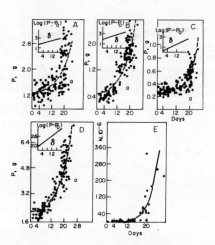

Fig. 43   Reticulum cell sarcomatosis in C57Bl mice.
(A) Liver weight;   (B) weight of mesenteric lymph nodes;
(C) weight of kidneys;   (D) total weight of infiltrated
organs;   (E) number of tumour cells in liver.

It did not seem possible to discover the kinetic regularities for the total number
of leucocytes in peripheral blood. Towards the terminal stage of the disease the
amount of neutrophil leucocytes in blood increased; the number of lymphocytes
remained within normal limits. Pathological cells in the spleen increased
exponentially; the total number of normal cells in the liver did not change.
This increase in the weight of the organs seems to be mainly due to the increasing
proportion of malignant cells.

From April 1969 to February 1970 the mean lifetimes of mice with reticulum cell
sarcomatosis shortened from 26.6 ± 1.9 to 19.6 ± 0.8 days under the same transplantation conditions. The doubling time of malignant cells decreased by one-third of
its original value. The values characteristic of the process development rate
later remained constant.

Leukaemia CL

A new strain of mouse leukaemia has been produced recently by inoculation of an
acellular culture of LL cells (leukaemic lymphoblasts) to newborn C57B1 mice
(Nikol'skaia et al., 1969). The line of LL cells produced a leukaemia virus in mice
in eight years of constant passages. The physico-chemical and morphological virus
characteristics can be found in Nikol'skaia and Lipchina (1968).

The development of leukaemia CL is accompanied by a marked increase in the size of
liver, spleen and lymph nodes. Intraperitoneal inoculation of a cell suspension of
spleen and lymph nodes from animals suffering from a leukaemia to C57B1 mice
resulted in the development of leukaemia in these mice. With an inoculum size
$4-10 \cdot 10^6$ cells the life-span of animals was 8-9 days. The kinetic regularities of
leukaemia CL were studied by Nikol'skaia et al. (1975). The increase in weight of
spleen (S), of inguinal (I) and mesenteric (M) lymph nodes and in the number of
blood leucocytes (L) (Figure 44) is described by autocatalysis equations:

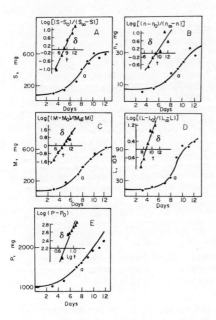

Fig. 44 Changes in certain character-
istics of leukaemia CL development
(Nikol'skaia et al., 1975).
(A) Spleen weight; (B) inguinal and
(C) mesenteric lymph nodes; (D) blood
leucocytes; (D) liver weight.

$$S = \frac{600}{1 + 287 \exp (-0.76t)} \text{ mg;} \qquad I = \frac{35}{1 + 455 \exp (-0.69t)} \text{ mg;}$$

$$M = \frac{650}{1 + 174 \exp (-0.67t)} \text{ mg;} \qquad L = \frac{1.1 \cdot 10^5}{1 + 3788 \exp (-0.94t)} \text{ 1/mm}^3$$

The increase in liver weight obeys the power law

$$P = 1044 + 6.3t^{2 \cdot 14}, \text{ mg.}$$

Lymphoid Leukaemia NKLy

This strain in an ascitic form was produced in 1960 from mice with spontaneous lymphoid leukaemia. The question of whether the lymphoid leukaemia NKLy was a sub-strain of the Ehrlich ascites carcinoma has been raised by Prigozhina and Vendrov (1971). However, there are distinct differences between these strains, in particular a different response to chemotherapeutic drugs.

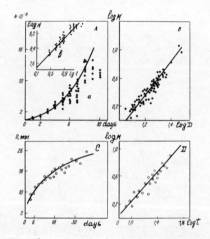

Fig. 45 Changes in characteristics of leukaemia NKLy development (Pelevina *et al.*, 1966). (A) Number of cells in ascitic fluid; (B) relation between mass and diameter of a solid tumour; (C) increase in tumour diameter; (D) logarithmic anamorphosis for changes in tumour mass.

The development of lymphoid leukaemia NKLy in both ascitic and solid forms was studied kinetically by Pelevina *et al.* (1966). The number of cells in the ascites N (Figure 45A) increases, obeying the power law

$$N = 2.8 \cdot 10^7 t^{1 \cdot 75}.$$

To evaluate the effective doubling time of ascitic cells, use was made of the expression

$$T_d^* = t \ln 2/b = 0.69 \ t/b, \text{ days.}$$

This doubling time, calculated in terms of the expression for $t = 3$ days, is

1.18 days. According to autoradiographic measurements to the 3rd day T_d is 0.94 days (Alesenko *et al.*, 1967), i.e. the agreement is quite close.

A power dependence of the tumour mass on its diameter was found for the solid form (Figure 45B):

$$\log M = -2.63 + 2.5 \log D.$$

A curve for increase in mass and its logarithmic anamorphosis (Figure 45D) were plotted from the kinetic curve for increase in the mean tumour diameter (Figure 45B) making use of this dependence. The increase in tumour mass obeys the power equation

$$M = 0.14t^{1.07}, \text{ g.}$$

Leukaemia LZ
_____

This strain was produced in 1961 by inoculating a chloroleukaemia virus into C3H mice. It represents acute haemocytoblastosis. The mean life-span of the diseased animals is 9 days.

The kinetics of leukaemia LZ development was studied by Dronova (1968). The kinetic curves for changes in liver weight (P), the number of leucocytes (L) and of haemocytoblasts in peripheral blood (H) and in bone marrow (M) are described by exponential functions (Figure 46):

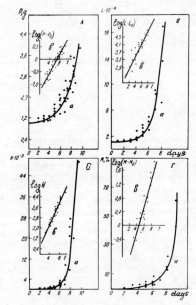

Fig. 46   Leukaemia LZ in C3H mice (Dronova, 1968).
(A) liver weight;   (B) blood leucocytes;   (C) haemocytoblasts in peripheral blood;   (D) haemocytoblasts
in bone marrow.

$P = 0.95 + 0.055 \exp (0.42t)$, g;

$H = 3.3 \exp (1.03t)$, $1/\text{mm}^3$;

$M = 1.85 + 1.03 \exp (1.53t)$, %;

$L = 12700 + 135 \exp (0.97t)$, $1/\text{mm}^3$.

Rat Erythroleukaemia

This strain was produced in 1957 by inoculation of an acellular filtrate of sarcoma BS into young Wistar rats (Svec *et al.*, 1957). Later on the strain was passaged in adult non-inbred animals. A subcutaneous tumour arises at the site of transplantation and it infiltrates the skin and underlying musculature of the abdominal wall. The number of blood leucocytes increases, young elements of the myeloid cells appear and erythroblasts increase to 20-40%. The development of leukaemia is accompanied by the appearance of anaemia with a decrease both of haemoglobin and of the total amount of erythrocytes. There is also a decrease in erythrocytes and thrombocytes. The lymph nodes, spleen and liver become larger, and are infiltrated by leukaemic cells. Swarms of pathological cells are also observed in the lungs. The tissue of the subcutaneous tumour consists of mononuclear mesenchymal cells.

The transplantability of erythroleukaemia, by both intraperitoneal and subcutaneous transplantation, is virtually 100%. No spontaneous resorption of the tumour is observed. The mean life-span of animals is 16.10 ± 0.33 days.

The kinetics of erythroleukaemia development were studied in non-inbred rats (Dronova *et al.*, 1966). The increase in the mean diameter of the subcutaneous tumour is described by an S-shaped curve (Figure 47A), which can be expressed by

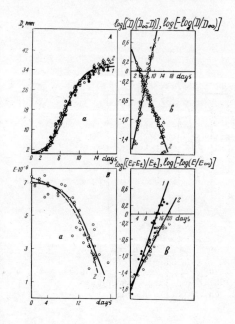

Fig. 47 Rat erythromyelosis (Dronova *et al.*, 1966). (A) Changes in mean diameter of the subcutaneous tumour; (B) erythrocyte count in blood: 1 — curves (a) and their anamorphoses (b) corresponding to the autocatalysis equation, and 2 — to the Gompertz equation.

the Gompertz equation

$$D = 38 \exp [-6.9 \exp (-0.32t)], \text{ mm}$$

or by the autocatalysis equation

$$D = \frac{36}{1 + 27 \exp (-0.4t)}, \text{ mm.}$$

The tumour weight increases exponentially (Figure 48a):

$$P = 0.24 \exp (0.37t), \text{ g.}$$

The kinetic differences when considering tumour diameter and tumour weight were discussed earlier (see page 34).

The decrease in blood erythrocytes (E) can also be described by an autocatalysis equation (Figure 47B):

$$E = \frac{1.5 \cdot 10^6}{1 - 0.8 \exp (-0.08t)}, \text{ } 1/\text{mm}^3$$

or by the Gompertz equation

$$E = 7.5 \cdot 10^6 \exp [-0.04 \exp (0.22t)], \text{ } 1/\text{mm}^3.$$

The kinetic curves for changes in other haematological parameters: the number of normoblasts (N), leucocytes (L), and spleen weight (S) are described by exponential functions over the whole time-span of leukaemia development (Figure 48a-d):

$$N = 12 \exp (0.47t), \text{ } 1/\text{mm}^3;$$
$$L = 13000 + 1800 \exp (0.21t), \text{ } 1/\text{mm}^3;$$
$$S = 0.45 + 0.01 \exp (0.34t), \text{ g.}$$

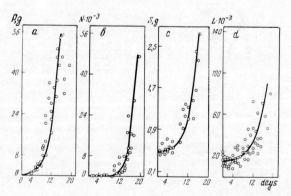

Fig. 48 Exponential kinetic curves for rat erythromyelosis development (Dronova *et al.*, 1966). (a) Tumour weight; (b) blood normoblasts; (c) spleen weight; (d) blood leucocytes.

Pliss Lymphosarcoma

This was produced in 1961 from a spontaneous tumour in a rat given the carcinogen 3.3-dichlorohydrobenzene in food from birth. The tumour consists of both small and large irregular lymphoid cells, swarms of which are observed in the liver and spleen. It is 100% transplantable subcutaneously; it is often accompanied by generalization of the process. The ascitic form also exists. The strain is sustained on non-inbred rats. The resistance of the Pliss lymphosarcoma to drugs makes the strain promising for the selection of effective antitumour drugs.

A detailed kinetic study of lymphosarcoma development and a generalization of the results reported by Lazarev and Miuller (1970) and Cherkaoova (1969) have been made by Gorkov and Vasileva (1973). The change in mean tumour diameter in 7-10 days after transplantation is linear:

$$D = b(t - t_0),$$

where t_0 is the crossing point of the straight line with the time axis, b is the rate of linear growth, and t is the time after transplantation (Figure 49).

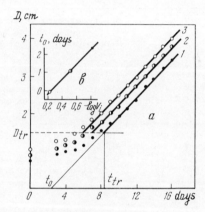

Fig. 49 Pliss lymphosarcoma (Gorkov and Vasileva, 1973).
(a) Change in tumour size upon inoculation of 0.15 (1), 0.3 (2) and 0.6 ml (3) of 50% tumour tissue suspension; (b) Latent period as a function of the inoculum volume.

The value b calculated by the least-squares procedure is independent of the inoculum and is 0.25 cm/day in all cases. As the inoculum size increases, t_0 diminishes (Figure 49, Table 12).

It was suggested that the increase in diameter and volume of the tumour at the initial stage was exponential. As a certain time t_{tr} was reached, there occurred a transition from exponential to linear growth, related to a change in the nutritional conditions of the tumour cells. Further on the growth rate attained at this time remains constant:

$$b = \frac{\phi}{3} D_{tr}$$

Here ϕ is the index of exponential growth, D_{tr} is the tumour diameter at time $t = t_{tr}$.

TABLE 12   Parameters of linear growth of Pliss lymphosarcoma
from various published data

Parameters of equations		Transplantation conditions			Factors studied	References
b cm/day	t_0 days	Animal weight, g	V_i^1 ml	Dilu-tion		
0.25	2.3	110-150	0.15	1:1		Gorkov and
0.25	1.0		0.30	1:1		Vasileva,
0.25	0.0		0.60	1:1		1973
0.25	1.6	90-110	-	-		
0.50	5.0	180-200	0.30	1:3		
0.28	1.6	150-200	-	-	Controls	Cherkasova,
0.28	1.8				Regular administration of ZnCl$_2$	1969
0.30	0.8	100-150	-	-	5th generation (controls)	Lazarev and
0.33	3.0				11th generation (controls)	Miuller,
0.32	4.4				Transplantation from rats	1970
0.30	2.0				treated with thiotepa	
0.36	1.1	not shown	0.24	5:1	Incubation of inoculum with physiological salt solution	
0.32	2.8		0.24	5:1	Incubation of inoculum with sodium citrate	
0.17	3.5	not shown	0.40	1:1	Incubation with physiological salt solution	
0.17	1.8		0.40	1:1	Incubation with trilon B	
0.19	4.0		0.40	1:1	Incubation with heparin	

Assuming that the summary volume of cell 'takes' depends linearly on the inoculum size V_i, we obtain

$$t_0 = A - \frac{1}{\phi} \ln V_i$$

where A is a constant.

The dependences obtained permit evaluation of the exponential growth phase parameters (which are difficult to evaluate with precision) from the values b and t_0 obtained experimentally for the linear growth phase. Here (Figure 49) ϕ and D_{tr} are 0.6 day^{-1} and 1.3 cm, respectively, and the tumour doubling time is 28 hours.

A large exponential region of tumour growth was observed. The relevant ϕ and T_d parameters (0.5 day^{-1} and 31 hours) are close to the calculated values (Gorkov and Vasileva, 1973).

The parameters b and t_0 were evaluated by Gorkov and Vasileva from the plots or from tabular data in Lazarev and Miuller (1970) and Cherkasova (1969) (Table 12). The factors discussed by Lazarev and Miuller (1970) and Cherkasova (1969) are seen to have no effect on tumour growth in the linear growth phase and to influence only the time of its attainment. The difference in values of b obtained from the results of Gorkov and Vasileva (1973) can be ascribed to different weights of the animals used.

A generalized linear mathematical model of transplanted leukaemia growth is given by Gorkov (1976). The system 'leukaemic cells — organism' is discussed for a model consisting of three inter-connected parts: (1) transplantation site, (2) peripheral blood, and (3) the set of organs infiltrated with leukaemic cells. The model structure is

$$N_1(\phi,k,t) \rightarrow N_2(\phi,k,t) \rightleftarrows N_3(\phi,k,t),$$

where N_1, N_2, N_3 are the number of cells in the above mentioned three parts, ϕ is the effective growth rate constant independent of cell localization, k stands for rate constants of cell exchange between the parts, and t is the time elapsed after transplantation.

In terms of the model, after intravascular transplantation ($N_1 = 0$) the changes in data of type N_2 and N_3 will be described by biexponential functions

$$N_2 = \frac{N_0}{K}[k_{32} \exp (\phi t) + k_{23} \exp (\psi t)]$$

$$N_3 = \frac{k_{23}N_0}{K} [\exp (\phi t) - \exp (\psi t)].$$

where $K = k_{23} + k_{32}$; $\psi = \phi - K$; N_0 is the number of transplanted cells. Approximation of the sum of two exponents by monoexponential functions should give underestimated apparent values of the pre-exponential factor N_0 and of the doubling time $T_d = \ln 2/\phi$. The difference in exponents would give over-estimated values of N_0 and T_d. This was actually so for the kinetic results when studying leukaemias La and LZ (Emanuel et al., 1964). The total number of leukaemic cells in the living body changes monoexponentially, as shown by summation of the above equations

$$N = N_2 + N_3 = N_0 \exp (\phi t).$$

The transport of cells from the site of transplantation into the blood occurs unidirectionally and in the general case obeys the equation

$$\frac{dN_1}{dt} = - \frac{aN_1}{b + N_1}$$

where a is the maximal transport rate, b is the parameters of the transport system 'affinity' to the transported cells. At $N_1 \ll b$ the transport equation reduces to a quasi-linear one

$$\frac{dN_1}{dt} \cong - \frac{a}{b} N_1$$

with an apparent rate constant $k_{12} = a/b$. For transport of L-1210 cells from a mouse abdominal cavity the estimated parameters a and b are: $a = 5 \cdot 10^7$, $b = 3.75 \cdot 10^7$. It follows that at $N_0 < 10^7$ the cell transport can be considered as pseudo-linear with a constant $k_{12} = 1.33$ day^{-1}. The time of 50% transport $T_{0.5} = \ln 2/k_{12} = 0.5$ days, corresponds to this value, and about 75% of the transplanted cells should be transported into the blood flow per day. This was actually so experimentally for $N_0 < 10^7$. The competing of nonlinear transport and linear proliferation at the site of transplantation in terms of the model is given by the equation

$$\frac{dN_1}{dt} = \phi N_1 - \frac{aN_1}{b + N_1}$$

Thus, when $dN/dt \leqslant 0$, we obtain the expression for the critical number of cells

$$(N_0)_{cr} = a/\phi - b,$$

below which a local tumour will not arise at the site of transplantation. Substituting into this expression the values $a = 5 \cdot 10^7$, $\phi = 1.5$ and $b = 3.75 \cdot 10^7$, we obtain $(N_0)_{cr} < 1$, which is consistent with the experimentally confirmed possibility of the arising of an ascites tumour upon transplantation of one cell of leukaemia L-1210.

3. SPONTANEOUS TUMOURS AND THEIR FIRST GENERATIONS

Spontaneously arising tumours are of great importance in experimental studies, since this class of tumours comes closest to human tumours.

Spontaneous tumours of various localizations arise in a number of animal species. These well-known and widespread tumours include Shoup papilloma in rabbits, the Rous hen sarcoma and cancer of the mammary gland in mice.

However, it is difficult to study the development of such tumours: the time of tumour incidence is not fixed and consequently the experimenter has to deal with tumours of various sizes and localizations. Only sparse studies on the kinetics of spontaneous tumour growth have been reported.

Certain studies dealt also with the kinetics of growth of the first tumour generation produced by transplantation of spontaneous neoplasms. The tumours of the first generation are close in their tissue specificity, immunological and biochemical properties to the original tumours, and it is expedient to discuss together the growth kinetics both of spontaneous tumours and of their first generations.

Spontaneous Tumours of Mouse Mammary Glands

These tumours arise as a rule in mice of high-cancer lines (C3H), 10-12 months old. Their life-spans are 1 to 4 months from the time of tumour appearance. This model involves a virus and depends on hormone action.

The growth kinetics of spontaneous tumours in C3H mice was studied by Matienko (1970). The increase in tumour weight P can be described by a power equation (Figure 50A):

$$P = 0.016t^{1 \cdot 35}, \text{ g.}$$

The results of changes in tumour volume are given in McCredie et $al.$ (1965). Though the kinetic curve is not distinctly S-shaped (Figure 50B), it was approximated by the Gompertz function

$$V = 4.5 \cdot 10^{-2} \exp \left[6.1(1 - \exp \left(-0.021t \right)) \right], \text{ cm}^3.$$

It will be noted that this expression is not compatible with experimental results: the theoretical curve given by MrCredie et $al.$ lies lower than all mean values V. A more accurate approximation is given by the exponential function with index $\phi = 0.044$ day^{-1} ($T_d = 15.8$ days). The pre-exponential factor cannot be evaluated here, as the time of tumour appearance is unknown. In Figure 50B the time of the first measurement is taken as the reference point.

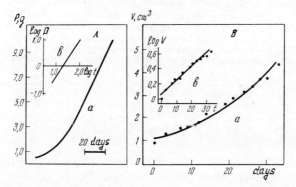

Fig. 50   Spontaneous mammary gland cancer in C3H mice.
(A) According to Matienko (1970);   (B) according to
McCredie *et al*. (1965).

The first generation of a spontaneous carcinoma of the mammary gland in a C3H
female mouse has been studied.   The tumour was transplanted subcutaneously to mice
of the same line 10-12 weeks old.   The inoculum size was 2×10^4 viable tumour cells.
The induction period varied for individual animals from 13 to 36 days.   From the
times the tumours arose their sizes ('areas') were estimated daily by measuring
two diameters.   The results are given for growth of tumours arising on the 14th,
21st, 28th and 35th days after transplantation (Figure 51, curves 1, 2, 3 and 4,
respectively.   The kinetic surves for the tumour area change S plotted from the
data are described by power equations in the form $S = at^3$.   The coefficients a for
curves 1 to 4 in Figure 51 are 5.9×10^{-5}, 2.9×10^{-5}, 1.0×10^{-5}, and 0.68×10^{-5} cm^2/day.

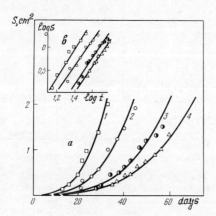

Fig. 51   Kinetic curves for changes in the effective tumour
area for the first generation of spontaneous mammary gland
cancer in C3H mice.   Induction period: 14 days (1), 21 days
(2), 28 days (3) and 35 days (4).

The effect of tumour localization on growth rate was studied by Eichten and
Maruyama in 1968. A spontaneous mammary gland adenocarcinoma which had arisen in
C3H(Z) mice and passed through five generations was transplanted subcutaneously
(inoculum 10^6 cells) to mice of the same line in various parts of the body. The
growth curve for a tumour transplanted subcutaneously in the tail, plotted from the
results in Eichten and Maruyama for a time span of 120-200 days is described by a
linear function

$$D = 0.10 + 0.016t, \text{ cm.}$$

The animals died about 200 days after transplantation;   pulmonary metastases were
observed in some cases. With other localizations the induction period was shorter
and the animals died in about 70 days.

Spontaneous Leukaemia in AKR Mice

Spontaneous leukaemias in mice have been described by Kassirskii (1964), Bergolts
and Rumyantsev (1966), Felistovich (1964), Stukov (1966) and Matienko et al. (1967)
These are used when studying aetiology, pathology and, less frequently, in chemotherapeutic investigations. This is due to the prolonged time of disease development and the existence of various leukaemia types in mice of this line.

A kinetic study of the lymphoid and myeloid forms in mice of the highly-leukaemiac
AKR line, 7-8 months old, was reported by Belich et al. (1972). The highest
frequency of the leukaemic disease (65-90%) in mice of this line was observed for
animals 7-11 months old (Krashilina, 1960). The total leucocyte count in blood,
the percentage of the differential blood cound in leucograms, the numbers of leukaemic cells, and neutrophils and lymphocytes in peripheral blood were measured
(Figure 52).

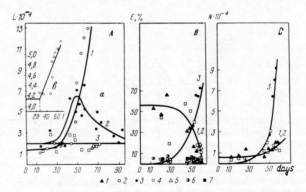

Fig. 52 Haematological indices for the lymphatic form of
spontaneous leukaemia in AKR mice (Belich et al., 1972).
(A) Total leucocyte count in blood of mice of various groups;
(B) differential blood count;   (C) blood cells responsible
for the increase in the total leucocyte count (1 — segmented
neutrophils, 2 — lymphocytes, 3 — undifferentiated cells,
4 — metamyelocytes, 5 — stab form neutrophils, 6 — eosino-
phils, 7 — monocytes).

An exponential increase in blood leucocyte count was observed in most animals
suffering from lymphoid leukaemia (Figure 52A, curve 1). For certain animals the
change in this parameter was of an extreme nature and at the time of death the
leucocyte count was reduced below normal values (Figure 52A, curve 2). The thymus
was enlarged. Some mice displayed an aleukaemic form of leukaemia (Figure 52A,
curve 3).

The kinetic curves for changes in certain other haematological parameters are also
of an exponential nature (Figure 52B,C, curve 3).

An exponential increase in the total blood leucocyte count, mostly due to neutrophils, is also characteristic for the myeloid leukaemia form (Figure 53). An
averaged curve (Figure 53D) was plotted by combining the experimental curves
obtained for individual animals. It is approximated by the equation

$$L = 16800 \exp\left[0.033(t - t_0)\right]$$

where t_0 is the time of the onset of the stable rise in the number of leucocytes.

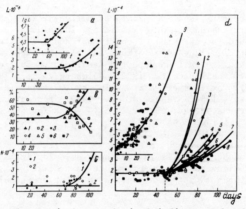

Fig. 53 Changes in haematological indices on development
of the myeloid form of spontaneous leukaemia in AKR mice
(Belich *et al.*, 1972). (a) Total leucocyte count; (b)
relative content of blood cells (denoted as in Fig. 52A);
(c) number of individual blood cells; (d) individual (1-8)
and normalized (9) kinetic curves for changes in leucocyte
count in 8 animals.

When plotting the averaged curve, the shift along the y-axis was taken to be the
difference between the mean normal number of leucocytes for the whole group of
animals L and the number of leucocytes normally present in each mouse L_i

$$\Delta L = \overline{L} - L_i$$

The shift along the x-axis δ_i was calculated using the equation

$$\delta_i = \overline{t}_0 - t_{0i}$$

where t_0 is the mean time for the start of the growth in leucocyte numbers for all
mice, and t_{0i} represents the start of this growth for an individual animal.

4. CRITICAL PHENOMENA IN THE DEVELOPMENT OF EXPERIMENTAL TUMOURS

A study of the kinetic regularities in the development of transplanted tumours is closely connected with the dependence of this process on the number of malignant cells in the inoculum.

The transplantation of one or several cells produces a tumour in only a few strains and then only in newborn or young animals. For instance, with intraperitoneal transplantation of a single cell of the Yoshida sarcoma, a tumour arises in 33-60% of involved animals, and with subcutaneous transplantation a tumour occurs in 19% of the animals. The Krebs-2 carcinoma is successful in only 4% of young mice, and in 2% of adult mice.

The tetraploid Ehrlich tumour transplanted by a single cell inoculum 'takes' in 14% of animals. Lymphoid and myeloid leukaemia 'take' when the inoculum contains from one to 100 cells (Furth, 1935; Furth *et al.*. 1933, 1937). In many other cases attempts to transplant experimental tumours by means of a small number of cells failed.

Transplantation of tumours, and the growth of malignant cell colonies *in vitro*, require a certain minimum number of cells in the inoculum or culture. This critical number depends on the kind of the tumour and the state of the host, on genetic characteristics of the animal line, and also on experimental conditions. For instance, according to various reported data for the Ehrlich carcinoma, this number is 10^4 to 5×10^6 cells (Costa, 1932; Goldberg *et al.*, 1950; Koenigsfeld and Prausnitz, 1914), for leukaemias it is 10^2 to 10^4 cells (Richter and McDowell, 1933; McDowell *et al.*, 1934; Vesely *et al.*, 1960), for sarcoma 37 it is 10^5 (Costa, 1932), for the mouse sarcoma it is 5×10^3, and for the linearly-specific sarcoma it is 10^5 (Phillips, 1966).

Not only the transplantability but also the metastasization of the tumour is connected with the number of cells in the inoculum. For instance, the transplantation of 10^5 Ehrlich ascites carcinoma cells resulted in the development of the process, but without metastasization; with a larger inoculum metastases were observed.

The threshold (critical) phenomena in experimental leukaemia were studied most extensively by Erokhin (1968), Emanuel *et al.* (1964) and Gorkov (1976) for leukaemia La in C57Bl mice and for erythromyelosis in non-inbred rats.

The leukaemia La cells of leukaemic mice were transplanted intraperitoneally. The curves for changes in spleen weight (S), in the leucocyte count (L), in peripheral blood haemocytoblasts (H), and in bone marrow (M) for inocula of various sizes are shown in Figure 54. The malignant process did not develop after transplantation of 10^4 cells and no signs of disease were observed for 6 months.

The kinetic parameter ϕ appeared to be always the same in the development of the process; the inoculum size influenced the latent period duration only.

The curves for leukaemia development can always be described by exponential equations of the form

$$F = F_n + F_0 \exp(\phi t).$$

The pre-exponential factor values F_0 are connected with inoculum size as follows: log F_0 are linearly dependent on log N_0 for $N \geqslant 10^5$ cells and on log $(N_0 - N_{cr})$ for all values of N_0 (Figure 54). The general equation can be written as

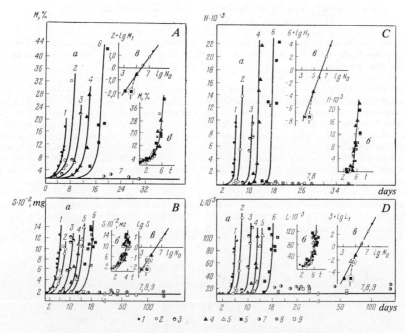

Fig. 54 Kinetic phenomena in the development of leukaemia La
in C57Bl mice (Emanuel *et al.*, 1964).   (A) Bone marrow haemocytoblasts;   (B) haemocytoblasts of peripheral blood;   (C)
spleen weight;   (D) leukocytes in peripheral blood: transplantation of 4×10^7 cells (1), 10^7 (2), 10^6 (3), 10^5 (4),
5×10^4 (5), 1.5×10^4 (6), 10^4 (7), 5×10^3 (8);   (a) individual
curves for each inoculum;   (b) curves normalized relative to
the standard one (4×10^7);   (c) the pre-exponential factor as
a function of inoculum size without correction and with
correction (dots) for the critical value.

$$\log F_0 = \log A + \alpha \log (N_0 - N_{cr})$$

or $$F_0 = A(N_0 - N_{cr})^{\alpha}.$$

For any of the parameters studied the equation are of the form

$$S_0 = 2 \cdot 10^{-5}(N_0 - N_{cr})^{0 \cdot 8}, \quad mg;$$
$$L_0 = 2 \cdot 10^{-15}(N_0 - N_{cr})^{2 \cdot 0}, \quad 1/mm^3;$$
$$H_0 = 10^{-23}(N_0 - N_{cr})^{2 \cdot 5}, \quad 1/mm^3;$$
$$M_0 = 10^{-4}(N_0 - N_{cr})^{0 \cdot 7}, \quad \%.$$

The value N_{cr} can be estimated from the difference between $\log N_0$ and $\log (N_0 - N_{cr})$
for the same value $\log F_0$

$$\delta = \log N_0 - \log (N_0 - N_{cr})$$
$$N_{cr} = N_0 [1 - \exp (-2.3\delta)]$$

For leukaemia La, $N_{cr} = 1.4 \times 10^4$ cells.

The assumption that the critical phenomenon of transplantation results from linear growth and non-linear losses (Gorkov, 1976) leads to a somewhat different dependence for the pre-exponential function, namely

$$F_0 = AN_0(1 - N_{cr}/N_0)^\alpha,$$

where A is the proportionality coefficient.

Comparing the above expressions for F_0 it will be noted that the latter seems to be more adequate, since when $N_{cr} \ll N_0$ we obtain for the second case $F_0 = AN_0$; whereas in the first variant, when $N_{cr} \ll N_0$, the value F_0 is connected with the inoculum value by the non-linear dependence $F_0 = AN_0{}^\alpha$, and this is incompatible with the definition of the pre-exponential factor as a value proportional to the number N_0 of transplanted cells.

Critical phenomena have also been observed for the Sveč erythromyelosis produced by subcutaneous transplantation of the leucosarcomatosis tissue of donor rats. The malignant process developed only with an inoculum containing $N_0 \gg 10^5$ cells (Figure 55). When the inoculum contained $10^5 - 10^6$ cells leukaemia did not appear in all animals.

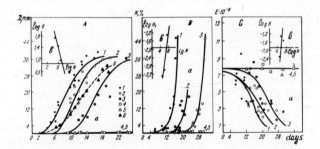

Fig. 55 Changes in the mean diameter of the subcutaneous tumour (A), in the count of normoblasts (B) and blood erythrocytes (C) for transplantation of erythromyelosis with different numbers of cells: (1) 1×10^7; (2) 1×10^6; (3) 1×10^5; (4) 1×10^4; (5) 1×10^3; (6) daily administration of ethoxene 2 mg/kg (a — kinetic curves, b — the Gompertz function parameters or the pre-exponential factor as a function of the inoculum size N_i).

The curves for changes in the mean diameter of a subcutaneous tumour are S-shaped (Figure 55A) and are described by the Gompertz equation in the form

$$D = D_\infty \exp[-b \exp(-ct)], \quad \text{mm}.$$

The inoculum size has virtually no effect on the value D_∞. Regression analysis showed that the kinetic parameter c is the same for curves 1–3 in Figure 55A, i.e. the process develops ar a rate independent of the number of transplanted cells. The inoculum size influences only the parameter b, i.e. the latent period duration.

The increase in the number of normoblasts (N) in the blood of rats after the end of the latent period is exponential with close kinetic parameters for all curves

(Figure 55B, curves 1-3). The decrease in the number of erythrocytes in blood is described by S-shaped curves that are well approximated by the Gompertz equation (Figure 55C, curves 1-3).

Analysis of these kinetic curves shows that in all cases the parameters characteristic of the latent period duration (b or H_1) are connected with the inoculum in that the logarithm of the relevant parameter has a linear relationship to log N_0 (Figure 55b).

In addition to the prolongation of the latent period when a small number of malignant cells are used in the inoculum, the erythromyelosis percentage of 'takes' decreases from 100% at $N_0 = 1 \times 10^7$ to zero at $N_0 = 1 \times 10^4$ (Figure 56a, curve 1). A similar phenomenon was observed on transplantation of ascites sarcoma 180 and of a Marsh-Simpson tumour (Figure 56b,c).

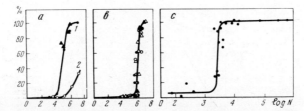

Fig. 56 Tumour transplantability as a function of the number of transplanted cells. (a) Erythromyelosis (1 — control, 2 — upon ethoxene administration); (b) sarcoma 180; (c) Marsh-Simpson tumour

The effect of ethoxene, an antitumour drug, on the critical inoculum value has been studied. With daily administration of ethoxene, the percentage of 'takes' markedly decreased starting from the second day after transplantation (Figure 56a, curve 2). Transplantation of 10^7 cells resulted in development of erythromyelosis only in 30% of animals (100% in controls). With an inoculum of 10^5 cells the tumour did not take. Animals treated with ethoxene developed tumours more slowly than untreated controls (Figure 55A, curve 6).

In the development of transplanted tumours, the threshold phenomena seem to be caused by the relationships between the rates of proliferation of transplanted cells and the immune reactions of the host. This explains the dependence of N_{cr} on the type of tumour and the state of the host. Administration of the antitumour drug seems to kill a certain part of the transplanted cells and to decrease the percentage of 'takes' below a certain critical value.

5. COMPARATIVE KINETIC ANALYSIS OF THE GROWTH OF PRIMARY TUMOURS AND THEIR METASTASES

One of the most characteristic features of malignant tumours is metastasization. At first tumour development is local, and later the malignant process spreads beyond the affected organ and then distant metastases appear.

According to some data, the start of metastasization coincides with the onset of the maximum rate of primary tumour growth. The metastases often grow faster than the primary tumour. Exponential growth of the number and size of metastases was reported in a number of papers. For instance, at the initial stage after transplantation, the increase in the number of Lewis tumour metastases in kidneys (Ferrer and Mihich, 1968), and in the weight of rat sarcoma metastases in lymph nodes (Brenk *et al*., 1971) were described by exponential equations. A similar type of dependence was found also when studying metastases in regional lymph nodes for the Walker carcinosarcoma inoculated in the testis, and for the Zaidel ascites hepatoma (Emanuel *et al*., 1975). This research compared the kinetic characteristics of primary and metastatic tumours.

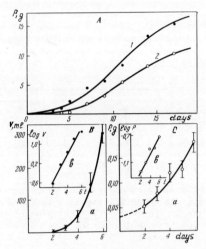

Fig. 57   Growth kinetics of primary tumours and of their metastases (Emanuel *et al*., 1975).   (A) Walker carcinosarcoma (1) and its metastases to retroperitoneal lymph nodes (2);   (B) Zaidel ascites hepatoma;   (C) metastases of Zaidel hepatoma to paratracheal lymph nodes.

Figure 57A shows the kinetic curves for the growth of the Walker carcinosarcoma and its metastases in the lymph nodes. The most satisfactory approximation of these data is attained by using the Gompertz equation with algebraic calculation of its parameters (see Chapter 1). Comparison of the numerical values of the parameters calculated from the data in Emanuel *et al*. (1975) shows that the growth rate of metastases is higher than that of the primary tumour.

Parameters of the Gompertz equation	Walker carcinosarcoma inoculated in the testis	Metastases in retro-peritoneal lymph nodes
P_0 10^{-3}, g	21	0.06
P_∞, g	17	11.5
α, day^{-1}	0.219	0.255
A, day^{-1}	1.46	3.1

Evaluation of the effective doubling time gives metastases a value T_d approximately half that of the tumour mass doubling, at initial growth stages. As the metastases and the primary tumour grow, the difference in the effective doubling time of the tumour mass to that of the metastases (T_t/T_{met}) becomes less. The results of histological and radioautographical studies are compatible with these data. The initial phase (4-7 days) is characterized by higher values of labelled thymidine incorporation and of the labelled cells index in metastases (Table 13).   Unlike

TABLE 13 Incorporation of labelled thymidine into cells of Walker carcinosarcoma metastases (in parts relative to the primary tumour) and the relation of the effective mass doubling time of tumour and metastases T_t/T_{met} (Emanuel et al., 1975)

Characteristic	Days			
	4	7	11	14
T_t/T_{met}	1.60	1.40	1.20	1.10
Relation of labelled cell index in metastases and tumour	1.10	1.40	1.00	1.00
Relation of incorporation intensity of labelled thymidine into metastases and tumour	1.25	1.20	0.95	1.00

the situation for primary tumours, necrosis is not observed in metastases at this stage, but at a later stage (11-14 days) necrosis develops in metastases as well, and this is accompanied by a less intense incorporation of thymidine. At this stage the difference between the primary and metastatic tumours becomes inappreciable.

The exponential growth of primary tumours and of their metastases for the Zaidel ascites hepatoma metastasizing to paratracheal lymph nodes and displaying a 100% transplantability is shown in Figure 57B,C. The increase in the ascitic fluid volume and in the weight of lymph nodes is described by equations in the form of

$$V = 0.03 \exp(1.23t), \text{ ml}; \quad P = 0.03 \exp(0.26t), \text{ g.}$$

It was also found by radioautography that the proliferation of malignant cells in metastases is faster than in the primary tumour. The apparent incompatibility of these data with the rate constants of V and P increase is because the amount of ascitic fluid increases faster than does the mass of malignant cells it contains. Indeed, an exponential dependence was found for the increase in the number of Zaidel hepatoma cells with an exponential index $\phi = 0.3 \text{ day}^{-1}$. In other words, the growth rate of the cell mass in the primary tumour does not differ much from the growth rate of metastases in lymph nodes, as could be expected from the exponential for V in Emanuel et al. (1975).

A comparison of the growth rate of metastases in various groups of regional lymph nodes was made by Brenk et al. (1971). A rapidly-growing rat sarcoma was inoculated into the gastrocnemius muscle and changes in the weights of the primary tumour and its metastases in popliteal and pelvic ganglia, and retroperitoneal lymph nodes were recorded. The curves for changes in weight of primary tumours and metastases are given for two inocula containing 10^7 and 5×10^6 malignant cells. Quantitative processing of these curves (Figure 58) shows that in both cases the kinetics of changes in weight of primary tumours and their metastases can be described by an equation of the form $(P)^{1/3} = a + bt$. The numerical values of coefficients a and b for all cases considered in Brenk (1971) are given in Table 14.

With 50% of the inoculum the coefficients a diminish approximately to the same extent; at the same time the coefficients b (linear growth rate) for identical groups of lymph nodes remain virtually the same. In other words, changes in inoculum size have no effect on the growth rate of primary tumours and metastases and result only in a shift of the kinetic curves, and this shows in the lower values of coefficients a. The functional relationship of b and a with the inoculum

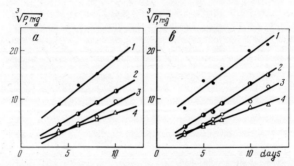

Fig. 58 Kinetic curves for rat sarcoma growth (1) and its
metastases to pelvic (2), retroperitoneal (3) and popliteal
(4) lymph nodes after intravascular transplantation of
$5×10^6$ (a) and 10^7 (b) tumour cells (Brenk *et al.*, 1971).

TABLE 14 Linear growth parameters of rapidly growing rat sarcoma and
its metastases in lymph nodes (calculated from data in Brenk *et al.*, 1971)

Inoculum size	Primary tumour		Pelvic lymph nodes		Retroperitoneal lymph nodes		Popliteal lymph nodes	
	a	b	a	b	a	b	a	b
5×10^6	2.79	1.55	-0.10	1.18	-1.46	1.03	0.60	0.65
1×10^7	5.24	1.38	0.60	1.20	-0.44	1.02	0.89	0.65

size was discussed in conducting a kinetic analysis of the Pliss lymphosarcoma
(see pp. 71-74). Comparison of the growth rates of metastases in different lymph
nodes shows that it decreases in the order: (1) pelvic ($b = 1.18$-1.20), (2) retroperitoneal ($b = 1.02$-1.03), and (3) popliteal ($b = 0.65$) lymph nodes. Unlike the
Walker carcinosarcoma, the growth rate of the primary tumour is considerably
higher than that of metastases ($b = 1.4$-1.5).

The metastasization of alveolar cell carcinoma in BALB/C mice was studied by Yukhas
and Pazmino (1974, 1975). Total irradiation with a 500 r dose two hours in advance
of subcutaneous tumour transplantation increases the frequency of metastasization
to the lungs, but the process was delayed two days when local thoracic irradiation
or no radiation at all was given (Yukhas and Pazmino, 1974). In Figure 59A the tin
dependence of metastases is plotted for two points only. A later paper by the same
authors in 1975 reports the effect of subcutaneous pre-transplantation of different
amounts of tumour cells on the metastasization process modelled artificially by
subsequent intravascular inoculation of cells of the same type. The problem was
to study the effect of specific (transplantation) immunity on the metastasization
process. A sub-strain giving no metastases when subcutaneously transplanted was
used. The dependence of the number of pulmonary metastases in BALB/C mice on
inoculum size and on the size of the subcutaneous tumour on the 21st day after
transplantation is as follows:

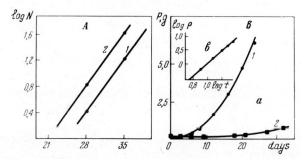

Fig. 59 Metastases development in lung. (A) Number of
metastases of alveolar cell carcinoma in BALB/C mice lungs
(1 — control and local pre-irradiation of the primary tumour,
2 — total pre-irradiation of animals) (Yukhas and Pazmino,
1974); (B) growth of the primary Lewis tumour (1) and
changes in lung weight (2) (De Wys, 1972).

Subcutaneous inoculum, cells	Weight of the subcutaneous tumour, g	Number of metastases
0.00	0.00	83 ± 8
5×10^4	0.41	84 ± 5
5×10^5	0.72	48 ± 8
5×10^6	2.95	31 ± 9
5×10^7	5.20	0

The smallest inoculum studied (5×10^4 cells) had virtually no influence on the
process of artificial metastasization: the numbers of pulmonary metastases on the
21st day after transplantation in controls and experimental animals did not differ
significantly. Ths only control here was the intravascular transplantation of
2×10^4 malignant cells. When the subcutaneous inoculum was 100 times larger, the
amount of metastases was approximately three times lower. Further increase of the
inoculum up to 5×10^7 cells completely impeded the appearance of pulmonary
metastases. A greater size of the tumour corresponded to the larger inoculum and
it was suggested that this was responsible for the intensity of the immunological
reactions.

Experimental studies of metastasization often use the Lewis tumour metastasization
to the lungs. Figure 59B shows the curves for gain in the weight of primary tumour
and of pulmonary metastases, plotted from tabular data in De Wys (1972). The
presence of pulmonary metastases was proved experimentally, but the technique for
observing the growth of metastases used by De Wys is very crude: the authors
recorded gain in total weight of the lungs. It will be seen from Figure 59 that
the weight of the lungs remains more or less constant for a long time (though
histological studies show the presence of metastases), and an increase in weight is
observed only at the 30th day (one point). A comparison of the growth rates of the
primary tumour and of its metastases using only one point is scarcely satisfactory.

The kinetic curve for development of the primary Lewis tumour can be described by
a power equation of the form

$$P = 7.6t^{2.13}, \text{ mg.}$$

Thus, the growth kinetics of metastases follow the same regularities as the primary tumour. The experimental data are insufficient for clearing up the quantitative differences in growth parameters. Further kinetic studies will have to yield the parameters needed for quantitative characteristics of the relationships in the system of 'tumour – metastases'.

6.   GENERALIZATION OF DATA ON THE KINETICS OF TUMOUR GROWTH

The data discussed in this Chapter show that all the transplanted, induced and spontaneous experimental leukaemias, solid tumours and their ascitic forms can be described by exponential, S-shaped and power functions.

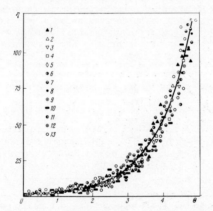

Fig. 60 Generalized kinetic curve for exponentially-growing experimental tumours. (1) Radiation-induced skin tumours in rats;   (2) adenocarcinoma 755;   (3) sarcoma 180;   (5) hepatomas;   (6) Ehrlich ascites carcinoma;   (7) Sveč erythromyelosis;   (8) Walker carcinosarcoma;   (9) reticulum cell sarcomatosis;   (10) leukaemia LZ;   (11) leukaemia L-1210; (12) spontaneous leukaemia in AKR mice;   (13) leukaemia La.

Figure 60 shows the data on exponentially-growing tumours in dimensionless variables,

$$\eta = \exp{(\theta)}$$

where $\eta = F/F_0$, $\theta = \phi t$. A similar generalization for tumour growing according to the power equation (Figure 61) gives

$$\eta = \theta(\eta = \log{\frac{F}{a}};\ \theta = b \log{t})$$

and according to the linear equation (Figure 62)

$$\eta = \theta(\eta = \frac{F}{a} - 1;\quad \theta = \frac{b}{a}\ t)$$

and also for cases corresponding to S-shaped curves (Figure 63)

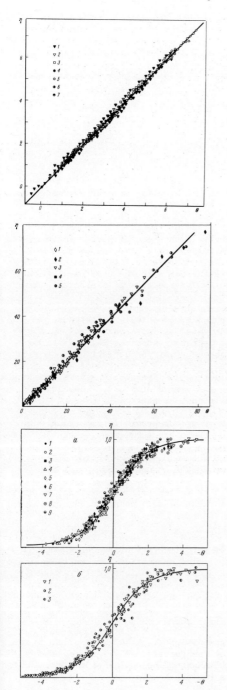

Fig. 61 Generalized logarithmic anamorphosis of kinetic curves for growth of experimental tumours approximated by a power function. (1) Sarcoma 37; (2) sarcoma 180; (3) spontaneous mammary gland tumours; (4) fibrosarcoma in mice; (5) Cuérin carcinoma; (6) Ehrlich ascites carcinoma; (7) lymphatic leukaemia NKLy.

Fig. 62 Generalized kinetic curve for linearly-growing experimental tumours. (1) Hepatomas; (2) Cloudman melanoma; (3) sarcoma 180; (4) sarcoma 45; (5) Ehrlich ascites carcinoma.

Fig. 63 Generalized S-shaped kinetic curves for growth of solid (a) and ascites (b) experimental tumours. a: (1) Walker carcinosarcoma; (2) Guérin carcinoma; (3) sarcoma 45; (4) adenocarcinoma 755; (5) hepatomas; (6) melanomas; (7) sarcoma 180; (8) other models (osteogenic Ridgway sarcoma, sarcoma T241, adenocarcinoma EO-771, carcinoma C1025); (9) Sveč erythromyelosis. b: (1) sarcoma 180; (2) Ehrlich ascites carcinoma; (3) leukaemia L-1210.

$$\eta = \frac{1}{1 + \exp\,\theta} \quad \left(\eta = \frac{F}{F_\infty};\ \theta = \ln\,a - bt\right).$$

Kinetic studies have become one of the dominant trends in experimental oncology. The literature on tumour growth kinetics contains many conflicting results; there is no standard approach to processing and analyzing experimental data. Further study of tumour growth kinetics needs to be conducted, whenever possible, in a standardized manner.

Statistical analysis of data obtained permits strict evaluation of the correctness of the values (experimental points) used in plotting the kinetic curves: in the absence of such an analysis even the form of a kinetic curve may appear to be incorrect.

In discussing the data obtained for sarcoma 45 (Figures 15A and 16) it was found that regular distribution of the end-points in the kinetic curve was violated and, strictly speaking, these points could not be used for plotting the curve. Since they were still taken into account, the experimenter had to plot an S-shaped curve. A more thorough approach would give a linear shape of the kinetic dependence. Violation of the normal distribution regularity in the initial parts of the curve was due to inaccurate (as a rule over-estimated) values of the values measured. This was caused by the indistinct shape of the tumour for a solid strain, and by the presence of a certain amount of non-malignant cells in the peritoneal region for ascites tumours. It was also influenced by the response of the animal to the administration of foreign material.

In the later stages of the process the lesions are connected with the onset of mortality. Animals with large tumours seem to die earlier: this leads to under-estimated values of the mean tumour size, if averaging of sizes is confined to surviving animals. Probably this is often the cause of the deflection of the curve at the latest stages. Many researchers do not take this into account when trying to follow the tumour growth kinetics to the very end. Frequently studies on growth kinetics present no data on mortality during the period of study; consequently correct processing of such experimental data cannot be precise.

The choice of the value for characterization of tumour growth is important. In counting the number of cells or in estimating the characteristics (weight and size) proportional to it, the curve only rarely has an exact S-shape (with the exception of certain ascites tumours); as a rule the S-shaped kinetic curve for diameter changes after transformation to the curve for volume changes 'loses' its S-shape. The cause of this was discussed earlier (see page 34). This certainly does not mean that S-shaped kinetic curves are unreliable in general. The setting up of a scheme for the planning and processing of the kinetic data obtained in experimental oncology is highly expedient.

A comparison of data on specific growth rates of various tumours discussed in this Chapter seems to be of interest. The maximum specific rate of tumour growth ϕ_{max} is a very important biological characteristic. The connection between the value ϕ and the cell kinetics was discussed in a monograph by Frankfurt (1975). Usually the specific rate reaches its maximum at relatively early stages of the tumour development, at which time the tumour can still be unobservable. Consequently the value ϕ_{max} referring to the observed part of the kinetic curve may appear to be lower than the true ϕ_{max}.

Table 15 (pp. 90–91) lists ϕ_{max} values for tumours obeying the exponential or the autocatalysis dependence, and also for one of the tumours (NKLy) growing in accordance with the power dependence. When measuring the number of malignant cells, the weight or volume of the tumour, $\phi_{max} = \phi$ for exponential growth $[F = F_0 \exp\,(\phi t)]$;

$\phi_{max} = b$ for autocatalytic growth $[F = F_\infty/1 + a \exp(-bt)]$, since the inequality $a \gg 1$ was always fulfilled. When the measured value was the tumour diameter, it was assumed that $\phi_{max} = 3\phi$ (or $\phi_{max} = 3b$).

To make the distribution of ϕ_{max} values more illustrative the tumours in Table 15 are numbered in the order of increasing ϕ_{max}, in the plot drawn accordingly the values of ϕ_{max} are given along the x-axis, and the number of tumours in Table 15 along the y-axis (Figure 64).

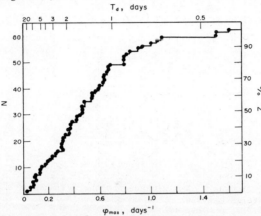

Fig. 64 Function of empirical distribution of maximum specific tumour growth rates (according to data in Table 15). N = number of tumours; Z = cumulative frequency; $T_d = \ln 2/\phi_{max}$ is the doubling time.

Figure 64 illustrates certain features of ϕ_{max} distribution in the sample obtained. At first, the empirical distribution function growth is virtually linear over the range $\phi_{max} = 0$ to $\phi_{max} = 0.7$ day^{-1}, i.e. the distribution of ϕ_{max} over this range is virtually uniform. It follows from such a distribution that the tumours can have any small value of ϕ_{max}. As seen from Table 15, the range with low ϕ_{max} embraces first of all the spontaneous and induced tumours, though certain transplanted tumours can also have low ϕ_{max} values. This refers first of all to minimally deviated hepatomas and to sub-lines of transplanted tumours resistant to chemotherapy.

About 80% of the tumour observed lie within the linearity range of 0 to 0.7 day^{-1}. There are many fewer tumours for which $\phi_{max} > 0.8$ day^{-1}. Ths upper limit for ϕ_{max} is 1.6 days^{-1}, which corresponds to a doubling time T_d of about 10 hours. The question whether this sample reflects the statistical properties of all tumours known in experimental oncology or of those arising in natural populations awaits further study.

TABLE 15   Maximum specific growth rates for experimental tumours

Number in Fig. 64	Tumour	max day^{-1}	T_d hour	References
1	Radiation-induced skin tumour	0.027	607	Albert et al., 1969
2	Spontaneous adenocarcinoma	0.044	380	McCredie et al., 1965
3	Morris hepatoma 7800	0.075	222	Knox et al., 1970; Tsou et al., 1974; Looney et al., 1973
4	Leukaemia L-1210, sub-line	0.075	222	Johnson et al., 1965, 1966
5	Sarcoma 37 solid	0.090	185	Minenkova et al., 1968
6	Morris hepatoma 7793	0.093	179	Knox et al., 1970; Tsou et al., 1974; Looney et al., 1973
7	Hepatoma 46	0.100	167	Bogdanov et al., 1973
8	Radiation-induced skin tumours	0.126	138	Albert et al., 1969
9	Morris hepatoma 5123c	0.129	129	Knox et al., 1970; Tsou et al., 1974; Looney et al., 1973
10	Morris hepatoma 7777	0.135	123	Knox et al., 1970; Tsou et al., 1974; Looney et al., 1973
11	Adenocarcinoma 755	0.170	98	Adams and Bowman, 1963
12	Sarcoma 180 solid	0.190	88	Minenkova et al., 1968
13	Morris hepatoma 3924A	0.207	81	Knox et al., 1970; Tsou et al., 1974; Looney et al., 1973
14	Morris hepatoma 3924A	0.231	72	Lo et al., 1973
15	Sarcoma 180 solid	0.260	64	Summers, 1966
16	Walker carcinosarcoma	0.270	62	Harding et al., 1964
17	Cloudman melanoma S-91	0.300	56	Summers, 1966
18	Zaidel ascites hepatoma	0.300	56	
19	Walker carcinosarcoma	0.300	56	
20	Adenocarcinoma 755	0.310	54	Wilcox et al., 1965
21	Morris hepatoma 3683F	0.315	53	Knox et al., 1970; Tsou et al., 1974; Looney et al., 1973
22	Carcinoma C1025	0.330	50	Schmid et al., 1966
23	Sarcoma 180 solid	0.360	46	Adams and Bowman, 1963
24	Adenocarcinoma 755	0.360	46	Laster et al., 1969
25	Sveč erythroleukaemia	0.370	45	Dronova et al., 1966
26	Sarcoma 180 solid	0.370	45	Wilcox et al., 1965
27	Sarcoma SSK	0.380	44	
28	Osteogenic Ridgway sarcoma	0.420	40	Schmid et al., 1966
29	Hepatoma solid	0.420	40	Taper et al., 1966
30	Adenocarcinoma 755	0.440	38	Laster et al., 1969

31	Ehrlich ascites carcinoma	0.460	36	Klein and Revesz, 1953
32	Hepatoma 60	0.470	35	Bogdanov *et al.*, 1973
33	Sarcoma 37 ascites	0.470	35	Minenkova *et al.*, 1967
34	Sarcoma 45, subline	0.480	35	Larionov, 1962
35	Sarcoma T241	0.480	35	Schmid *et al.*, 1966
36	Adenocarcinoma 755	0.530	31	Summers, 1966
37	Melanoma B-16	0.540	31	Vasileva *et al.*, 1974
38	Walker carcinosarcoma	0.540	31	Schmid *et al.*, 1966
39	Sarcoma 45, sub-line	0.570	29	Larionov, 1962
40	Lymphatic leukaemia NKLy, ascites form	0.620	28	Pelevina *et al.*, 1966
41	Pliss lymphosarcoma	0.600	28	Gorkov and Vasileva, 1973
42	Sarcoma 180 solid	0.620	27	Wilcox *et al.*, 1965
43	Adenocarcinoma 755	0.630	26	D'iachkovskaia and Konovalova, 1973
44	Melanoma B-16	0.630	26	Schmid *et al.*, 1966
45	Hepatoma 22a	0.630	26	Bogdanov *et al.*, 1973
46	Ehrlich ascites carcinoma	0.650	26	Ilina and Markle, 1973
47	Harding-Passey melanoma	0.660	25	Vasileva *et al.*, 1969
48	Adenocarcinoma E0771	0.660	25	Schmid *et al.*, 1966
49	Ehrlich ascites carcinoma	0.680	25	Baserga, 1963; Tannock and Steel, 1970
50	Hepatoma ascites	0.790	21	Taper *et al.*, 1966
51	Adenocarcinoma 755	0.800	21	D'iachkovskaia and Konovalova, 1973
52	Leukaemia L-1210, sub-line	0.800	21	Johnson *et al.*, 1966
53	Ehrlich ascites carcinoma	0.810	21	Laird, 1964
54	Leukaemia La	0.830	20	Baserga, 1963
55	Guérin carcinoma	0.900	18.5	
56	Sarcoma 45	0.930	18	Kiseleva *et al.*, 1969
57	Leukaemia L-1210, ascites form	1.00	17	Kiseleva *et al.*, 1969
58	Leukaemia La	1.05	16	Gorkov and Ostrovskaia, 1977
59	Leukaemia L-1210, ascites form	1.08	15	
60	Leukaemia L-1210, ascites form	1.50	11	Johnson *et al.*, 1965, 1966
61	Leukaemia L-1210, ascites form	1.50	11	Shelton and Rice, 1958
62	Leukaemia L-1210, brain tumour	1.60	10	Skipper *et al.*, 1964

CHAPTER 3

KINETIC PARAMETERS OF VARIOUS ANTITUMOUR EFFECTS

The basic problems challenging current experimental cancer chemotherapy are the investigation of the principles for a rational approach to the search for new antitumour drugs, the development of methods for unbiassed quantitative evaluation of their effectiveness, the development and optimization of combined treatment methods, and ways of applying these experimental results clinically. The search for new anticancer drugs is conducted along two lines: (1) the study of the derivatives and analogues of known drugs, and (2) the screening of new drugs from synthetic and natural compounds.

The kinetic approach to the investigation of chemotherapeutic efficiency allows us to obtain strictly quantitative parameters of the antitumour effects of various compounds, an unbiassed evaluation of the inhibition effect, the description of tumour regression, remission, recurrence, and metastatic spreading processes.

Information on some established and some new antitumour drugs, and their kinetic parameters of action of a number of experimental tumours is given below. The authors used various criteria for evaluation of the drug's antitumour efficiency. This Chapter attempts to discuss the data on the chemotherapy of experimental tumours, making use of the kinetic criterion $\varkappa^*$ (activity coefficient)

$$\varkappa^* = 1 - \frac{\phi_e}{\phi_c} = \frac{\phi_c - \phi_e}{\phi_c} \, ,$$

where ϕ_e and ϕ_c are specific rates of tumour growth in experimental animals and controls (see Chapter 1).

When the tumour growth is exponential both in experimental animals and in controls, the specific growth rates ϕ_e and ϕ_c represent appropriate exponential indices. The same refers to exponential regression of tumours but here the exponential indices will be negative. When the tumour growth in controls, especially after chemotherapeutic treatment, is described by kinetic rules which are not exponential, the method of equivalent exponents is used to determine the values ϕ_c and ϕ_e needed for calculation of $\varkappa^*$. According to this method:

$$\phi = \frac{\ln F(t_2) - \ln F(t_1)}{t_2 - t_1} = \frac{\Delta \ln F}{\Delta t} \, ,$$

where t_1 is the time of starting therapy, t_2 is the end-time of the averaging interval, $F(t_1)$ and $F(t_2)$ are tumour sizes corresponding to times t_1 and t_2. The averaging time intervals for control and experimental curves can be either different or similar, depending on the kind of kinetic curves compared.

Thus there is no limitation on the types of kinetic curves for tumour growth in control and experimental animals, and it is possible either to compare the data on various drugs obtained by different researchers for the same tumour model, or to correlate the data on the action of the same drug on different tumour strains.

The efficiency of chemotherapy depends on many factors including the time of starting treatment, the doses and intervals between administrations, etc. Therefore, strictly speaking, the value $и^*$ obtained by analysis of kinetic curves might appear to be not the optimal one, since it depends on the technique used in the specific experiment.

It will be remembered that the values $и^* > 1$ correspond to tumour regression; when the tumour growth is stopped by chemotherapy, $и^* = 1$; the values $0 < и^* < 1$ refer to stronger or weaker inhibition of tumour growth; $и^* = 0$ when there is no effect, and negative $и^*$ values pertain to stimulation of growth.

The types of kinetic curves for tumour growth when subjected to various treatments are given in Chapter 1 (Figure 1). The most complicated curve is that with two extremes: one maximum and one minimum. This type of curve corresponds to a period of tumour regression followed by repeated growth or recurrence. Here is the sequence of calculations by the method of equivalent exponents:

TABLE 16   Method for calculation of the activity coefficient $и^*$
for averaging over different points of the control and
experimental curves for tumour growth given in Figure 65

t	F_K	$\ln F_K$	$\Delta\ln F_K$	F_3	$\ln F_3$	$\Delta\ln F_3$	Δt	ϕ_c	ϕ_e	$и^*$
4.0	3.3	1.19	–	3.3	1.19	–	–	–	–	–
5.0	4.6	1.52	0.33	4.0	1.38	1.19	1.0	0.33	0.19	0.4
8.5	6.5	1.87	0.68	1.8	0.58	-0.61	4.5	0.15	-0.13	1.9
9.0	6.6	1.88	0.69	–	–	–	5.0	0.14	–	
16.0	–	–	–	6.6	1.88	0.69	12.0	–	0.06	0.6

Table 16 shows the intermediate calculations needed for obtaining the values of $и^*$ on averaging to the maximum point ($t_2 = 5$), to the minimum point ($t_2 = 8.5$) or to the end points of the controls (K; $t_2 = 9$) and of the experimental (curve 3; $t_2 = 16$) kinetic curves. The tumour sizes (F) and appropriate time values (t) in conditional units are presented in Figure 65a; the time of therapeutic treatment start is $t_1 = 4$.

As seen from Table 16, the activity coefficient $и^*$ depends on the choice of the averaging interval (t_1; t_2). The changes in the therapeutic treatment efficiency can naturally be followed over the whole length of the experimental kinetic curve, assigning arbitrarily the time values t_2. The nature of changes in $и^*$ with time for different types of experimental kinetic curves is shown in Figure 65b. The curves 1, 3 and 4 correspond to treatment of a developed tumour ($t_1 = 4$; $F_1 = 0.5F_\infty$), and curve 2 to start of treatment immediately after transplantation ($t_1 = 0$; $F_1 = F_0$).

Evaluation of efficiency by means of kinetic criteria is a very valuable guide to choosing a rational approach to the elucidation of an optimal treatment schedule. A case can be readily conceived when one drug, providing the maximal value $и^*$

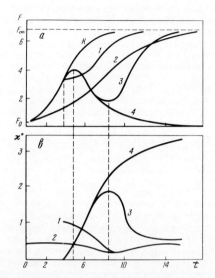

Fig. 65 Changes in the activity coefficient $\varkappa^*$, with time
(b) for different types of kinetic curves (a) in chemotherapy.

during a certain period of time and giving, for example, the possibility of obtaining profound regression is chosen from the number of drugs studied. Let the regression be followed by a recurrence, then for the time following $\varkappa^*$ will start reducing, and considering this specific case only it might seem that the drug is of no interest (Figure 65b, curve 3). If we discuss treatment efficiency, and not drug characteristics, the possibilities opened up by repeated administration of the drug after the start of the recurrence will not be encouraging. However, another drug which would effectively retard the tumour process, would cause a recurrence, etc., could be administered from this time.

Thus, a set of data giving quantitative characteristics of drug effects at various stages of tumour growth and the administration of these drugs in various sequences and combinations can be the basis of a rational optimized chemotherapy programme. At present experimental chemotherapy is still in its infancy in respect to this problem, and the treatment of data in this chapter aims only at showing the possible approaches to evaluation of the drugs' efficacy for various cases of their application.

These approaches can be used also for creating a unified system for screening antitumour compounds. The examples here show a possible approach to the screening problems and to defining rational treatment schedules.

The experimental work must demonstrate how good the drug is going to be, i.e. the conditions for obtaining the highest value of $\varkappa^*$. Such values are obtained for complete and partial regression, when $\varkappa^* > 1$, since

$$\varkappa^* = \left(1 - \frac{-|\phi_e|}{\phi_c}\right) = \left(1 + \frac{|\phi_e|}{\phi_c}\right) > 1,$$

where $|\phi_e|$ is the absolute value of the rate constant of tumour regression.

A summary evaluation of chemotherapy efficiency is obtained by averaging out over the whole time of follow-up. The $\varkappa*$ value obtained is often not a decisive characteristic of the drug's possibilities and a conclusion that its efficiency is low might be wrong. Such errors can be avoided by analyzing the kinetic curve and selecting out sections corresponding to the highest drug effect. Different versions of averaging are used in processing the data given below, but each version is specifically stipulated and correlated with the peculiarities of kinetic curves for tumour growth under chemotherapy. For comparative evaluation of different drug effects on the same tumour, and taking into account that the experimentalist has to make a conclusion as to which of the drugs is more active than the other, and by how much, the averaging intervals must be chosen so as to ensure strictly comparable conditions.

Obviously the kinetic curves will be unbiassed only with absolute standardization of the experiment schemes. However, this applied also to any other quantitative criterion.

The existing classification of antitumour drugs is to some extent conditional since it is based on the molecular mechanisms of the drug's effect (alkylating agents, antimetabolites) on the one hand and on their belonging to this or that class of chemical compounds (N-nitrosocarbamides, phenolic compounds) on the other. The conventional classification of antitumour drugs is used in this chapter. Certain molecular mechanisms of the action of individual drugs are discussed separately (see Chapter 5).

1. ALKYLATING COMPOUNDS

This class of chemical compounds has been used in the chemotherapy of tumours since the nineteen-forties, when nitrous analogues of mustard gas (chloroethlyl-amines) were first used as antitumour drugs (Larionov, 1962; Ross, 1964; Chernov, 1964). By now more than 40 drugs are available to the clinician and are assigned in their mechanism of action to the alkylating group. B-chloroethylamines, ethyl-enimines, esters of disulphonic acids, some antibiotics and some other compounds belong to this group.

Sarcolysine [n-bis-(β-chloro-ethyl)amino-d,1-phenylalanine hydrochloride]

$$ClCH_2CH_2\diagdown$$
$$\quad\quad\quad N-\langle\bigcirc\rangle-CH_2-CH-COOH$$
$$ClCH_2CH_2\diagup \cdot$$
$$\quad\quad\quad HCl \quad\quad\quad\quad NH_2$$

Sarcolysine was synthesizes taking into account Larionov's suggestion that it might be possible to use natural metabolites, in particular amino acids, as 'carriers' of cytotoxic groups into tumour tissue (Larionov, 1962). Sarcolysine at doses of 1.5 to 2.0 mg/kg/day induces resolution of the Walker carcinosarcoma, sarcoma 45, the Yoshida sarcoma, the Jensen sarcoma, inhibits the development of leukaemia L-1210, melanoma S-91, lymphosarcoma L10-1 and adenocarcinoma 755 (Larionov, 1962). The drug proves to be effective for treatment of seminoma, the Ewing sarcoma and multiple myeloma (Blokhin et al., 1958).

A kinetic study of the antileukaemic activity of sarcolysine was carried out for transplated leukaemia La in C57Bl mice (Emanuel et al., 1962). The drug was injected intraperitoneally at a dose of 1.5 mg/kg/day for a week after inoculation with 10^8 leukaemic cells. The exponential indices decreased under the action of sarcolysine (Figure 66a-d). The treatment had a different effect on the kinetics of changes in the main characteristics of the leukaemic process.

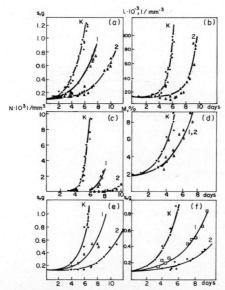

Fig. 66   The action of alkylating agents on the development
of transplanted leukaemia La in mice.
(a) Spleen weight;   (b) leucocytes;   (c) blood haemocytoblasts;   (d) bone marrow haemocytoblasts (K — control, 1 —
Thiotepa, 2 — sarcolysine) (Emanuel *et al.*, 1962);   (e)
1 — Thiotepa, 2 — PAT-1 (Konovalova *et al.*, 1973);   (f)
1 — N,N-bis(β-chloroethyl)pinocamphylamine hydrochloride or
N,N-bis(β-chloroethyl)pinylamine hydrochloride, 2 — 3,5-di-
tert.butyl-4-hydroxy-N,N-bis(β-chloroethyl)benzylamine
(Konovalova *et al.*, 1964).

The increase in spleen weight (S) and in the haemocytoblast count in blood (H) was
inhibited to a higher extent ($\varkappa^*_S = 0.50$; $\varkappa^*_H = 0.55$) than that of the leucocyte
count in peripheral blood (L) and in the relative haemocytoblast count (M) in
bone marrow ($\varkappa^*_L = 0.4$; $\varkappa^*_M = 0.3$).

At a summary dose of 7-10 mg/kg the drug induced partial inhibition of the sarcoma
SSK growth in rats.   After treatment with sarcolysine the exponential nature of
growth persisted, but the rate constant became 0.23 days^{-1} compared to 0.38 days^{-1}
in controls ($\varkappa^* = 0.4$, Figure 67a).

Multiple intraperitoneal administration of sarcolysine at a dose of 2 mg/kg/day to
rats with transplanted sarcoma 45, starting from the 5th day after transplantation,
resulted in complete inhibition of tumour growth for approximately 5 days (Kiseleva
et al., 1970).   Then, despite continuous drug injections, the growth recommenced,
though at a rate lower than in controls (see Figure 67b).   A comparison of the
appropriate sections in the experimental and control curves yields the average
values for specific growth rates $\phi_c = 0.22$ and $\phi_e = 0.14$ day^{-1}.   Thus, the kinetic
criterion value $\varkappa^*$ decreases from $\varkappa^* = 1$ for the section of complete inhibition to
$\varkappa^* = 0.4$ for growth recurrence (on the 10-18th day).   The decrease in treatment
effectiveness with time can be due to development of resistance to sarcolysine in
some tumour cells (Syrkin, 1965);   a substrain of sarcoma 45 displaying higher
resistance to alkylating agents was used by Syrkin.

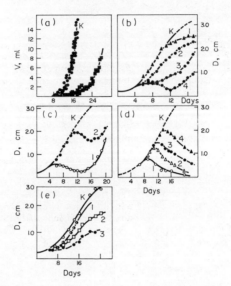

Fig. 67   Chemotherapy of various solid tumours by alkylating agents.
(a) Sarcolysine for sarcoma SSK;   (b) sarcoma 45: spirasidine (1),
mitomycin C (2), sarcolysine and dopane (3), cyclophosphamide (4);
(c) sarcoma 45, cyclophosphamide administered on the 5th (1) or 10th (2)
day (Kiseleva, 1971);   (d) Guérin carcinoma, cyclophosphamide on 7th,
9th, 11th or 13th day (1 to 4, respectively) (Emanuel *et al.*, 1970);
(e) adenocarcinoma 755: PAT-2 (1), Thiotepa (2), PAT-1 (3).

The Walker carcinosarcoma and the Sveč erythroleukaemia are more responsive to
alkylating agents, in particular to sarcolysine (Figures 68 and 69). With certain
doses and a sufficient number of administrations (usually 10-15) one can succeed in
obtaining complete tumour regression, whereas insufficient chemotherapy results in
reproducible recurrences. For instance, the incomplete regression of a developed
Walker tumour in rats occurs after administration of sarcolysine at a dose 2 mg/kg/
day for 5 days (Parkanskii *et al.*, 1973). The mean tumour diameter decreases
exponentially from 2-5 to 1.5 cm on the 8th to 18th day with a rate constant
$\phi_e = -0.06$ day^{-1}. After this, the tumour starts growing again (Figure 69). The
mean growth rate of a recurring tumour (0.16 cm/day) is considerably lower than
that in controls (0.34 cm/day). When the growth curve is averaged to a minimum
$\varkappa^* = 1.85$, an assessment of the whole follow-up range gives $\varkappa^* = 0.73$.

The administration of the same summary dose, but by 1 mg/kg/day to rats with
developed erythroleukaemia, results in complete resolution of the subcutaneous
tumour node (see Figure 68a) (Emanuel *et al.*, 1970). Tumour regression is also
exponential, but with a rate constant almost three times higher in absolute
magnitude (-17 day^{-1}) than that for the section of incomplete regression of the
Walker carcinosarcoma. This difference in constants seems to be due to simultaneou
removal of the dead cells and proliferation of the tumour cells which survived
chemotherapy.

Since the average specific tumour growth rate in controls is 0.07 day^{-1}, and the
regression rate constant is 0.17 day^{-1}, the criterion value will be
$\varkappa^* = 1-(-0.17)/0.07 = 3.4$.

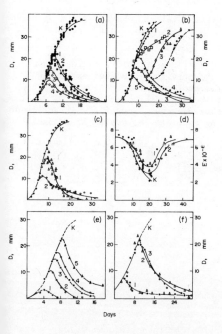

Fig. 68 Effect of alkylating agents on Sveč erythromyelosis. (a) 1 — sarcolysine, 1 mg/kg on 5th day after transplantation; 2,3,4 — ethoxene, 5 mg/kg on 6th (2), 5th (3) and 4th (4) day; (b) spirasidine — 1, 3, 5, 10 mg/kg administered on 5th or 6th day (4,5); (c) and (d) changes in subcutaneous tumour diameter (c) and in the blood erythrocyte count (d) under the action of ethoxene (1) and spirasidine (2); (e) imiphos on 1, 4, 5, 6 and 7th day (1 to 5) after transplantation (Emanuel et al., 1970); (f) Thiotepa (1,2) and PAT-1 (1,3), single administration on 3rd day and multiple administrations starting on 8th day.

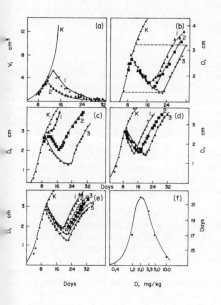

Fig. 69 Chemotherapy of Walker carcinosarcoma. (a) Thiotepa, 1 mg/kg/day (1) and 3 mg/kg/day (2) for tumour transplanted in the tail; (b) 1 — cyclophosphamide by 20 mg/kg, 2 — sarcolysine by 2 mg/kg, 3 — Thiotepa by 2 mg/kg on 8th to 12th day (Parkanskii et al., 1973); (c) administration of five Thiotepa doses of: 0.4 mg/kg/day (1), 0.8 mg/kg/day (2), 2.0 mg/kg/day (3); (d) Thiotepa, administration of a single total dose of 10 mg/kg (1) on 2nd or 3rd day (2,3); (e) administration of a single dose of Thiotepa of 2 mg/kg on 1st, 2nd, 3rd, 4th and 5th day (1-5); (f) time of start of recurrence as a function of Thiotepa single dose (Parkanskii and Konovalova, 1973).

Thus, the effect of sarcolysine on the Sveč erythromyelosis characterized by value $\varkappa^* > 1$ places this drug in the category of highly active therapeutic agents (see Figure 12).

Naturally, when under certain conditions the drug causes complete regression of the tumour, this is in itself characteristic of its activity. Numerous experiments show that the regression constant of a tumour, completely resolved as a result of single administration, is a fairly constant value depending on the type of drug, the time of its intake, and on a number of other factors. Thus the most active of the compound series studied is the drug causing complete regression at a dose lower than those needed with other drugs.

Dopane   [4-methyl-5-bis-(2-chloroethyl)-aminouracil]

When used clinically, the drug has a certain therapeutic effect on chronic myeloid leukaemia, lymphogranulomatosis and reticulosarcoma (Chernov, 1964).

The efficiency and kinetic features of the action of dopane (0.3 mg/kg/day intra-peritoneally) for a sub-strain of sarcoma 45 highly resistant to alkylating agents are practically the same as those of sarcolysine: after a relatively short period of complete inhibition the growth recommences with a mean specific rate 1.5 times lower than in the control (see Figure 67b) (Kiseleva et al., 1970).

Spirasidine   [N,N'-(β,β'-bis-chloroethyl)-N'',N'''-dispirotripiperazinium dichloride]

This drug is used clinically for the treatment of bladder cancer, reticulosarcoma-tosis and chronic lymphoid leukaemia. Experimentally it exerts a considerable therapeutic effect: it inhibits the growth of sarcomas 45, M-1, 180, mammary aden carcinoma in mice, and other tumours, even when administered at doses much lower than the maximum well-tolerated dose.

Multiple administration of spirasidine at small doses of 2 mg/kg/day to rats with a sarcoma 45 sub-strain resistant to alkylating agents had only a small effect ($\varkappa^* = 0.14$; see Figure 67b) (Kiseleva et al., 1970). The same refers to developed Sveč erythromyelosis treated with spirasidine at doses close to the above ($\varkappa^* = 0.1$ to 0.4). Increase in the dose up to 5-6 mg/kg/day gave a greater effect: partial tumour regression for some animals, and complete regression for others (Figure 68b A higher extent of regression and a delayed start of the growth of recurring tumours were observed at a dose of 6 mg/kg, compared to that of 5 mg/kg. The regression rate constants for doses of 5 and 6 mg/kg did not essentially differ ar were about 0.2 day^{-1}. A further increase in the dose up to 10 mg/kg caused death of some of the animals and complete regression of the subcutaneous tumour node anc

the return to normal of erythropoiesis (Figure 68c-d) in live individuals. The
activity coefficient $\varkappa^*$ for maximum doses increased to 1.7.

Cyclophosphamide [Cyclophsphane, endoxane; N,N-bis(β-chloroethyl)-N-γ-hydroxypropyldiamide of phosphoric acid (cyclic ester)]

$$(ClCH_2CH_2)_2N-P=O \begin{array}{c} NH-CH_2 \\ \diagup \\ \diagdown \\ NH-CH_2 \end{array} CH_2$$

This drug converts to its most active form directly in the body; compared to other
drugs, its toxicity is low.

Clinically, it is used for the treatment of lymphosarcoma and reticulosarcoma and
for prevention of recurrences and the appearance of metastases in the post-
operational chemotherapy of tumours, in particular, pulmonary cancer (Larionov,
1962). Experimentally it displays a wide spectrum of antitumour activity; it
causes regression of the Walker carcinosarcoma, of Jensen and Yoshida sarcomas,
even when the tumour is some way developed, and it inhibits development of leukaemia
L-1210 in mice, etc.

In the case of a sarcoma 45 sub-strain with elevated resistance to alkylating
compounds, four administrations of 80 mg/kg of cyclophosphamide induced partial
tumour regression which lasted for 7 days from the start of treatment (Kiseleva
et al., 1970). The growth recurrence proceeded in accordance with the exponential
dependence, at a rate constant 0.22 day^{-1} which did not differ from controls.
Averaging to the minimum point in the growth curve (in the regression section)
$\varkappa^* = 2.1$, evaluation over the whole range of measurements gave the value $\varkappa^* = 0.5$.

The nature of the drug's effect on sarcoma 45 was independent of the time of
starting treatment (Figure 67c) (Kiseleva et al., 1970). The absolute extent of
regression (~0.3 cm) and its duration (6-7 days) upon administration of the drug
5 or 10 days after transplantation did not differ essentially. However, the
relative effects for earlier administration were more distinct: at the minimum
point $\varkappa_5^* = 2.1$, $\varkappa_{10}^* = 1.5$; over the whole range $\varkappa_5^* = 0.8$, $\varkappa_{10}^* = 0.5$ (the subscripts
5 and 10 denote the times of administration).

A single large dose of 100 mg/kg induced complete resolution of tumours in rats
with transplanted Guérin carcinoma for any time of administration (Figure 67d)
(Kiseleva et al., 1970). The recurrence rate constants for administration on the
9th, 11th and 13th day after transplantation were virtually no different (the
absolute values were $0.13 - 0.14$ day^{-1}) and only in the case of very early administration (on the 7th day) the recurrence occurred at a somewhat higher specific
rate ($\phi_e = -0.20$ day^{-1}). The activity coefficient $\varkappa^*$ also depended insignificantly
on the time of treatment and was $1.7 - 1.9$.

Fractional five-time administration of the same dose on the 8th to 12th day after
subcutaneous transplantation of the Walker carcinosarcoma led to only partial
tumour regression with growth recurrence in 9 days after start of treatment (Figure
69b) (Parkanskii et al., 1973). The value $\varkappa^*$ averaged to the minimum point was
1.5, the value averaged to end points was 0.7.

It is characteristic that practically all cases of both complete and incomplete
tumour regressions under consideration were preceded by a certain period of
continuous growth with intensity and duration in some way dependent on the time of
starting treatment and drug dose.

Thiotepa (N,N',N"-triethylenimide of thiophosphoric acid)

$$\begin{array}{ccc}
H_2C & S & CH_2 \\
& \| & \\
& N-P-N & \\
H_2C & N & CH_2 \\
& \wedge & \\
& H_2C-CH_2 &
\end{array}$$

This drug has been widely studied both experimentally and clinically (Larionov, 1962; Chernov, 1964; Sugiura and Stook, 1955). The kinetics of changes in the haematological parameters for transplanted leukaemia La under the action of Thiotepa was studied by Emanuel et $al.$ (1962). The drug was administered as 2.5 mg/kg daily for a week, starting 3 hours after transplantation. Thiotepa administered in this way was rather less effective than sarcolysine: the mean coefficient $\varkappa^*$ was 0.3 for all characteristics (spleen weight, leucocyte and haemocytoblast counts). For sarcolysine it attained 0.5 - 0.6 (Figure 66a-d).

Detailed kinetic studies of the Thiotepa effect under various regimens of administration were carried out for Walker carcinosarcoma. Multiple injections into the tail at doses of 1 or 3 mg/kg daily from the 8th to the 17th day after transplantation caused complete resolution of the tumour. When the dose was lower, regression began six days after the start of treatment, and in four days at a dose of 3 mg/kg daily (Figure 69a). In the latter case the period of continuous growth was shorter and the maximal tumour volume to the moment of the start of regression was considerably less than for small doses (3.3 and 5.3 cm^3 respectively). The regression rate constants were the same for both cases (ϕ_e = -0.16 day^{-1}). Since ϕ_c = 0.3, the $\varkappa^*$ value was 1-(-0.16)/0.3 = 1.5

The effect of Thiotepa on a tumour transplanted subcutaneously into an animal flank has been studied. At a dose of 10 mg/kg daily the drug induced only partial regression with subsequent tumour recurrence in all animals (Figure 69b) (Parkanskii et $al.$, 1973). The regression period was rather long (it lasted from 2 to 14 days after the start of treatment). The tumour size in the course of regression diminished approximately by half (from 2.6 to 1.3 cm). The regression rate constant (ϕ_V = 3; ϕ_D = -0.18 day^{-1}) was close to that determined previously (-0.16 day^{-1}). The mean growth rate of the recurring tumour (0.2 cm/day) was 1.7 times lower than in controls. The coefficient $\varkappa^*$ on averaging to the minimum point of the curve was 1.7, on averaging to the end points it was 0.8.

Other administration schedules and drug doses resulted in considerable changes in the extent of regression and in the time at which recurring tumour growth began (Parkanskii and Konovalova, 1973). A single administration of the drug at a dose of 2 mg/kg caused prolonged regression with recurrences appearing much later (Figure 69e). The same dose injected in five instalments caused only an insignificant decrease in the growth rate (Figure 69c); large doses administered several times were more effective. The regression extent and especially the start of tumour growth were markedly lower after a single 10 mg/kg injection, compared to the same dose administered by fractions three or four times (Figure 69d-e). Thus the optimal single dose seems to be 2 mg/kg (Figure 69f.

The data obtained are presented in Table 17. The constants for regressions and recurring growth were calculated by straightening of the appropriate sections of kinetic curves in co-ordinates log $D/(D_\infty - D)$ vs t. The final value 4.6 of the tumour diameter in controls was taken as D_∞. The criterion $\varkappa^*$ was evaluated by averaging the control and experimental curves to their end points. The activity coefficient $\varkappa^*$ was 1.3 to 1.5 for the regression sections up to the minimum points.

TABLE 17   Rate constants of regression and recurrence growth of the
Walker carcinosarcoma for various administration schedules

Curve number in Fig. 69	Single dose, mg/kg	Number of injections	Summary dose, kg/kg	Time of recurrence beginning, days	ϕ_e, day^{-1} regressions	ϕ_e, day^{-1} recurrence	$\varkappa^*$
c, 1	0.4	5	2	–	–	0.37	0.27
c, 2	0.8-1.6	5	4-8	17	-0.13	0.18	0.38
c, 3	2.0	5	10	22	-0.12	0.18	0.79
d, 3	3.3	3	10	20	-0.12	0.18	0.80
d, 2	5.0	2	10	17	-0.18	0.16	0.77
d, 1	10.0	1	10	14	-0.19	0.20	0.72
e, 1	2.0	1	2	18	-0.12	0.17	0.72
e, 2	2.0	2	4	20	-0.11	0.18	0.78
e, 3	2.0	3	6	21	-0.11	0.16	0.80
e, 4	2.0	4	8	22	-0.11	0.16	0.84
e, 5	2.0	5	10	22	-0.13	0.17	0.87
K	0.0	0	0	–	–	0.40	

The rate constants of recurring tumour growth were close, irrespective of the
administration schedule. Only large single doses of 5 and 10 mg/kg caused more
rapid regression. Single administration of the drug at a dose of 2 mg/kg was more
effective than that at 10 mg/kg. With equal values of the $\varkappa^*$ coefficient in the
first case the growth recurrence started later.

It can be seen from Table 17 that the regimen of drug administration is of great
importance in obtaining the best therapeutic effect.

In this case the tumour recurrence after the end of the therapy is characterized by
a considerably lower growth rate, compared to the control group. The origin of
this phenomenon is not clear. A lower growth rate of the Walker carcinosarcoma
(compared to controls) was observed also after treatment with sarcolysine and cyclophosphamide (Figure 69b) (Parkanskii *et al.*, 1973). It was also stated that the
development of sarcoma 45 after incomplete regression under the action of cyclophosphamide (Figure 67b-c) (Kiseleva *et al.*, 1970; Kiseleva, 1971), as well as
the recurrent growth of subcutaneous tumours of Sveč erythromyelosis after treatment
with spirasidine (Figure 68b) (Emanuel *et al.*, 1970), progressed at a rate equal to
that of tumour growth in controls.

Paramagnetic Analogues of Thiotepa (PAT)

It is known that structural modification of chemotherapeutic drugs can induce
marked changes in their biological activity and in the appearance of new properties.
The incorporation of certain chemical groups into a drug molecule gives an insight
into the mechanism of the drug action on a molecular level and gives the possibility
of determining their affinity to certain body systems. For instance, the incorporation of stable free radicals as a molecular structure fragment permits using the
spin-labelled compounds obtained in studying the interaction of drugs with enzymes,
nucleic acids and proteins, and also for detection of the drug and of its metabolites in blood, tissues and body eliminations.

The antitumour activity reported earlier for some stable free radicals stimulated
the synthesis of two paramagnetic Thiotepa analogues by substitution of an iminoxyl
radical for one of the ethylene imine groups in its molecule.

Such chemical modifications of known anticancer drugs may result in the creation of novel antitumour agents.

Thiotepa   PAT-1   PAT-2

TABLE 18 Toxic and therapeutic doses (in mg/kg) of Thiotepa
and its paramagnetic analogues (Konovalova *et al.*, 1973)

Drug	LD$_{50}$		MPD	
	Single administration	Seven-dose administration	Single administration	Seven-dose administration
Thiotepa	18	6	12	2
PAT-1	187	32	150	10
PAT-2	40	15	20	10

The results of comparative studies on the toxicity of these compounds are given in Table 18. The toxicity of PAT-1 is lower than that of Thiotepa, but an insignif-icant modification of the structure, such as incorporation of the CH_2 group, results in an increase in toxicity (Konovalova *et al.*, 1973).

Investigation of the antitumour effect of these compounds demonstrated that PAT-1 is more active than Thiotepa and PAT-2 for solid tumours, while the difference in their effect on ascites forms of tumours is less marked (Table 19).

TABLE 19 Comparative antitumour activity of Thiotepa
and of its paramagnetic analogues

Drug	Inhibition of tumour growth, %					
	Ascites tumours		Solid tumours			
	EAC	S-180	Ca-755	WCS	Guérin carcinoma	Sarcoma 45
Thiotepa	44	64	75	98	79	80
PAT-1	67	47	94	100	100	99
PAT-2	65	57	30	93	54	56

PAT-1 also exhibits a more pronounced antileukaemic activity than Thiotepa. The activity coefficients ϰ* calculated by the curves for changes in the spleen weight were 0.5 and 0.3, respectively, for transplanted leukaemia La in mice (Figure 66e).

Figure 67e shows the kinetics of changes in the mean diameter of adenocarcinoma 755 in untreated tumour-bearing animals (controls) and in those for whom treatment started on the 5th day after transplantation, when the tumour is already advanced and its mean diameter is 0.4 cm. The highest activity was displayed by PAT-1 ($\varkappa^* = 0.47$), next was Thiotepa ($\varkappa^* = 0.36$), and PAT-2 was less active ($\varkappa^* = 0.05$).

A small but statistically significant difference in the effect of Thiotepa and PAT-1 was observed for rats bearing transplanted Sveč erythroleukaemia and treated at doses equivalent in their ethyleneimine group contents (2 and 5 mg/kg/day, respectively) during 10 days starting on the 8th day after transplantation. Complete resolution of tumours was observed in both cases, but after injection of PAT-1 the period of continuous growth was half that after administration of Thiotepa, and regression occurred with a somewhat higher mean specific rate (0.11 and 0.15 day^{-1}) correspondingly. Single injections of similar quantities of drugs 8 days after transplantation caused regression with a higher rate constant (0.21 day^{-1}), the same for both drugs (Figure 68f). Complete tumour resolution in animals treated with Thiotepa occurred later than in those treated with PAT-1. It was shown by means of the autoradiography technique that PAT-1 caused more pronounced disturbances in the vital activity of Ehrlich ascites carcinoma cells than did Thiotepa (D'iachkovskaia, 1973).

The antitumour activity of PAT-1 which can be regarded as a drug of combined action seems to be due not only to the ethyleneimine groups but also to one more active fragment present in its molecule — the iminoxyl radical.

Drugs of the bis-(β-chloroethyl)-amine Group with no Effect on Haemopoiesis

The antitumour properties of three drugs of the bis-(β-chloroethyl)amine group were studied by Konovalova et al. (1964): N,N-bis-(β-chloroethyl)pinocamphylamine hydrochloride (I); N,N-bis(β-chloroethyl)pinylamine hydrochloride (II); and 3,5-di-tert.butyl-4-hydroxy-N,N-bis(β-chloroethyl)benzylamine (III).

The experiments were conducted for leukaemia La, Ehrlich ascites carcinoma, and sarcoma 180 in mice, Guérin carcinoma and sarcoma 45 in rats. The drugs were administered intraperitoneally at doses of $0.2 - 0.3$ LD_{50} for solid tumours and leukaemias and subcutaneously for ascites tumours. The values of toxic and therapeutic doses, of the inhibition coefficients (in %) for ascites and solid tumours and those of activity coefficient $\varkappa^*$ for various haematological parameters of the leukaemic process are given in Table 20. The kinetic curves for changes in the spleen weight in controls and under chemotherapeutic action are presented in Figure 66d.

Comparison of drugs I and II, which are close chemical analogues, showed that the less toxic drug II possessed a higher activity for leukaemia La and solid tumours. For the Ehrlich ascites carcinoma, drug II is ineffective.

The absence of a toxic effect on haemopoiesis is a characteristic of the above compounds compared to most other β-chloroethylamines. When drugs I, II and III

TABLE 20   Toxicity and the therapeutic activity parameters of drugs from the bis(β-chloroethyl)-amine groups for experimental tumours (Konovalova *et al.*, 1964)

Drug	LD_{50} mg/kg	TD mg/kg	Leukaemia La			EAC S-180 inhibition %		TD mg/kg	Guérin carcinoma inhibition %	Sarcoma 45 inhibition %
			$\varkappa^*_S$	$\varkappa^*_L$	$\varkappa^*_H$					
I	20	6	0.4	0.3	0.2	33	100	3	–	0
II	27	4	0.4	0.4	0.3	0	100	6	90	52
III	85	25	0.5	0.3	0.4	83	80	15	50	–

were administered to rats in therapeutic doses none of these compounds substantially affected the quantitative morphological composition of blood (Konovalova *et al.*, 1964). Only a slight increase in the neutrophil count was observed under the action of drug II.

Ethoxene [N-(2-hydroxybutene-3-yl)ethylenimine]

$$H_2C \overset{\displaystyle}{\underset{\displaystyle H_2C}{\diagdown\hspace{-0.3em}\diagup}} N-CH_2CHCH{=}CH_2 \atop \hspace{3em} OH$$

Clinical assays showed a low tolerance of the drug in patients with tumours of the digestive organs and therefore it was not widely used (Larionov, 1962).

The drug caused 80–90% inhibition of growth of many experimental tumours in mice and rats. The capacity of ethoxene to polymerize due to opening of the C=C bonds with persistence of the ethyleneimine cycle stimulated attempts to study the antitumour activity of ethoxene polymers with a different content of the ethyleneimine cycles (61.3 – 68.6%).

$$\left[\begin{array}{ccc} -CH_2{-}CH{-}CH_2{-}CH{-}CH_2CH_2N{-} \\ | \hspace{3em} | \hspace{3em} | \\ CHOH \hspace{1em} CHOH \hspace{1em} CH_2 \\ | \hspace{3em} | \hspace{3em} | \\ CH_2 \hspace{1.5em} CH_2 \hspace{1.5em} CHOH \\ | \hspace{3em} | \hspace{3em} | \\ N \hspace{2em} N \hspace{2em} CH \\ \diagup\diagdown \hspace{1em} \diagup\diagdown \hspace{2em} \| \\ H_2C\ CH_2\ H_2C\ CH_2 \hspace{1em} CH_2 \end{array} \right]_n$$

Polyethoxenes were considered to display a lower toxicity and a prolonged effect compared to monomers. However, a comparative study of the effects of ethoxene and of its polymers on leukaemia La showed no advantage of the polymer form of the drug (Figure 70, Table 21) (Dronova *et al.*, 1966).

Multiple injections of a maximum therapeutic dose markedly increase the polyethoxene activity ($\varkappa^*_S = 0.6$; $\varkappa^*_L = 0.4$). The monomer injected at similar doses suppresses normal haemopoiesis (Figure 70d). The effects of ethoxene and of its polymer given as multiple injections of small doses are similar and do not differ from results obtained with a single injection.

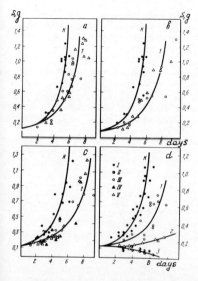

Fig. 70 Effectiveness of ethoxene and its polymer for leukaemia La (Dronova *et al.*, 1966). (a), (b), (c) Single doses of 8 mg/kg (a), 16 mg/kg (b) and 20 mg/kg (c); (d) multiple doses injected by 8 mg/kg/day (1) and 20 mg/kg/day (2,3) (I — controls; II, III — ethoxene; IV, V — polyethoxene).

TABLE 21 Toxicity and therapeutic activity of ethoxene and of its polymers with respect to transplanted leukaemia La in mice (Dronova *et al.*, 1966)

Drug	LD_{50} mg/kg	TD mg/kg	$\varkappa^*_S$	$\varkappa^*_L$
Ethoxene	40	20	0.33	0.23
		16	0.31	0.29
		8	0.20	0.20
Polyethoxene (68.6%)	42	20	0.33	0.23
		16	0.29	0.29
		8	0.20	–
Polyethoxene (61.3%)	45	20	0.33	–

Ethoxene was considerably more effective for Sveč erythroleukaemia than for leukaemia La. Multiple injections of only 5 mg/kg/day in the exponential growth phase resulted in complete resolution of subcutaneous tumours in all animals (Figure 68a). The regression rate constants (-0.2 day^{-1}) and the activity coefficients (3.2 – 3.9) depended only slightly on the time of starting treatment (on the 4th, 5th or 6th day). As well as in the case of spirasidine, the tumour regression was accompanied by normalization of erythropoiesis (Figure 68c,d).

Imiphos (Diethylenimide of 2-methylthiazolidyl-3-phosphoric acid)

This drug induces marked inhibition of many experimental tumours in mice and rats. Kinetic studies of the antitumour activity was carried out for Sveč erythroleukaemi (Emanuel *et al.*, 1970). Imiphos was administered at a dose of 10 mg/kg/day for a period of 10 days starting from the 1st, 4th, 5th, 6th or 7th day after transplantation. Complete resolution of the tumour was observed in all cases (Figure 68e). The kinetic curve corresponding to the earliest time of treatment slightly differs from the others: the phase of continuous growth lasts longer in this case, and the regression rate constant ($\phi_e = -0.5$ day^{-1}) is higher in absolute magnitude than for all other times of starting treatment for which this value is always $\phi_e = -0.3$ day^{-1}. The ϰ* values calculated from the regression constants and the mean specific growth rates of the control tumour ($\phi_c = 0.3$ day^{-1}) range from 2.0 (injection on 7th day) to 2.6 (injection on 1st day).

2. N-NITROSOCARBAMIDES

This class of compounds occupies a special place among the drugs proposed in the last twn years for the treatment of malignant neoplasms. The derivatives of N-nitrosourea, N-nitrosoguanidine and N-nitrosobiuret are the best known:

Alk—N—C—NH$_2$ N-alkyl-N-nitrosoureas
     | ‖
     NO O

Alk$=$ — CH$_3$; —C$_2$H$_5$; —C$_3$H$_7$.

ClCH$_2$CH$_2$—N—C—NH—CH$_2$CH$_2$Cl   N,N'-bis(chloroethyl)-N-nitrosourea (BCNU)
              | ‖
              NO O

ClCH$_2$CH$_2$—N—C—NH—⟨   ⟩   N-chloroethyl-N'-cyclohexyl-N-nitrosourea (CCNU)
              | ‖
              NO O

ClCH$_2$CH$_2$—N—C—NH—⟨   ⟩—CH$_3$ N'-methylcyclohexyl-N-chloroethyl-N-nitrosourea
              | ‖   (MeCCNU)
              NO O

C$_2$H$_5$—N—C—NH—C$_2$H$_5$ N,N'-diethyl-N-nitrosourea (DENU)
        | ‖
        NO O

CH$_3$—N—C—NH—C—NH$_2$ N-methyl-N-nitrosobiuret (MNB)
      | ‖   ‖
      NO O   O

      NO
      |
CH$_3$—N   N-methyl-N-nitrosoguanidine
      \
       C=NH
      /
   H$_2$N

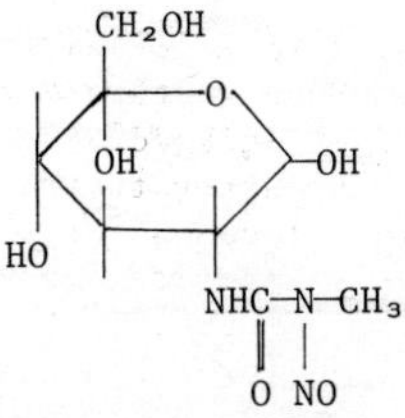

Streptozotocin

N-alkylnitrosoureas possess an extremely high and versatile biological activity. In particular they exert marked antitumour and anti-mutagenic effects. These compounds have the capacity to penetrate through the haemato-encephalic barrier and this provides the possibility of their application in chemotherapy of patients with brain tumours.

These compounds demonstrated a high antitumour activity not only experimentally but also clinically. Systematic experimental studies of the homologous series of N-alkylnitrosoureas carried out in the USSR since 1963 (Ostrovskaia *et al.*, 1964, 1968; Emanuel *et al.*, 1966, 1970; Kukushkina *et al.*, 1972; Ostrovskaia, 1968) resulted in the adoption of a new active antitumour drug, the N-methyl-1-nitrosourea, in oncological practice. This drug is used for the treatment of undifferentiated lung cancer and lymphogranulomatosis (Vermel *et al.*, 1970).

American researchers proposed four drugs of this type: streptozotocin (antibiotic), BCNU, CCNU and MeCCNU: some have already been used in clinical practice (Schabel *et al.*, 1963; Comis *et al.*, 1972; Wheeler and Alexander, 1974).

Table 22 presents data (in per cent inhibition) on the antitumour activity of the first four members of the homologous series of N-alkylnitrosoureas: N-methylnitrosourea (MNU), N-ethylnitrosourea (ENU), N-propylnitrosourea (PNU), N-isobutylnitrosourea (BNU) and on two other derivatives — N,N-diethyl-N-nitrosourea (DENU) and N-methylnitrosobiuret (MNB). The drugs were administered six times intraperitoneally (i.p.) and subcutaneously (s.c.) in the maximum tolerated doses. The drugs were administered to ascites tumour-bearing animals a day after transplantation. For solid tumours the treatment was started at the period of complete tumour formation (when the tumour attained a palpable size).

All drugs were highly active towards ascites forms of Ehrlich carcinoma (EAC), sarcoma 180 (S-180) and sarcoma 37 (C-37) in mice. The inhibition attained 90-100% for maximally tolerated doses, and 70-85% for therapeutic doses. The development of ascites lymphoma NKLy was suppressed by 70-100% under the action of MNB, DENU, MNU and BNU. The effects of ENU and PNU were lower for this strain (40-70%). A high effect was obtained for solid tumours such as sarcoma 45 and Walker carcinosarcoma, as well as for the first generation of spontaneous mammary gland tumour (MC) in C3H/He mice. The latter tumour model is characterized by resistance to chemotherapeutic agents of other classes. The Lewis tumour and adenocarcinoma 755 (Ca 755) appeared to be most resistant: only BNU and MNB in their maximum tolerated doses inhibited their development by 70-85%. The effectiveness of these drugs was approximately the same for both intraperitoneal and subcutaneous injections.

Figure 71 presents the kinetic curves for changes in ascites volume and tumour cell number of sarcoma 180 and Ehrlich carcinoma in controls and when treated with N-alkylnitrosoureas. The changes in the two characteristics of the process for sarcoma 180 are of an extreme nature. However, for a considerable period of time (up to 12 days) the kinetic curves can be described by an exponential dependence with $\phi_c = 0.39$ day^{-1}. Six subcutaneous administrations of the drugs at therapeutic doses (MNU, 20 mg/kg/day, and PNU, 100 mg/kg/day) considerably inhibit the process

TABLE 22   Antitumour activity of nitrosocarbamides (Ostrovskaia, 1968)

Drug	Dose mg/kg/day	Route of administration	EAC	S-180	C-37	NKLy	Lewis tumour	Ca755	MGC	WCS	C-45
							inhibition, %				
MNU	20	i.p.	90	90	90	85	70	60	95	95	95
	10	i.p.	80	80	70	40	60	55	85	90	90
	50	s.c.	95	85	70	90	75	65	90	-	-
	20	s.c.	80	75	60	70	60	60	85	95	90
ENU	200	i.p.	100	95	100	65	65	50	70	80	85
	100	i.p.	95	90	80	50	-	-	65	60	50
	200	s.c.	100	95	90	60	60	55	65	95	80
	100	s.c.	80	80	35	40	-	-	50	60	65
PNU	200	i.p.	90	100	95	65	50	50	65	60	75
	100	i.p.	90	85	80	50	-	-	55	40	20
	200	s.c.	100	95	95	70	55	50	70	55	75
	100	s.c.	75	70	85	60	-	-	65	0	40
BNU	20	i.p.	95	80	70	90	85	70	80	95	90
	10	i.p.	70	60	60	80	60	40	65	80	80
	50	s.c.	90	75	70	90	-	-	75	95	90
	20	s.c.	80	50	60	85	-	-	-	70	70
DENU	25	i.p.	90	95	100	100	65	40	-	85	70
	12.5	i.p.	80	80	90	60	-	-	-	65	-
MNB	25	i.p.	100	95	100	100	70	70	-	70	-

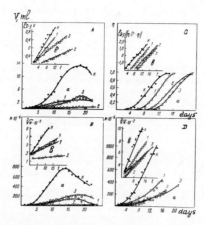

Fig. 71 The effect of N-alkylnitrosoureas on ascitic forms of tumours.
(A), (B) Sarcoma 180: changes in ascitic fluid volume (A) and number of
tumour cells present in fluid (B) under the action of MNU (1), ENU (2)
and PNU (3); the drugs were injected subcutaneously at doses: 20 mg/kg
of MNU, and 100 mg/kg of ENU and PNU within 6 days. (C), (D) Ehrlich
carcinoma: change in the relative volume of ascitic fluid (C) and the
number of cells (D) under the action of ENU: single dose of 200 mg/kg
on 1st and 7th day (1); single dose of 400 mg/kg (2); by 100 mg/kg
from 1st to 6th day (3).

development. The exponent index is reduced in this case to $\phi_e = 0.10$ under the
action of ENU ($\varkappa^* = 0.7$) to $\phi_e = 0.18$ under the action of PNU ($\varkappa^* = 0.5$) and to
$\phi_e = 0.29$ day^{-1} ($\varkappa^* = 0.3$) under the action of MNU (Figure 71A, Table 23). ENU also
greatly affects the kinetics of changes in cell numbers (Figure 71B).

The effects of various administration schedules were studied for the Ehrlich
ascites carcinoma. Figure 71C,D presents kinetic curves for development in controls
and under the action of single injections (400 mg/kg), and of twice injected (by
200 mg/kg on 1st and 7th day) and six-times injected (by 100 mg/kg daily) doses of
ENU. The experimental data obtained are given in Table 23.

TABLE 23 Antitumour effect of alkylnitrosourea (Ostrovskaia, 1968)

Drug	Dose mg/kg	Number of doses given	$\varkappa^*_V$		$\varkappa^*_N$	
			EAC	S-180	EAC	S-180
MNU	120	1	0.31	–	0.55	–
	20	6	0.21	0.26	0.26	0.51
	20	2	0.22	–	0.08	–
ENU	400	1	0.39	–	0.44	–
	200	2	0.21	–	0.25	–
	100	6	0.43	0.74	0.45	0.81
PNU	400	1	0.37	–	0.44	–
	200	2	0.22	–	0.25	–
	100	6	0.21	0.53	0.22	0.43

The drug causes a parallel shift of the kinetic curves for ascitic fluid accumulation (Figure 71C). The shift value varies from 5 to 10 days, depending upon the
drug type and the administration schedule. However, the maximum rates of increase
in the ascites volume ($\phi_e = 0.6 - 0.7$ day^{-1}) remain approximately the same as in
controls ($\phi_c = 0.64$ day^{-1}). In Figure 71C the corresponding curves are given in
normed co-ordinates. This case will be considered in detail, since with a parallel
shift of the S-shaped kinetic curves the calculation of the coefficient strongly
depends on the choice of the averaging interval, especially for the end sections of
the kinetic curves. The inflection points in the kinetic curves or the times of
attaining similar reliably determined tumour sizes for controls (t_c) and experimental animals (t_e) can be better used as end points of the averaging intervals.
Then

$$\varkappa^* = (t_e - t_c)/t_e.$$

The criterion $\varkappa^*_V$ in Table 23 was calculated making use of this equation.

In all cases the increase in cell number was described by the equation

$$(N)^{1/3} = a + bt$$

(Figure 71D). The drugs had an effect mainly on parameter b characterizing the
rate of development. The b value varied from 63 day^{-1} in controls to 17 day^{-1} for
maximum inhibition induced by a single injection of MNU at a dose of 120 mg/kg.
The coefficient $\varkappa^*_N$ was calculated by averaging to the end point of the control
kinetic curve (14 days) (Table 23). It follows from Table 23 that in order to
obtain the best effect the drugs must be introduced in large doses. For example,
for ENU and PNU such an administration schedule was more effective than the
fractional treatment by summary doses 1.5 times higher.

Comparison of the drug effect on sarcoma 180 and EAC demonstrated that under
similar schedules of administration the effect of MNU, ENU and PNU on EAC was
smaller. This was supported by comparison of coefficients $\varkappa^*_V$ and $\varkappa^*_N$. MNU was
found to be most effective against EAC, and ENU against sarcoma 180. These
conclusions on the specific antitumour action of alkylnitrosoureas on ascitic
tumour models could be made only after having used the kinetic criterion $\varkappa^*$
(Table 23). For instance, the inhibition percent used for the evaluation of antitumour activity (Table 22) gives practically indistinguishable high values of the
drug's effectiveness (70-80%). That is one more example of the advantage of
kinetic criteria for evaluation of a drug's antitumour effects.

The drug's effects on certain characteristics of the process are different. A
conclusion about comparative drug effectiveness will depend on the tumour characteristic chosen. Therefore in setting up the treatment regimen it is possible to
choose drugs acting in the most effective way on this or that characteristic of the
tumour process.

A high antileukaemic activity was found for N-alkylnitrosoureas experimentally as
well. Five subcutaneous injections of MNU at a dose of 10 mg/kg on the 1st to 5th
day after transplantation of leukaemia L-1210 inhibited the process development for
about 4 days. Double doses induced a decrease in the tumour cell number in the
ascites (Figure 72a). The coefficient $\varkappa^*$ increased from 0.35 to 1.0 with the dose
doubling (virtually complete stopping of the process).

In experiments with leukaemia La the drugs were injected intraperitoneally at doses
of 30 (MNU), 100 (ENU) and 200 (PNU) mg/kg/day (Emanuel et $al.$, 1966). These doses
considerably inhibited spleen growth and the increase in the haemocytoblast count
in the blood of mice (Figure 72b-d). The antitumour activity increased with the
alkyl chain length: for MNU $\varkappa^*_S = 0.58$; for ENU $\varkappa^*_S = 0.64$, $\varkappa^*_H = 0.57$; for PNU
$\varkappa^*_S = 0.78$, $\varkappa^*_H = 0.76$. Under the action of drugs the leucocyte count fell below

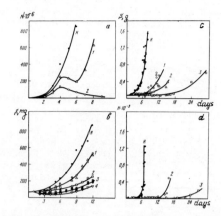

Fig. 72 N-alkylnitrosourea effect on leukaemias.
(a) Leukaemia L-1210, five subcutaneous injections of MNU at
doses of 10 (1) and 20 (2) mg/kg/day (Ostrovskaia, 1968);
(b) leukaemia La, injection of the drugs on 1st and 7th day,
CNNU and MeCCNU (1) by 24 and 38, BCNU (2) by 27, BNU and
DENU (3) by 100, MNU (4) by 80 mg/kg (Ostrovskaia *et al.*,
1977); (c), (d) change in spleen weight (c) and the haemocytoblasts in blood (d) for leukaemia La under the action of
five-dose administration of 20 mg/kg of MNU (1), 120 mg/kg
of ENU (2) and 200 mg/kg of PNU (3) (Emanuel *et al.*, 1966).

normal but gradually returned to normal after the treatment was discontinued.

Similar results were obtained for subcutaneous injections. The toxicity in the
homologous series of N-alkylnitrosoureas decreased with increase in the alkyl
chain length and this shows the possibilities that are opened up by a search for
active antileukaemic compounds among the closest homogues of the series.

Like the ascites tumours, the leukaemic processes are more strongly suppressed when
N-alkylnitrosoureas are introduced in discrete large doses. The activity of other
nitrosourea derivatives diminishes in the order: MNU and DENU ($\varkappa^*_S = 0.6$), BCNU
($\varkappa^*_S = 0.5$), CCNU and MeCCNU ($\varkappa^*_S = 0.2$) (Figure 72b). MNU, BNU, DENU and BCNU were
injected intraperitoneally in a 25% solution of dimethylsulphoxide (BCNU in 10%
ethanol solution), and CCNU and MeCCNU in oil solution were administered orally
(Ostrovskaia *et al.*, 1977). Development of leukopaenia was observed in experiments,
especially with MNU and BNU. In all cases the survival times did not differ from
those in controls.

The study of the antitumour effects of nitrosourea derivatives on Walker carcinosarcoma revealed that a higher activity was displayed by drugs containing chloroethyl groups (Figure 73a). Under the action of CCNU and MeCCNU complete tumour
resolution was observed in 40%. The life-span of the other animals doubled
compared to controls, and in this case, $\varkappa^* = 0.84$. BCNU caused an incomplete curve,
and the coefficient $\varkappa^*$ was 0.8. The average life-span for animals treated with
BCNU more than doubled. The activity of a BCNU analogue with no chloroethyl groups
in its structure is lower: $\varkappa^*_{DENU} = 0.47$. CCNU and MeCCNU were highly effective
against solid tumours resistant to the action of other drugs. Single doses of
CCNU (57 mg/kg) or of MeCCNU (36 mg/kg) administered to mice with well-developed
Lewis carcinoma caused a decrease in the tumour size 7 days after administration

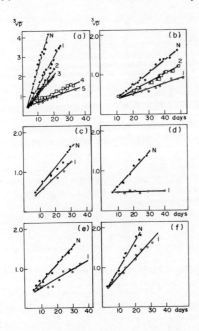

Fig. 73 N-alkylnitrosourea effect on
solid tumours. (a) Walker carcinosarcoma,
injection of BNU (1), DENU (2), MNU (3),
BCNU (4), CCNU and MeCCNU (5) (Ostrovskaia
et al., 1977). (b), (c) — 1 (b) and 21 (c)
generations of spontaneous mammary gland
tumours in C3H mice, injections of MNU (1),
ENU and PNU (2). (d) to (f) — 1 (d), 29,
41 (e), 48 (f) generations of spontaneous
mammary gland tumours in A mice, injections
of MNU (1) (Ostrovskaia and Vermel, 1975).

($\varkappa^* = 1.5$) (Wheeler and Alexander, 1974). Alkylnitrosoureas having no chloroethyl
groups exerted a lesser effect on this tumour (Table 22).

The effect of N-alkylnitrosoureas on successive generations of spontaneous tumours
has been studied (Ostrovskaia and Vermel, 1975). It is generally accepted that
slow-growing tumours in animals most closely simulate the development of solid
malignant tumours in humans. In this connection spontaneous tumours, preferably in
their first generation, are used in experimental oncology whenever possible.

Later generations were derived from spontaneous tumours which arose in A and C3H
mice at the age of 8-10 months. The chemotherapy was started at time t_0 when the
tumour weight attained approximately 100 mg. The drugs were injected intraperitoneally six times at 2-day intervals, by single doses of 20 mg/kg (MNU) and 100 mg/kg
(ENU and PNU). The kinetic curves for changes in tumour weight were satisfactorily
described by a cube root equation.

The values of parameter b characterizing the tumour growth rate are given in
Table 24.

The linear growth rate in the first-generation tumour in C3H mice decreased under
the action of MNU by a factor of 3, $\varkappa^* = 0.5$. ENU and PNU are considerably less
effective: the growth rate decreases under their action by only 30%, the value
$\varkappa^*$ — to 0.2 (Figure 73b). In the 21st generation the tumour growth rate markedly
increases in controls and the MNU effectiveness greatly decreases ($\varkappa^* = 0.2$; Figure
73c).

Tumours of the first generation in A mice grow a little faster than the equivalent
generation in C3H mice, and are characterized by a higher response to MNU. For
example, the linear growth rate decreases by a factor of eight, and the corresponding $\varkappa^*$ value is 0.8 (Figure 73d). The response to MNU drops in the 29th and
41st generations ($\varkappa^* = 0.2$), though the kinetic parameters of control tumours in

TABLE 24   Effect of N-alkylnitrosourea on the growth kinetics of generation series of spontaneous mammary gland tumours in mice (Ostrovskaia and Vermel. 1975)

Strain of mice	Tumour generation	Drug	t_0, day	t_f, day	P_{max}, r	b	$\varkappa*$
A	1	Controls	7	29	2.4±0.6	0.40	0.8
		MNU	7	40	0.3±0.1	0.05	
	29,41	Controls	5	32	4.0±0.8	0.35	0.2
		MNU	5	35	2.0±0.6	0.30	
	48	Controls	3	24	7.0±1.2	0.60	0.3
		MNU	3	31	5.0±1.9	0.40	
C3H	1	Controls	12	48	4.2±1.4	0.30	0.5
		MNU	12	52	1.0±0.4	0.10	
		ENU, PNU	12	48	1.6±0.8	0.20	0.2
	21	Controls	8	31	4.6±1.2	0.50	0.2
		MNU	8	31	2.4±0.8	0.40	

t_f = the time corresponding to the start of animal deaths;
P_{max} = the maximum tumour weight by time t_f.

these generations do not change substantially (Figure 73e, Table 24). In the 48th generation the control tumour growth rate markedly increases, the life-span diminishes and the response to MNU becomes low (Figure 73f).

The above results refer to monofunctional compounds with only one nitrosamine group >N—NO in its structure. The activity of the bifunctional analogues of N-alkylnitrosourea had to be studied, since the presence of two functional groups was needed in order that the alkylating type drugs (chloroethylamines and ethyleneamines) display antitumour properties (Ross, 1964).

Three drugs of this type described by the general formula

$$H_2N—CO—N—NO$$
$$|$$
$$(CH_2)_n \quad n = 1, 2, 3.$$
$$|$$
$$H_2N—CO—N—NO$$

have been studied (Vasileva et al., 1973).

A comparison of the toxic and therapeutic properties of MNU, ENU and PNU, with the appropriate bifunctional derivatives, is made in Tables 25 and 26.

As seen in Table 25, the toxicity of monofunctional compounds drops with increase in the length of alkyl groups in the order: MNU, ENU, PNU. No such dependence is seen for bifunctional derivatives. There is also no clear-cut dependence of cumulative properties and chemotherapeutic parameters of the above compounds on their structure. It can only be stated that PNU and its bifunctional analogue — BPNU — show the highest cumulative capacity and the narrowest range of therapeutic effect.

TABLE 25   Comparison of toxic and therapeutic characteristics of
N-alkylnitrosoureas and their bifunctional analogues (Vasileva *et al.*, 1973)

Drug	MNU	BMNU	ENU	BENU	PNU	BPNU
LD_{50}, mg/kg	150	535	380	75	1375	190
Cumulation index	100	43	22	25	120	68
Chemotherapeutic index	16	2	10	3	5	2

TABLE 26   Antitumour activity (in % inhibition) of N-alkylnitrosoureas
and their bifunctional analogues (Vasileva *et al.*, 1973)

Drug	EAC	S-180	NKLy	Ca 755	Harding-Passey melanoma	Walker cs	C-45	Erythro-leukaemia
MNU	95	90	90	65	50	95	95	–
BMNU	95	55	45	75	–	95	60	51
ENU	100	95	65	55	–	95	85	–
BENU	50	30	45	65	–	75	30	0
PNU	100	95	70	50	20	60	75	90
BPNU	85	85	50	75	65	98	95	90

The antitumour activity of these compounds compared for several transplanted
tumours (Table 26) gives ground to the conclusion that addition of a second
functional group usually does not result in higher drug effectiveness. Exceptions
are the increased general response of adenocarcinoma 755 (Ca 755) to the bifunctional derivatives, and the greater effect of BPNU on the Harding-Passey melanoma,
Walker carcinosarcoma and sarcoma 45, compared to that of its monofunctional
prototype — MNU.

Moreover, the bifunctional derivatives of N-alkylnitrosoureas display a relatively
high antileukaemic effect (Figure 74).

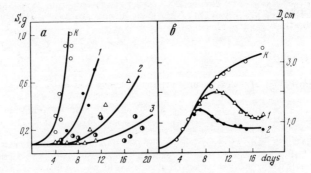

Fig. 74. Bifunctional analogues of N-alkylnitrosourea
(Vasileva *et al.*, 1973). (a) BENU (1), BPNU (2) and BMNU (3)
for transplanted leukaemia La; (b) effect of PNU (1) and
BPNU (2) on s.c. tumour development for Sveč erythroleukaemia.

In experiments with leukaemia La, BMNU was more effective than MNU ($\varkappa^*_{MNU} = 0.52$, $\varkappa^*_{BMNU} = 0.78$). At the same time the activity coefficients of PNU and BPNU were close ($\varkappa^* = 0.78$ and 0.72 respectively) while ENU activity ($\varkappa^* = 0.64$) exceeded that of its bifunctional analogue ($\varkappa^* = 0.45$). The possible reasons for the high anti-leukaemic activity may be the difference between toxic and cumulative properties, which permits injection of BMNU at larger single and summary doses, compared to MNU, as well as the increased lipophil nature related to molecular weight. Antileukaemic activity in the series of monofunctional derivatives increases with molecular weight and lipophil nature.

The activities of PNU and of its bifunctional analogue were different for various times of starting treatment. However, when the drug was injected one day after transplantation of rat erythroleukaemia, both drugs inhibited the process to the same extent (Table 26). With a more advanced process (injections started on the 6th day), BPNU exerted a more distinct antitumour effect than PNU (Figure 74b). The period of continuous growth was virtually absent under BPNU treatment and the tumour size remained smaller than in the case of PNU throughout the follow-up interval. In experiments *in vitro* BPNU selectively suppressed the growth of cultures of human tumour cell strains — the angiosarcoma and HeLa — that have passed through many generations. The first passage of a human embryo tissue was considerably more resistant to this drug (Vasileva *et al.*, 1973).

Thus, virtally all compounds of the nitrosocarbamide class display antitumour activity to some extent. Therefore N-nitrosoureas appear to be a promising group of drugs for which profound studies of the correlation between chemical structure and biological activity are very important. These studies can obviously lead to the creation of new active antitumour agents.

3. ANTIMETABOLITES

Compounds representing structural analogues of cell metabolites and possessing the capacity to block separate links of metabolic processes are included in the anti-metabolites (Vulli, 1954).

Antimetabolites were first used in cancer chemotherapy in the late nineteen-forties, when the effect of these compounds on human leukaemias was discovered. Later this trend was widely developed. At the present time three groups of anti-metabolites are used preferentially in oncological practice: the antagonists of folic acid, purines, and pyrimidines.

Antagonists of Folic Acid

The best known drugs of this group are aminopterin and methotrexate (amethopterin).

Folic acid

COOH
|
NH₂ ... CH₂ —NH—〈 〉—C(O)—NH—CH
|
Aminopterin
|
H₂N   (CH₂)₂
|
COOH

Aminopterin

COOH
|
NH₂ ... CH₂N(CH₃)—〈 〉—C —NH—CH
|
Methotrexate
‖
H₂N   O   (CH₂)₂
|
COOH

Methotrexate

Methotrexate was found to be less toxic than aminopterin and has been more widely
used clinically and experimentally. It was used as the reference drug in primary
studies on new antitumour agents for transplanted leukaemia L-1210. The drug activity
for this strain is usually evaluated by comparing the average life-span of tumour-
bearing animals treated with methotrexate with the life-span of mice treated by the
new drug under assay. This method of comparative evaluation was used, for example,
by Goldin *et al.* (1964) in studying the dose-dependence of the antileukaemic effect
of methotrexate administered daily starting from the third day after tumour transplantation to the time of the animal's death. The dose of 1.56 mg/kg/day appeared
to be optimal, since it doubled the animal's life-span (Figure 75a).

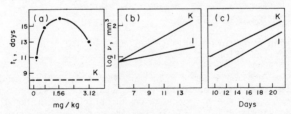

Fig. 75   Effect of methotrexate on the life-span of mice
with leukaemia L-1210 (a) (Goldin *et al.*, 1964) and on the
growth of human thyroid gland cancer cells (b) and melanoma
cells (c), transplanted into cheek pouches of hamsters.

Since the generally accepted method for evaluating the antimetabolite's effectiveness is the study of the antimetabolite's effect upon survival, the appropriate
kinetic curves naturally are not numerous. An example of such data is given in
the results obtained for the methotrexate effect on the kinetics of growth of two
experimental tumours in hamsters: cells of thyroid gland cancer and human
melanoma were implanted in their cheek pouches (Friedell *et al.*, 1961). Injections
of the drug began on the 8th to 9th day for a melanoma and on the 4th to 6th day
after transplantation of thyroid gland cancer and these injections were repeated
every two days. The inhibition of tumour growth was only observed after injections
of methotrexate at doses exceeding 10 mg/kg. Figure 75b,c presents semilogarithmic
anamorphoses of the curves for changes in tumour volumes in controls and under the
action of methotrexate (20 mg/kg/day) taken from the original paper. The tumour
volumes increased exponentially both in controls and in experimental animals. A
distinct inhibition of tumour growth was observed in the thyroid gland cancer under

the action of methotrexate (Figure 75b);   the mean specific growth rate decreased by a factor of 3 compared to controls ($\phi_c = 0.3$, $\phi_e = 0.1$ day^{-1}; $\varkappa^* = 0.65$). The drug action on melanoma caused a delay in the beginning of tumour growth, and as a result of it the experimental kinetic curve shifted relative to the control curve by a value $\Delta t = 4.5$ days. The mean coefficient $\varkappa^*$ was 0.3. Thus, these tumours are characterized by a different response to methotrexate.

Pyrimidine Antagonists (Fluorinated Pyrimidines)

In 1954, Rutman *et al.* reported that induced hepatoma in rats incorporates labelled uracil to a much higher extent than the normal rat liver. Later, similar observations were made for transplanted carcinomas, and then for other transplanted tumours. This peculiarity of tumour biochemistry can be used for the creation of appropriate drugs, blocking synthesis in tumour cells and thus inhibiting tumour growth. It follows from certain facts, such as the increase in biological activity of fluorinated steroids, that the substitution of fluorine for the hydrogen atom in the pyrimidine ring can raise the biological activity of compounds (Peters and Buffa, 1949). 5-Fluorouracil is the most studied and efficient compound of this class (Haggmark, 1962; Reichard *et al.*, 1962; Heidelberger, 1958). The effects of fluorouracil and of 5-fluoro-orotic acid on certain transplanted tumours have been discussed by Heidelberger (1958).

5-fluorouracil (5-FU)   5-fluoro-orotic acid (5-FOA)

The toxicity of these compounds under different administration schedules is compared below (from Heidelberger, 1958):

LD$_{50}$, mg/kg	5-fluorouracil	5-fluoro-orotic acid
Intravenously	250	94
Intraperitoneally	188	188
Subcutaneously	233	190
Orally	189	532

Ten tumour strains were used when Heidelberger studied the antitumour activity of 5-FU and 5-FOA. Figure 76A shows the curves for changes in tumour sizes of mice with solid sarcoma 180 in controls and under the action of 5-FU and 5-FOA injected subcutaneously on the first to eighth day after transplantation at doses of 25 and 12 mg/kg/day, respectively. It follows from the semilogarithmic anamorphoses of the curves that the tumour growth in controls and in experimental animals is close to the exponential for 14 days. The rate constant for the control tumour is $\phi_c = 0.38$ day^{-1} and the doubling time of the volume $T = 1.8$ days. Under the action of 5-FU the rate constant decreases by a factor of 2.5 ($\varkappa^* = 0.6$); 5-FOA is less active ($\phi_e = 0.28$ day^{-1}; $\varkappa^* = 0.3$).

The effect of 5-FU on an established tumour is greater. Injections of the drug following the same regimen, but started on the ninth day after transplantation, virtually completely inhibited the process in 23 days (Figure 76B). Rapid ulcer-

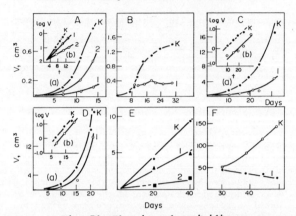

Fig. 76   Fluorinated pyrimidines.
(A) Sarcoma 180, early administration of 5-FU (1), 5-FOA (2);
(B) 5-FU effect on developed sarcoma 180;   (C) 5-FU, early
administration in adenocarcinoma 755;   (D) 5-FU for Flaxner-
Gobling carcinoma (Heidelberger, 1958);   (E) 5-FU for induced
adenocarcinoma in rats (1 — injections on 21st day, 2 — from
1st day) (Gropper and Shimkin, 1967);   (F) rabbit carcinoma
regression after 5-FU perfusion (Knoepp *et al.*, 1964).

ation of tumours and regressions in individual animals were observed later.   It was
found that multiple injections of 5-FU at small doses were more effective than a
single large dose of the drug;   for 5-FOA changes in the treatment regimen affected
its performance only slightly.

Somewhat different results for the 5-FU effect were obtained for the solid
sarcoma 180 (Humphrey, 1963).   Five drug injections at a dose of 20 mg/kg/day
starting from the second day after transplantation resulted in an insignificant
shift (about 2 days) of the initial section of the curve for growth of treated
tumours, compared to controls.   The less potent effect of 5-FU in this case could
be caused by the shorter period of treatment (5 days) and the lower total dose
(100 mg/kg).

Both 5-FU and 5-FOA had an approximately similar effect on adenocarcinoma 755.
Curves for changes in tumour volume in controls and for treatment by 5-FU are
presented in Figure 76C;   similar results were obtained for 5-FOA.   As in the case
considered above (Figure 75b,c) the effect of 5-FU on adenocarcinoma 755 differs
from that observed for sarcoma 180:   tumour growth inhibition is manifest in a
6-day shift of the experimental curve relative to the control curve.   The mean
value of the activity coefficient $\varkappa^*$ is 0.6.   However, it will be noted that
recurrence of the growth of melanoma implanted in hamsters took place against
continuous methotrexate administration (Figure 75c), whereas recurrence of adenocarcinoma 755 was a result of discontinuing the drug administration.   A similar
effect was observed for the action of 5-FU on tumour growth in rats having Flexner-
Gobling carcinoma.   The shift of the experimental curve in this case was 3 days,
while the mean value of the activity coefficient was $\varkappa^* = 0.3$ (Figure 76D).

Comparison of the effects of 5-FU and 5-FOA with the effect of a metabolite of
another group — 6-mercaptopurine — was made for Swiss strain mice bearing
sarcoma A-1 (Heidelberger, 1958).   The tumours were measured only twice: on the
11th and 18th day of the experiment;   therefore it was impossible to plot the

kinetic curves. Evaluation of the criterion for the time interval between the 11th and 18th days shows that the activity of the compounds studied was reduced in the order: 6-mercaptopurine ($\varkappa^* = 0.6$), 5-FU ($\varkappa^* = 0.3$), 5-FOA ($\varkappa^* = 0.1$). However, a study of survival of mice bearing Ehrlich ascitic carcinoma and leukaemia L-1210 showed that the activity of 5-FOA and, especially, of 5-FU exceeded that of 6-mercaptopurine for these strains.

Dependence of the 5-FU effect on the start and times of treatment was studied for rats having mammary gland carcinoma induced by methylchloroanthrene (Gropper and Shimkin, 1967). Treatment was started on the first or 21st day after the tumour attained the size of 6 mm to 10 mm, and was discontinued on the 42nd day: the measurements are given in Figure 76E. The number of points is insufficient for reliable setting up of rules for tumour growth in controls and experimental animals. Nevertheless, it can be seen from the data obtained that the drug was more effective when injected from the first day than on the 21st to 42nd day ($\varkappa^* = 0.5$ and 0.1, respectively).

The method of regional perfusion is one of the routes for increasing the effectiveness of chemotherapeutic drugs. This method was used for treating carcinoma-bearing rabbits with 5-FU (Knoepp *et al.*, 1964). The tumour was transplanted in the muscles of both thighs: one of the tumours was the control. Perfusion of 5-FU at a dose of 7.5 mg/kg for 30 minutes resulted in a decrease in the tumour size ($\varkappa^* = 1.60$) (Figure 76F). The effectiveness of the assayed drugs in treating malignant tumours was high. Methotrexate was very effective for metastasizing chorionepithelioma, and fluoroacetyl was effective for stomach cancer. At present antimetabolites in combination with other drugs are used for leukaemia treatment, and less frequently used for treatment of solid tumours.

4. ANTIBIOTICS

More than 100 antibiotics possessing the ability to supress the growth of experimental tumours have been studied. Many of these are clinically successful on a number of malignant neoplasms.

The antitumour antibiotics differ significantly in their mechanism of action. Some antibiotics disturb RNA and DNA metabolism, suppress protein biosynthesis, inhibit respiration and oxidative phosphorylation. Other antibiotics damage the structure and function of membranes (Lippman *et al.*, 1975). The action of antibiotics effective on experimental tumour processes are considered in this section in terms of kinetics.

Olivomycin

Olivomycin

This agent belongs to the group of antibiotics selectively disturbing RNA synthesis in bacterial and animals cells. Since the antitumour properties of phenolic compounds will be considered later, attention will be paid here to the two hydroxy-aromatic groups present in the olivomycin structure. An important specific feature of this antibiotic is its capacity to form a complex with metals. The biological activity of olivomycin is due to suppression of the DNA-dependent synthesis of RNA as a result of formation of a complex of the antibiotic Mg-chelate with DNA. Olivomycin exerts a marked antitumour effect *in vivo* and *in vitro*. For example, it inhibits the growth of the Harding-Passey melanoma which is characterized by a high resistance to therapy. In these experiments olivomycin was injected six times at a dose of 6 mg/kg at 4-day intervals starting from the 9th, 14th or 20th day after tumour transplantation. The curves for melanoma growth under the action of olivomycin injected starting from the 20th day after transplantation are presented in Figure 77a. A marked inhibition of tumour growth attaining 40% ($\varkappa^* = 0.4$) is even seen for a later start of treatment. For early administration of the drug, the inhibition of melanoma growth was 80%.

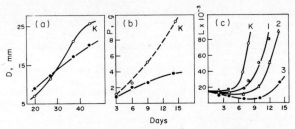

Fig. 77 Kinetic characteristics of antibiotics action.
(a) Olivomycin effect on Harding-Passey melanoma growth;
(b) inhibition of HEp-3 tumour in mice by actinomycin D
(Merker and Hurley, 1962);   (C) leucocytes in transplanted
leukaemia La in controls (K) and under the action of mitomycin C with 0.5 (1), 1.0 (2) and 1.5 (3) mg/kg/day.

DON and Azaserine

$$N_2CH—\overset{\overset{\textstyle O}{\|}}{C}—CH_2—CH_2—CH—COOH \qquad \text{6-Diazo-5-oxo-I-norleucine (DON)}$$
$$\underset{\textstyle NH_2}{|}$$

$$N_2CH—\overset{\overset{\textstyle O}{\|}}{C}—O—CH_2—CH—COOH \qquad \text{Diazoacetyl-P-serine (Azaserine)}$$
$$\underset{\textstyle NH_2}{|}$$

The antibiotics DON and azaserine represent derivatives of amino acids and inhibit purine exchange in the cell. The structures of both compounds are close to that of glutamine and are capable of competing with the latter in various metabolic processes. It was found, in particular, that these antibiotics are capable of irreversible bonding with sulph-hydryl groups of the enzyme catalyzing the conversion of formylglycin-amide-ribonucleotide to formylglycinamidine-ribonucleotide.

The antitumour effects of azaserine and DON have been studied in detail (Clarke *et al.*, 1957; Sugiura, 1962; Tarnowski and Stock, 1957). The activity of DON with respect to experimental tumours and cellular cultures was higher than that of azaserine, but no marked therapeutic difference was observed clinically.

The effects of DON and of certain other antibiotics were studied in terms of kinetics for leukaemia La. Their antitumour activity was compared with that of sarcolysine. The specific results of the antileukaemic action of antibiotics are given in Table 27. The activity coefficients $\varkappa^*_L$ were calculated making use of the plot for changes in the blood leucocyte counts with time; the $\varkappa^*$ values were calculated with respect to the animal life-span in controls and in experimental animals.

As can be seen from Table 27, the antileukaemic activity coefficients $\varkappa^*$ and $\varkappa^*_L$ for each drug were in good agreement.

TABLE 27   Comparative characteristics of the action of antibiotics on leukaemia

Drug	Dose mg/kg/day	Number of mice	Life-span, days	$\varkappa^*$	$\varkappa^*_L$
Controls	–	141	8.0±0.14	–	–
Sarcolysins	1.5	83	15.6±1.6	0.49	0.47
Mitomycin C	1.0	30	15.5±1.80	0.48	0.42
DON	0.1	20	11.1±1.38	0.28	0.31
Actinomycin C	0.2	16	10.9±0.84	0.27	0.23
Levomycetin	1000.0	15	10.5±0.80	0.24	0.23

Actinomycins

A peculiar feature of this group of antitumour antibiotics is the presence of poly-peptide fragments in their structure:

Actinomycin D

The biological action of actinomycins is accounted for by their selective complexing with DNA (Dingman and Sporn, 1965; Reich, 1963). These antibiotics react solely with polydeoxynucleotide molecules involving guanine. They inhibit the proliferation of DNA-containing viruses and have no effect on RNA-containing viruses (Reich, 1963). Clinically actinomycins are applied together with X-ray irradiation for treating Wilms tumour with metastases.

Actinomycins exhibit a wide range of antitumour action experimentally. Small doses of these antibiotics inhibit the growth of adenocarcinoma 755, melanoma S-91, glio-blastoma and other tumours.

The data on the effect of actinomycins on the kinetics of experimental tumour growth are sparse. The effects of certain antibiotics on leukaemia La are given in Table 27.

The effect of actinomycin D on human epidermal carcinoma transplanted to Swiss mice was observed (Figure 77b). Daily injections of the drug on the first to eighth day inhibited tumour growth; the activity coefficient was $\varkappa^* = 0.24$.

Judging by the data reported, antibiotics of the actinomycin series have a low antitumour effect in experimental tumour models.

Mitomycin C

This drug is one of the best investigated antitumour antibiotics. The chemical properties and the wide spectrum of mitomycin C's biological action are due to the presence of several (ethyleneimine, urethane and quinoid) functional groups in its structure, which makes possible selective suppression of DNA biosynthesis (Sekiguchi and Takagi, 1959, 1960; Kersten, 1962).

Mitomycin C is used clinically for the treatment of stomach cancer, pulmonary cancer and osteosarcoma (Larionov, 1962). Experimentally the drug completely inhibits the growth of Ehrlich ascites, sarcoma 180, Walker carcinosarcoma, mammary gland adenocarcinoma, etc. (Sugiura, 1959). The curves for the increase in the total leucocyte count in the peripheral blood of mice with transplanted leukaemia in the control group and under the action of various doses of mitomycin C are presented in Figure 77C. When the dose of the drug is increased from 0.5 mg/kg to 1.5 mg/kg the activity coefficient $\varkappa^*_L$ increases linearly from 0.31 to 0.55. However, the highest dose generates toxicity accompanied by a decrease in the median life-span of the experimental animals.

Administration of mitomycin C at a dose of 7 mg/kg to rats with a transplanted sarcoma 45 sub-strain on the 5th to 8th day after transplantation resulted in moderate inhibition of the tumour growth (Figure 67b, curve 2); the activity coefficient was $\varkappa^* = 0.23$ (Kiseleva et al., 1970).

Adriamycin and Daunomycin

These antibiotics of the anthracyclin series, resembling in structure and containing quinoid and hydroxyaromatic groups, are highly active antitumour drugs.

The antitumour activity of adriamycin is greater than that of daunomycin (see Carter et al., 1972). Clinically adriamycin produces longer remission of lymphoid and myeloid leukaemias, and reticulocellular sarcoma. Experimentally the treatment of Ehrlich ascites carcinoma with adriamycin results in longer survival; for sarcoma 180 it gives 80% inhibition, while daunomycin gives only 50%.

Though adriamycin displays greater antitumour activity, its suppressive effect is

Adriamycin   Daunomycin

weaker than that of daunomycin. This is seen from the effect of this antibiotic on
mice sarcoma induced by the Moloni virus (see Carter *et al.*, 1972). As a rule, the
control tumour suffers spontaneous regression 48-50 days after initiation. The
administration of antibiotics 3 to 10 days after the tumour has become measurably
large prevents regression. Moreover, under the action of daunomycin the recurrence
of the tumour starts much earlier (Figure 78a). In experiments with preliminary
administration of the drug (before tumour induction) the immunosuppressive effects
of the drug were highly variable: adriamycin somewhat retarded the commencement of
regression, while daunomycin completely prevented it (Figure 78b).

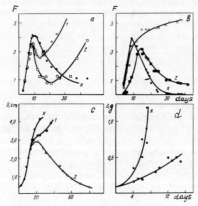

Fig. 78   Antitumour and immunosuppressive effects of adriamycin
and daunomycin.
(a) Action of daunomycin (1) and adriamycin (2) on development
of sarcoma MSV induced in mice;   (b) the same with preliminary
administration of the drugs before induction (Carter *et al.*,
1972);   (c) alternative effects of adriamycin on Guérin carcinoma
growth;   (d) adriamycin on leukaemia La (Konovalova, 1975).

Konovalova and Vasilieva have recently conducted kinetic studies of adriamycin
antitumour activity against the Guérin carcinoma. The drug was administered at a
dose of 1 mg/kg/day on the first to 16th day after subcutaneous transplantation of
the tumour. Complete regression was observed in 50% of the animals which remained
healthy 4 months later ($\varkappa^* = 1.11$), while only partial inhibition of tumour growth
was observed for the others ($\varkappa^* = 0.43$) (Figure 78c). The latter effect might have

been due to the immunosuppressive properties of the drug. Adriamycin was also
found to display a high antileukaemic activity in a model transplanted leukaemia La
in mice ($\varkappa^* = 0.71$) (Figure 78d), whereas tumours such as the Walker carcinosarcoma,
Harding-Passey melanoma and Sveč erythromyelosis showed no response to it.

Macromycin B

This new antibiotic of a polypeptide nature was isolated from *Streptomyces macro-*
myceticus. The mechanism of its antitumour action is connected with the absorption
of the drug by membranes and cell damage in the G_2 phase. As a rule the antibiotic is most effective in contact with tumour cells (Lippman *et al.*, 1975). A
moderate activity of the drug for leukaemias L-1210 and P388 ($\varkappa^* = 0.3 - 0.4$) was
observed after 3-9 intraperitoneal injections at doses of 4-8 mg/kg/day starting
on the first day after transplantation.

In experiments with melanoma B-16 transplanted intraperitoneally, administration of
macromycin B by 20 mg/kg led to complete regression of the tumour process in 10% of
the animals, and in other cases the inhibition of tumour growth was insiginficant
($\varkappa^* = 0.1$).

With increase in the macromycin B dose to 30 mg/kg the activity coefficient $\varkappa^*$
increased to 0.5, complete tumour regression was observed in 40% of animals. At
the same time intraperitoneal administration of the drug to mice with developed
subcutaneous Lewis carcinoma had no effect on the kinetics of tumour growth and the
survival of animals. Subcutaneous injection of the drug at the site of tumour
transplantation induced complete growth inhibition in 10 days after the start of
the treatment ($\varkappa^* = 1$). Later on growth was restored, and averaging over the whole
period of observation yielded an activity coefficient $\varkappa^* = 0.7$.

5.   PHENOLIC COMPOUNDS

The changes in the free radical content specific for certain phases of tumour growth
stimulated many studies of antitumour properties of inhibitors of free radical
processes, in particular of the low-toxicity phenolic compounds.

These studies were first carried out in 1958 using ionol (2,6-di-tert.butyl-4-
methylphenol), butyloxyanisol (mixture of two isomers of 2- and 3-tert.butyl-4-
hydroxyanisol) and propylgallate (n-propyl ester of gallic acid).

Ionol   Butyloxyanisol   Propylgallate

These drugs in therapeutic doses inhibited the increase in leucocyte and leukaemic
cells in the peripheral blood of mice with transplanted acute leukaemia LIV (Figure
79). The life-span of treated mice increased by a factor of $1.2 - 2.0$.

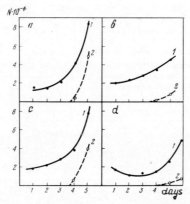

Fig. 79 Changes in leucocyte (1) and leukaemic cell count
(2) for leukaemia LIV in afb mice in controls (a,b) and for
three-dose injections of propylgallate (c,d).

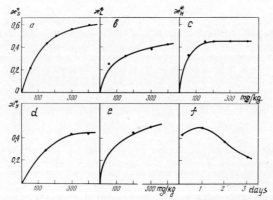

Fig. 80 Dose-effect relationship for ionol administered
intraperitoneally (a,b,c) and orally (d — in Tween 80
solution, e — in linetol solution) to mice with leukaemia La;
(f) relation between ionol efficiency and the time of
starting treatment.

The antileukaemic action of ionol has been studied in detail for transplanted leukaemia La. Intraperitoneal and oral administration of ionol at doses of 50 mg/kg
to 400 mg/kg inhibited the increase in spleen weight, leucocyte count and leukaemic
cells in blood (Figure 80a-e).

With an increase in the dose of ionol up to 300 mg/kg the antileukaemic action
attained a certain limiting value. The drug was administered at 3 day intervals
starting 3 hours after transplantation. The drug was less active when administered
orally than by intraperitoneal injections (cf. Figure 80a,d,e). A stronger effect
was observed for Tween-80 solution (10%) than for the linetol solution (cf. Figure
80d,e). The effectiveness of ionol was markedly lower when treatment was started
on the third day (Figure 80f).

The values obtained for the antileukaemic activity of ionol ($\varkappa^* = 0.6$) characterize it as an active antitumour agent. Even in maximum doses ionol does not induce the leucopenia observed in using many cytotoxic compounds.

The high activity of ionol stimulated further studies of the antitumour properties of other low toxicity phenolic compounds. Two water-soluble analogues of ionol: 4-hydroxy-3,5,-di-tert.butyl-benzylamine hydrobromide (IRP-1) and 4-hydroxy-3,5-di-tert.butyl-N,N-(β-hydroxyethyl)benzylamine hydrochloride (ambunol) have been studied

OH

$(CH_3)_3C$⸺⸺$C(CH_3)_3$

CH_2NH_2 • HBr

IRP-1

OH

$(CH_3)_3C$⸺⸺$C(CH_3)_3$

$H_2C-N\begin{smallmatrix} CH_2CH_2Cl \\ \\ CH_2CH_2Cl \end{smallmatrix}$

• HCl

Ambunol

Both agents displayed antileukaemic activity for leukaemia La (Emanuel *et al.*, 1962)

	IRP-1 (50 mg/kg per day)	Ambunol (30 mg/kg per day)
$\varkappa^*_S$	0.33	0.39
$\varkappa^*_L$	0.19	0.24
$\varkappa^*_H$	0.23	0.12
$\varkappa^*_M$	0.34	0.40

Further studies of water-soluble ionol analogues such as amine hydrochloride and sodium salts of carbonic acids, did not yield other drugs exceeding ionol in activity (Table 28) (Dronova, 1968).

The 2,6-dialkyl-4-bis(β-hydroxyethyl)-aminophenol hydrochloride, differing in the extent of spatial screening of hydroxyl groups, was studied in order to evaluate the relation between the antitumour activity and the structure of phenolic compounds (Konovalova *et al.*, 1966; Bogdanov *et al.*, 1968). Table 29 lists the activity coefficients characterizing the effects of five compounds of this series administered at close-to-equimolar doses on various characteristics of transplanted leukaemia La.

The data in Table 29 show that 2,6-di-tert.butyl-substituted phenol possesses the highest activity. A number of 2,6-di-tert.butyl-4-substituted phenols (Table 30) were assayed in this connection.

Besides ionol which was studied earlier ($R = -CH_3$), a high antitumour action is possessed by phenols with aromatic substituents which inhibit the development of leukaemia at relatively low doses. The effectiveness of hydroxydiphenyl derivatives is higher than that of phenol derivatives: this is seen from a comparison of the drugs in pairs of 1 and 6, 2 and 7, 3 and 8, in Table 30.

The effects of ionol and of a number of its water-soluble analogues on the haematological parameters and life-span of AKR mice bearing various forms of spontaneous leukaemias have also been studied.

TABLE 28   Toxicity and therapeutic characteristics of water-soluble ionol analogues

$$HO-\underset{C(CH_3)_3}{\overset{C(CH_3)_3}{\bigcirc}}-R$$

(Dronova, 1968)

R	LD$_{50}$ mg/kg	MTD mg/kg	TD mg/kg	u^*_S	u^*_L	u^*_H
−CH$_2$NH$_2$·HCl	90	75	50	0.33	0.17	0.33
−CH$_2$CH$_2$CH$_2$NH$_2$·HCl	75	40	30	0.09	0.00	0.00
−CHNH$_2$·HCl | CH$_3$	100	80	30	0.23	0.17	0.09
			60	0.50	0.29	0.29
−CHNH$_2$·HCl | C$_2$H$_5$	110	75	30	0.17	0.17	0.09
			60	0.33	0.17	0.23
−CH$_2$COONa	500	400	300	0.29	0.17	0.23
−CH$_2$CH$_2$COONa	320	275	150	0.17	0.09	0.09
			250	0.38	0.17	0.17

TABLE 29   Activity of phenolic compounds as a function of the extent of spatial screening of the hydroxyl group
(Konovalova *et al.*, 1966;   Bogdanov *et al.*, 1968)

$$HO-\underset{R_2}{\overset{R_1}{\bigcirc}}-CH_2-N\underset{HCl}{\overset{CH_2CH_2Cl}{\underset{CH_2CH_2OH}{}}}$$

R$_1$	R$_2$	Dose mg/kg	mmol/kg	u^*_S	u^*_L	u^*_H
−⬡	−⬡	20	0.05	0.09	0.09	0.17
−CH$_3$	−C(CH$_3$)$_3$	25	0.06	0.23	0.17	0.23
−⬡	−C(CH$_3$)$_3$	40	0.10	0.17	0.23	0.09
−C(CH$_3$)$_3$	−C(CH$_3$)$_3$	25	0.07	0.38	0.23	0.33
−C(CH$_3$)$_3$	−C(CH$_3$)$_2$C$_2$H$_5$	20	0.05	0.33	0.17	0.23

The frequency of leukaemia in AKR mice is about 70%. The first symptoms of leukaemia were observed at the age of 8-9 months, and development took 1.5 - 2.0 months. Haematological parameters of the leukaemic process were often equivocal: for example, the relative content of blast cells at a leucocyte level of 67 and 60 thousand/mm^3 was 92 and 2.5%, respectively; conversely, at almost equal high contents of blast forms (91 and 94%) the leucocyte counts differed markedly (12 and 48 thousand/mm^3).

For most mice with haemocytoblast and lymphoid forms of leukaemia the administration

TABLE 30   Effect of substituted 2,5-di-tert. butyl phenols $HO-\underset{C(CH_3)_3}{\overset{C(CH_3)_3}{\diagdown}}\!\!\!\diagup\!\!\!\diagdown\!\!\!\diagup-R$

on development of transplanted leukaemia La   (Bogdanov et al., 1968)

Number	R	Dose mg/kg	Dose mmol/kg	$\varkappa^*_S$	$\varkappa^*_L$	$\varkappa^*_H$
1	-H	100	0.48	0.17	0.09	0.17
2	-CH₃	100	0.45	0.33	0.29	0.38
		130	0.59	0.41	0.29	0.41
		400	1.82	0.58	0.41	0.45
3	-OCH₃	100	0.42	0.17	0.17	0.23
4	-CH₂OCH₃	110	0.44	0.45	0.17	0.29
5	-CH₂-⟨ ⟩	130	0.44	0.33	0.23	0.29
6	-⟨ ⟩	125	0.44	0.53	0.23	0.33
		230	0.78	0.45	0.23	0.41
7	-⟨ ⟩-CH₃	130	0.44	0.23	0.17	0.29
		175	0.56	0.50	0.23	0.41
8	-⟨ ⟩-OCH₃	135	0.43	0.47	0.17	0.33
		175	0.56	0.47	0.23	0.33
9	(naphthyl)	150	0.47	0.29	0.29	0.38
		180	0.56	0.47	0.29	0.38

of antioxidants resulted in complete haematological remission: the leucocyte count
and the number of blast cells decreased almost exponentially to the normal level.
Examples of normalization of haematological parameters under the action of ionol
($\varkappa^*_L = 4.0$) and of ambunol ($\varkappa^*_L = 8.0$) are given in Figure 81.   A reduction of lymph
nodes and a decrease in the amount of pathological forms in myelograms were
observed simultaneously.

The myeloid forms of spontaneous leukaemias were less responsive to the inhibitors:
only a temporary decrease in the leucocyte count and blast cell number was observed
followed by an increase on continuing administration of the drug.   The average life-
span of mice treated with ionol increased from 10.8 ± 0.13 months in the control
group to 11.5 ± 0.16 in the experimental animals.   This the prolongation of life-
span was about 20 days.   This means that the life-span of experimental animals
treated with phenolic inhibitors are 30-50% longer ($\varkappa^*_t = 0.23 - 0.33$) relative to
the average duration of the leukaemic process in untreated control animals (1.5 -
2.0 months).

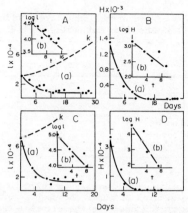

Fig. 81   Normalization of haematological parameters for
haemocytoblast and lymphatic forms of spontaneous leukaemias
in AKR mice treated with ionol (A,B) and ambunol (C,D)

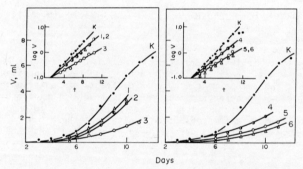

Fig. 82   Effect of oxychalcone on kinetics of changes in the
ascitic fluid volume in Ehrlich ascites carcinoma:
(1) m-oxychalcone;   (2) n-oxychalcone;   (3) o-oxychalcone;
(4) 4',2,4,6-tetra-oxychalcone;   (5) 2',4'2-trioxychalcone;
(6) 2',4',4-trioxychalcone.

The antitumour action of some natural phenols was studied for Ehrlich ascites
carcinoma.   The oxychalcones were found to inhibit the increase in tumour cell
number and ascitic fluid volume (Figure 82).

The greatest effect was shown by chalcones with a hydroxyl group in the o-position
(Table 31);   moreover, the oxychalcone activity increased with the number of oxy-
groups.   It will be noted here that gossipol belonging to the class of natural
polyphenols also exerts an antitumour effect.

TABLE 31   Effectiveness of hydroxychalcones for Ehrlich ascites carcinoma
as a function of location and number of hydroxyl groups

Compound	Dose mg/kg	$\varkappa^*_V$	$\varkappa^*_N$
o-Hydroxychalcone	50	0.33	0.23
m-Hydroxychalcone	80	0.09	0.17
p-Hydroxychalcone	50	0.17	0.09
2',4',2-Trihydroxychalcone	80	0.29	0.23
2',4',4-Trihydroxychalcone	80	0.33	0.33
4',2,4,6-Tetrahydroxychalcone	100	0.17	0.38

Thus, many synthetic and natural low toxicity phenolic compounds display antitumour
activity. After extensive studies of their therapeutic properties a new effective
drug — dibunol (ionol) was recommended for the clinical treatment of malignant
tumours of the urinary bladder (Erukhimov, 1966), as well as of trophic (Disvetova
et al., 1968a) and radiation skin damages (Disvetova *et al*., 1968b).

6.   DRUGS DISPLAYING VARIOUS MECHANISMS OF ACTION

Stable Free Radicals

It has been found that stable free radicals formed in the oxidation of phenol
antioxidants possess antimitotic activity and are capable of inactivating enzymes
(Garsou, 1956). At the same time the cytotoxic effects of radiation and radiomimetic agents is known to be due to free radicals inactivating the biosynthesis of
enzymes and degrading biologically important macromolecules (Pietro and Giacomelli,
1954). For this reason certain stable free radicals of the 4-substituted 2,2,6,6-
tetramethylpiperidine oxide series were assayed as potential antitumour drugs
(Neiman *et al*., 1962;   Konovalova *et al*., 1964).

Table 32 shows the data on the effect on these compounds on various parameters of
the leukaemia La process. All compounds are of relatively low toxicity. The dose
dependence of the antitumour effect of the nitroxyl radical I shows that this
effect is restricted to a rather narrow range: the drug is inactive below
200 mg/kg/day, and above 400 mg/kg/day its activity does not increase. A similar
tendency is observed for other drugs of this series.

Comparison of the toxicity and antitumour effectiveness for compounds III and IV
shows that a combination of nitroxyl and urethane groups enhances the therapeutic
effect. It is important also that stable radicals are more effective in inhibiting
the increase in haemocytoblast count in the peripheral blood and in bone marrow.
This fact can be of significance for chemotherapy of leukaemias.

TABLE 32 Antileukaemic activity of 4-substituted 2,2,6,6-tetramethylpiperidine oxides (Konovalova *et al.*, 1964)

Drug	LD_{50} mg/kg	TD mg/kg	$\varkappa^*_S$	$\varkappa^*_L$	$\varkappa^*_H$	$\varkappa^*_M$
I	800	110	0.00	0.00	0.00	0.00
		200	0.09	0.09	0.17	0.23
		250	0.09	0.17	0.17	0.17
		300	0.17	0.23	0.23	0.27
		400	0.23	0.23	0.38	0.27
		500	0.23	0.23	0.38	0.27
II	400	75	0.00	0.00	0.00	0.00
		150	0.09	0.09	0.09	0.09
		200	0.17	0.17	0.23	0.09
III	215	125	0.23	0.09	0.27	0.23
IV	260	100	0.17	0.09	0.17	0.09

The possibilities that would be opened up by further studies of the antitumour properties of stable nitroxyl radicals, in particular of paramagnetic analogues of known antitumour drugs, will be emphasized.

Polymers with conjugate bonds

Investigation of the antitumour activity of phenol antioxidants and of a number of stable free radicals stimulated the study of some polymers with conjugate bonds (PCBs).

PCBs are known to involve paramagnetic centres exhibiting an ESR signal — a narrow band at g = 2.00 and an intensity $10^{15} - 10^{19}$ spin/g. The activating action of paramagnetic centres conditions the PCB capacity to inhibit some free radical processes.

The antileukaemic effects of the polymer produced by the combination of benzidine-3,3-dicarboxylic acid with symmetric xylenol (I), polysulphophenylene quinone (II), and polysulphophenylene semiquinone (III) have been studied.

Polymers I and II exhibited an EPR signal specific for PCB and corresponding to approximately 10^{17} spin/g. The concentration of unpaired electrons in polymer III attained about 10^{19} spin/g.

Table 33 demonstrates the PCB effects on various parameters of leukaemia La development.

As seen from Table 33 the effectiveness of the PCBs studied is close to the activity of stable free radicals (Table 32). However, PCBs inhibit spleen growth, while stable radicals retard the increase in haemocytoblast count in blood and bone marrow.

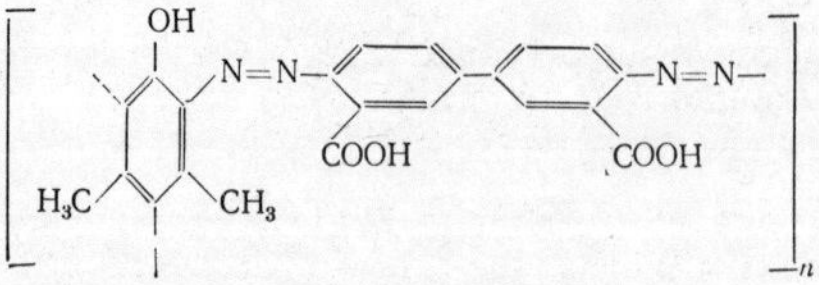

I

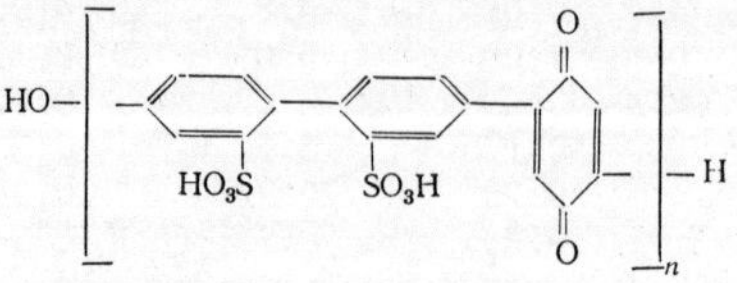

II

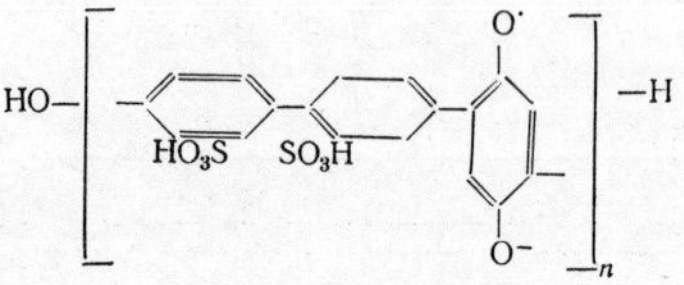

III

TABLE 33   Antileukaemic activity of PCB   (Berlin *et al.*, 1971)

Drug	Dose mg/kg	$и^*_S$	$и^*_L$	$и^*_H$
I	75	0.33	0.09	0.17
II	40	0.28	0.00	0.17
	75	0.33	0.09	0.23
III	75	0.37	0.09	0.23

Drugs of the Phenoxazine Dye Series

The antitumour activity of four compounds of this series were studied (D'iachkov-skaia *et al.*, 1969).

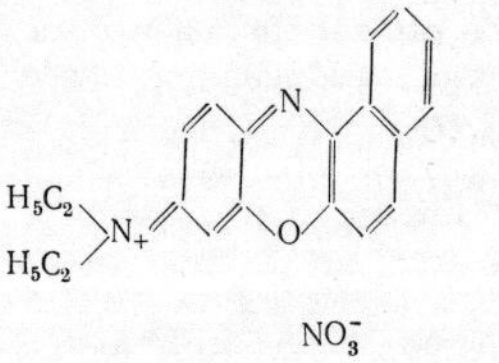

I

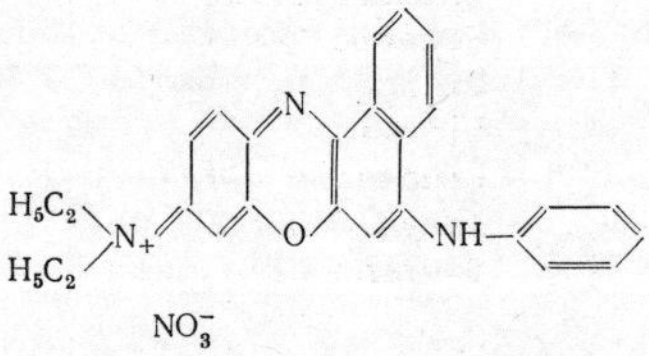

II

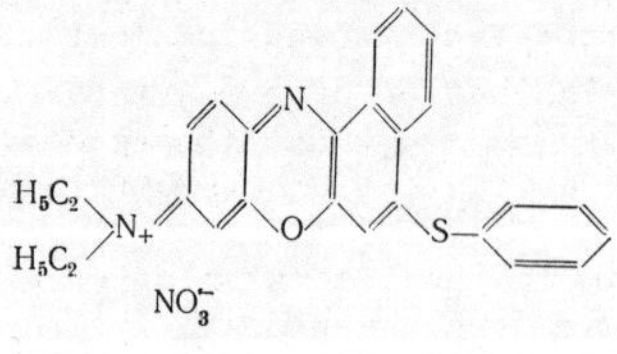

III

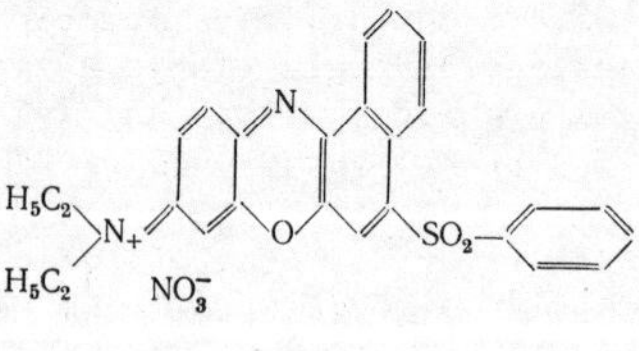

IV

Drugs I, III and IV were administered in aqueous solution, drug II in a 10% Tween-80 solution; subcutaneous injections were used for ascites tumours, and intraperitoneal injections for leukaemia La and sarcoma 45.

These drugs showed no significant activity against Ehrlich ascites carcinoma; the activity parameters for other tumour strains are listed in Table 34.

TABLE 34   The antitumour activity of compounds of the phenoxazine dye series
(D'iachkovskaia *et al.*, 1969)

Drug	LD_{50} mg/kg	Leukaemia La			Sarcoma 180	Sarcoma 45
		$\varkappa^*_S$	$\varkappa^*_H$	$\varkappa^*_L$	Inhibition, %	
I	40	0.45	1.00	0.23	75	55
II	400	0.37	0.17	0.23	62	23
III	50	0.29	1.00	0.23	90	31
IV	500	0.09	0.09	0.17	70	32

Polyunsaturated Fatty Acids

The biological activity of higher polyunsaturated fatty acids (UFA) manifests in their immunostimulating and anticarcinogenic action (Nakahara, 1925). This was observed, in particular, for linolenic acid and its ethyl ester which displayed antitumour activity *in vitro* (Tolnai and Morgan, 1962). Fractions of UFA from the livers of irradiated rabbits had an antitumour effect on certain transplanted tumours such as the Brown-Pearce tumour, Yoshida sarcoma, Ehrlich ascites carcinoma and on some lymphosarcomas in mice (Dennosuke *et al.*, 1961; Vatanebe, 1967). Skin cancer in man has also been treated with UFA. It induced necrosis of tumour tissue without damaging the surrounding sound tissues (Dennosuke *et al.*, 1961).

Kinetic studies of the effects of fatty acid drugs LK and AK on ascites sarcoma 37 and lymphoid leukaemia NKLy have been carried out. These drugs represented a mixture of higher fatty acids of the following compositions (in weight %):

Acid	LK	AK
Palmitic	2.9	5.4
Palmiticoleic	0.2	–
Stearic	1.0	–
Oleic	5.3	25.8
Linolic	14.0	25.7
Linolenic	76.7	2.1
Arachidonic	–	41.0
Content of double bonds, %	89	61

The drugs were administered intraperitoneally for 5 days as a fine disperse emulsion in Tween-80. Doses of 25 mg/kg/day and lower were ineffective. The administration of 100 mg/kg/day completely inhibited tumour growth. Intermediate doses exerted a selective effect: complete inhibition of tumour growth for some animals, and a rather low effect on others ($\varkappa^*_{N,V}$ = 0.0 - 0.2, Figure 83). The AK drug was less active, probably due to the lower content of unsaturated bonds.

Effective doses (100-200 mg/kg) increased the median life-span of sarcoma 37-bearing animals from 27 days in controls to 45 days experimentally. By the end of this time the ascitic fluid disappeared, but a solid tumour started developing at the site of transplantation, causing the death of the animal. The AK and LK drugs

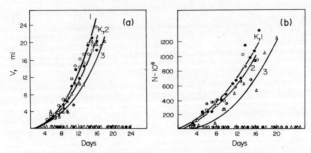

Fig. 83 Changes in ascitic fluid volume (a) and tumour cell
number (b) in sarcoma 37 bearing mice under five-dose administration of the drugs: Arachidonic acid at a dose of 50 mg/kg
(1) and 75 mg/kg (2) and linolenic acid at a dose of 50 mg/kg (3).

administered orally were practically non-toxic but they had no effect on tumour
development.

Diazane (1,2 bis-diazoacetylethane)

The presence of diazoacetyl groups in the structures of certain effective antitumour antibiotics such as azaserine, DON, etc., invited research on the biological
activity of aliphatic diazocompounds, in particular on mono- and bi-functional
diazoketones (Gumanov et al., 1966). Much work was carried out at the Institute
of Chemical Physics, Academy of Science, USSR (Plugina et al., 1971; Emanuel et
al., 1968; D'iachkovskaia, 1973; Goncharova et al., 1976; Konovalova et al.,
1968). The 1,2-bis-diazoacetylethane (diazane) was proposed and studied in
detail.

$$N_2CH-C-CH_2-CH_2-C-CHN_2$$
$$\quad\ \ \| \qquad\qquad \|$$
$$\quad\ \ O \qquad\qquad O$$

A specific feature of the drug is the well-defined dependence of its toxic properties on the treatment regimen: the lethal and maximum tolerated doses administered
daily are half those administered at intervals of three days, and one-third those
for a single administration (Table 35).

TABLE 35 Toxicity characteristics of diazane under various regimes of
administration to non-inbred animals (D'iachkovskaia, 1973)

Toxicity index	Mice			Rats		
	single	daily	at intervals of 3 days	single	daily	at intervals of 3 days
LD_{50}, mg/kg	760	1.3	90	150	3.0	12
MTD, mg/kg	625	0.5	75	100	1.6	5
CI		9720	124		816	190

An unusually high rate of accumulation under daily administration and a considerable decrease with an increasing interval between administrations are characteristics of treatment with diazane. The high cumulative properties of diazane might be due to formation of an active metabolite in the living body. In experiments the drug was administered at intervals of 3 days and more in order to decrease the cumulative toxic effect.

The antitumour effect of diazane was first observed for transplanted leukaemias. A single intraperitoneal injection at a dose of 150 mg/kg considerably inhibited spleen growth in mice with transplanted leukaemia La (Figure 84a).

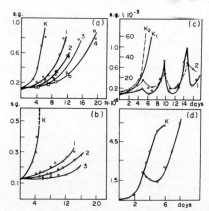

Fig. 84   Effect of diazane on the kinetics of development of
              transplanted leukaemias.
a: (1) 150, (2) 2×150, (3) 3×150, (4) 4×150 mg/kg intra-
    peritoneal injections for leukaemia La;
b: (1) intraperitoneal, (2) subcutaneous, (3) periodic oral
    administration at a dose of 20 mg/kg for leukaemia La
    (Emanuel *et al*., 1968);
c: (1) spleen weight, (2) blood leucocyte count after
    injection of a dose of 150 mg/kg at intervals of 5 days
    (D'iachkovskaia, 1973);
d: single intraperitoneal injection at a dose of 70 mg/kg
    three days after leukaemia L-1210 transplantation
    (Goncharova *et al*., 1976).

The effectiveness of treatment increases linearly with the number of injections, from $\varkappa^* = 0.45$ for a single injection to $\varkappa^* = 0.68$ for four injections of the same dose at intervals of three days. The antileukaemic activity of diazane remains high also with another administration regimen (at a dose of 20 mg/kg/day). The value $\varkappa^*_s$ is 0.83 for intraperitoneal injections, 0.72 for doses taken orally, and 0.78 for subcutaneous administrations (Figure 84b). It must be emphasized that the leucocyte count remains normal up to the 17-18th day, and single haemocyto-blasts appear in blood even later.

It was found in further studies on the kinetics of changes in haematological parameters that when the drug was given infrequently each new dose retarded the process development for 4-5 days (Figure 84c). The kinetic curves for changes in the spleen weight and the leucocyte count are seen to consist of regularly altern-ating sections of rise and fall dependent on the time of drug administration. Comparison of the numerical values of specific rates in different sections of the kinetic curve for spleen weight changes shows a regular increase in the rise and fall rates with every consecutive administration of diazane. The specific rates of change in spleen weight for different sections of the kinetic curve after unjecting diazane at a dose of 150 mg/kg at intervals of 5 days to mice with leukaemia La were studied by D'iachkovskaia (1973) and are given below:

Curve section	1st rise	2nd rise	3rd rise	1st fall	2nd fall	3rd fall
ϕ, day^{-1}	0.35	0.86	1.47	-0.98	-1.73	-2.06

Considerably inhibition of the increase in the total number of tumour cells in ascitic fluid was observed also after a single treatment of developed leukaemia La with diazane (at a mean и* value 0.4) (Figure 84d) (Goncharova *et al.*, 1976). In all cases the antileukaemic action of diazane was accompanied by a considerable increase in the life-span of tumour-bearing animals (Table 36).

TABLE 36   Effect of diazane on the mean life-span of mice with leukaemias (Konovalova *et al.*, 1968)

Leukaemia strain	Summary dose mg/kg	Start of administration, hour	Average life-span	
			days	% to control
Leukaemia La	100	48	14.0±2.4	215
	140	24	14.3±1.2	220
	220	3	22.4±2.0	345
Leukaemia L-1210	140	24	13.2±0.9	203

Note: The drug was injected intraperitoneally at a dose of 20 mg/kg at intervals of 3 days; the mean life-span in controls was 6.5±0.2 days in both cases.

TABLE 37   Antitumour activity (in inhibition %) of diazane for various transplanted tumour models (Frankfurt, 1975)

Tumour	Summary dose, mg/kg		Administration route	Inhibition, %	
	Early injections	Late injections		Early injections	Late injections
Solid					
Sarcoma 45	16	35		91	86
Guérin carcinoma	20	40		71	72
Walker carcinosarcoma	60	40		92	89
Pliss lymphosarcoma	–	15	i.p.	–	93
Erythroleukaemia	–	40		–	93
Hepatoma 22a	85	100		90	70
Carcinoma 755	100	75		70	29
Harding-Passey melanoma	–	120		–	52
Ascites					
Lymphatic leukaemia NKLy	100	–		97	
Sarcoma 180	120	–	s.c.	100	
Ehrlich carcinoma	150	–		100	

Diazane possesses a wide spectrum of antitumour activity. Table 37 shows that the drug markedly inhibits the growth of most tumours both as early injections and as treatment of a developed tumour. Exceptions are the adenocarcinoma 755 and Harding-Passey melanoma, against which the drug has moderate activity.

It was found in pharmacological and histological studies that diazane at therapeutic doses caused no persistent organic and functional changes in the body.

The Pharmacological Committee of the USSR Ministry of Health gave permission to carry out the second phase of clinical assays of this drug.

7. COMPARISON OF THE EFFEFECTIVENESS OF VARIOUS ANTITUMOUR DRUGS

The choice of systems for screening and standardization of tumour models which would make possible a comparison of the results obtained in many laboratories has long been discussed in experimental oncology. This problem can be solved only by using unique quantitative criteria for evaluation of the treatment effectiveness. The kinetic approach to results of chemotherapeutic experiments permits comparison from the same standpoint the effectiveness of various antitumour drugs for different experimental tumours, using the activity coefficient $\varkappa^*$ as a criterion.

The data on the effectiveness of antitumour drugs of the basic classes are given below for comparison of their activity towards solid tumours and transplanted leukaemias. The maximum values of the activity coefficients for antimetabolites, antibiotics, nitrosocarbamides are close both for solid tumours and leukaemias. In other words, solid tumours and transplanted leukaemias possess approximately the same responsiveness and both seem to be useful for selection of these active antitumour drugs; for chloroethylamines and ethyleneamines these dependences appear to be different.

Class of antitumour drugs	Solid tumours	Transplanted leukaemias
Antimetabolites	0.30-0.65	0.5
Antibiotics	0.25-0.70	0.2-0.7
Chloroethylamines	0.5-2.0	0.5
Ethyleneimines	0.5-1.5	0.2-0.6
Phenols	-	0.3-0.6
Nitrosocarbamides	0.5-0.8	0.2-0.8

As follows from the above data, solid tumours are slightly more responsive to drugs of the alkylating type than are the transplanted leukaemias. Leukaemia La, extensively studied in terms of kinetics, is moderately responsive to drugs of various chemical classes acting by different mechanisms (Table 38). Leukaemia La might serve as a reference system for comparison of various antitumour drug activities, alongside leukaemia L-1210 recommended at present. Unfortunately, the amount of experimental data on kinetic evaluation of chemotherapy is insufficient for making decisive conclusions about the comparative effectiveness of antitumour compounds of various classes and about rational choice of unique screening systems.

TABLE 38   Activity coefficients for the most effective drugs used
for treatment of some experimental tumour strains

Drug	Mammary gland cancer	Walker carcino-sarcoma	Leukaemia L-1210	Melanoma B-16	Leukaemia La
Cyclophosphamide	0.6	0.74	0.66	0.55	0.5
Sarcolysine	-	0.70	-	-	0.55
Thiophosphamide	0.4	1.5	-	-	0.3
Methylnitrosourea	0.8	0.5	-	-	0.58
Dibunol	-	-	-	-	0.6
Diazane	-	-	0.5	.	0.8
Adriamycin	0.65	0.41	-	0.33	0.70

8.   COMBINED CHEMOTHERAPY

Combined chemotherapy has become the basic method of treating tumours. Success
depends on correct choice of drugs and optimal regimen of administration. The
choice of combined drugs must be based on the specificity of each drug on the
cellular cycle (Frankfurt, 1975).

Antitumour drugs are classified with respect to the phase specificity of their
action. Scheme 1 contains additional data on the effects of sarcolysine, adriamycin (Tobey, 1972), alkylnitrosoureas (Ostrovskaia and Frankfurt, 1977) and diazane
(Goncharova et al., 1976) on cellular cycles.

Naturally, the selection of individual components for combined chemotherapy must
take into account the differences in molecular mechanisms of their action, as well
as the specificity of the drug's toxic effect. The problem of a rational regimen
of treatment with the given drug is no less complex. Information has appeared
recently on combined treatment regimens, taking into account the daily rhythm of
normal cell and tumour cell proliferation: however, as a rule these were empirical.

The antileukaemic action of the combinations of diazane with adriamycin and sarcolysine was studied within these terms of reference by Konovalova in 1975. These
drugs are known to have a different effect on separate phases of the cellular
cycle. For instance, diazane blocks cell transition from the presynthesis phase
to the phase of DNA synthesis, adriamycin retards the entry of cells into mitosis,
and sarcolysine decreases DNA synthesis and blocks for 24 hours the entry of cells
into mitosis (Scheme 1).

The most promising data come from the combination of diazane with adriamycin. The
effect of diazane on leukaemia La was that the kinetic curve for the process
development presented regularly alternating rise and fall sections related to the
times of drug administration (Figure 84c). Adriamycin alone only slight inhibited
the development of leukaemia ($\varkappa* = 0.33$) (Figure 85a, curve 1). Chemotherapy with
diazane combined with adriamycin prolonged the process inhibition ($\varkappa* = 1$, Figure
85b). This indicates synergism of the antileukamic action under combined use of
the drugs. In this case the time of adriamycin injection was determined by the
kinetic curve for changes in spleen weight under the action of diazane alone:
adriamycin was injected twice at the beginning of each upward trend in the kinetic
curve.

In order to ensure minimum toxicity, low doses were used when studying the effects

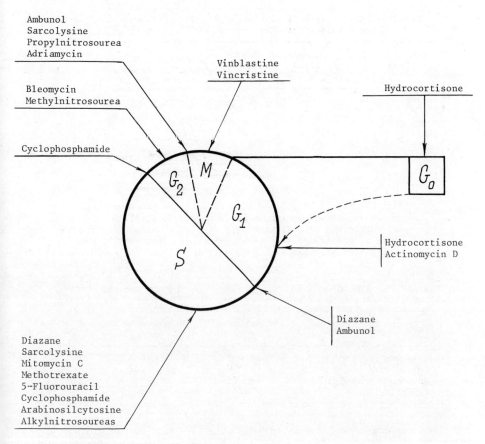

Scheme 1. Phase specificity of the effects of antitumour
drugs on the cellular cycle from the data of Tobey (1972)
and Ostrovskaia and Frankfurt (1977).

of combined drugs. Diazane was injected at a dose of 2 mg/kg, and sarcolysine at
a dose of 1 mg/kg. The two drugs were unjected simultaneously every 72 hours. The
kinetic curves for changes in the spleen weight in controls, under the action of
diazane alone, sarcolysine alone, and a combination of these drugs are given in
Figure 85c. The therapeutic synergism of diazane and sarcolysine is clearly seen:
the activity coefficients $\varkappa^*$ are 0.14, 0.26 and 0.81 for sarcolysine, diazane, and
the combination, respectively. The combined action of sarcolysine and diazane at
higher doses were also studied against leukaemia L-1210: the mean animal life-span
was doubled (Table 39).

The phenomenon of synergism observed with diazane together with adriamycin and
sarcolysine shows the potentiality of combined treatment for clinical use.

The antitumour effects of cyclophosphane, 6-mercaptopurine, vincristine, actinomycin D and daunorubicin, as well as their combinations, on first-generation

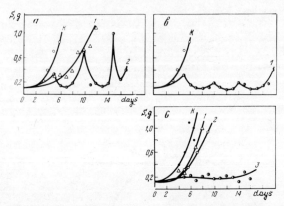

Fig. 85 Effect of diazane in combination with other drugs
on development of leukaemia La (Konovalova, 1975).
(a) Adriamycin (1), diazane (2); (b) combination of adriamycin with diazane; (c) sarcolysine (1), diazane (2), and
combination of diazane with sarcolysine (3).

TABLE 39   Effects of combined treatment by diazane and sarcolysine
on life-span of animals with leukaemia L-1210 (Konovalova, 1975)

Drug	Summary dose, mg/kg	Mean life-span, days	$\varkappa_t^*$
Diazane	450	13.5 ± 0.8	0.29
Sarcolysine	15	12.0 ± 0.9	0.20
Diazane + sarcolysine	450 + 15	20.0 ± 1.9	0.57
Controls	–	9.6 ± 1.5	–

spontaneous mammary gland tumours in Swiss mice have been studied (Cain et al.,
1974). The activity coefficients ϰ* for each experimental point were calculated
using Cain et al.'s plots. The curves for changes in inhibition coefficients ϰ*
with time are presented in Figure 86 for separate and combined use of the drugs.
6-Mercaptopurine, vincristine and oxyurea administered separately exhibit an almost
similar activity with this tumour model (they are represented by one curve in
Figure 86a). Vinblastine and antibiotics possess a slightly lower activity. Figure
86a shows that after these drugs are terminated, the effectiveness of treatment
sharply decreases.

A single injection of cyclophosphamide (Figure 86b) was only slightly effective.
An additional single injection of each of the above drugs resulted in increased
activity. The administration of cyclophosphamide together with 6-mercaptopurine,
vincristine or hydroxyurea was more effective when these drugs were used in combination with antibiotics.

The chemotherapeutic effectiveness was even higher in the case of a four-component
combination of the drugs (Figure 86c, curve 1). Cyclophosphane, oxyurea, vincristine and 6-mercaptopurine were injected in succession at early stages of tumour
development. A similar therapeutic cycle gave an even higher effect (Figure 86c,
curve 2). When the drugs were unjected at an advanced stage of tumour development,
the effectiveness of combined therapy was lower (Figure 86c, curve 3).

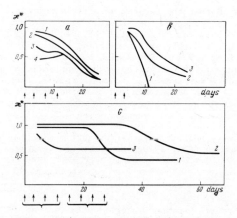

Fig. 86 Kinetic control of the effectiveness of antitumour
drugs and their combinations for first-generation spontaneous
mammary gland tumour in C3H/HeJ mice (Cain *et al.*, 1974).
a: (1) 6-mercaptopurine, vincristine and hydroxyurea;
    (2) vinblastine; (3) actinomycin D; (4) daunorubicin
    at separate administration.
b: cyclophosphamide (1) and its combination with anti-
    biotics (2), vincristine, hydroxyurea or 6-mercapto-
    purine (3).
c: Four-component chemotherapy of small (0.3 - 0.4 cm³ —
    1, 2) and developed (1.2 cm³ — 3) tumours.

The combination of cyclophosphamide and adriamycin appeared to be highly effective
for a wide spectrum of experimental tumours, such as the mammary gland adenocarcinoma,
melanoma B-16, osteogenic sarcoma and leukaemia P-388 (Corbett *et al.*, 1975). The
drug doses in experimental combined treatment were as a rule lower than on separate
administration of these drugs in optimal doses.

The life-span prolongation of animals was chosen as the activity characteristic
for osteogenic sarcoma and leukaemia P-388. It represents the difference between
the mean times for attaining a tumour weight of 500 mg ($t_e - t_c$) for adenocarcinoma
and melanoma B-16. The values of t_e and t_c given in Corbett *et al.* (1975) were
used for calculation of criterion $\varkappa^*$ (Table 40).

TABLE 40 Activity coefficients for cyclophosphamide, adriamycin
and their combination for various tumour models (Corbett *et al.*, 1975)

Tumour	Cyclophosphamide	Adriamycin	Cyclophosphamide + adriamycin
Mammary gland adenocarcinoma	0.64	0.65	0.73
Melanoma B-16	0.55	0.33	0.69
Osteogenic Ridgway sarcoma	0.32	0.34	0.48
Leukaemia P-338	0.66	0.42	0.67

It follows from Table 40 that the antitumour activity of the combination of adria-mycin and cyclophosphamide exceeds the effect of each drug used separately. An exception was observed only for leukaemia P-388. In this case the combined action gave a result similar to that of cyclophosphamide alone. It was noted that the greater antitumour effect was not accompanied by an increase in the toxic action. Combinations of various nitrosocarbamides with other antitumour drugs have been widely studied recently. For example, the antitumour effects of a combination of methylnitrosourea (MNU) with adriamycin and cyclophosphamide was investigated for Walker carcinosarcoma and the sixth generation of spontaneous mammary gland adeno-carcinoma in mice (Ostrovskaia and Emanuel, 1976). The drug doses for the groups of animals receiving combined treatment were 0.25 - 0.50 of the optimal ones used separately. The activity coefficients к* for adriamycin (AM) methylnitrosourea (MNU) and cyclophosphamide (CPh) are given below for separate, paired and combined injections.

Tumour	AM	MNU	CPh	AM+MNU	AM+CPh	MNU+CPh	AM+CPh+MNU
Adenocarcinoma	0.11	0.19	0.06	0.05	0.19	0.29	0.43
WCS	0.41	0.50	0.74	0.47	0.79	0.90	0.91

The three drugs used separately are seen to be only slightly effective for mammary gland adenocarcinoma. MNU inhibits tumour growth only 1.2 times ($к = 0.19$), and the combined use of MNU and adriamycin results in an even lower effect. The combin-ation of adriamycin and cyclophosphamide exerts cumulative antitumour effect.

A considerable synergistic effect was observed on combined use of the three drugs. Combined injection of MNU, adriamycin and cyclphosphamide decreased by half the tumour growth rate ($к* = 0.43$) and increased the average life-span of animals by 35%

Similar results were obtained for combined chemotherapy of the Walker carcino-sarcoma. MNU and adriamycin and combination considerably exceeded the antitumour effects of each drug administered alone. The dependence of the effect on the treatment regimen should also be noted. Injection of MNU (20 mg/kg × 6) before adriamycin had more than double the effect of giving adriamycin before MNU.

A sharp increase in activity occurs with a combination of the three drugs. The synergism of combined treatment with MNU, cyclophosphamide and adriamycin results in cure of 40% animals, in an 11.3-fold retardation of tumour growth in other rats ($к* = 0.91$), and in an almost three-fold increase in the life-span of treated animals, compared to controls. It will be noted that this effect is to a consid-erable extent due to the synergism of the combined action of MNU and cyclophos-phamide ($к* = 0.90$).

Thus, the combined use of two highly active antitumour drugs, adriamycin and MNU, does not increase the effect of either taken separately, but when these drugs are used in combination with cyclophosphamide, the antitumour action is synergistic.

Various immunological systems are suppressed in the course of the tumour process. Chemotherapy and radiation therapy also frequently exert an immunosuppressive action and this increases the general toxic effect. In order to decrease the toxicity of antitumour drugs and to stimulate the protective action of the body, the chemotherapeutic drugs are often combined with various stimulating and protective agents, in particular with biologically active polysaccharides and hormones.

For example, polysaccharide complexes (prodigiosane) were found to stimulate the reticuloendothelial and endocrine systems. The combined effect of cyclophospha-mide with prodigiosane and prednisolone on the growth kinetics of solid sarcoma 37 has been studied. Daily administration of prednisolone alone had no effect on

tumour growth. Treatment with prodigiosane alone resulted in weak inhibition
($\varkappa* = 0.8$). Combined use of prednisolone and cyclophosphamide also had no effect
on the activity of the latter ($\varkappa* = 0.45$). Prodigiosane slightly increased the
cyclophosphamide activity, but had virtually no effect on its toxicity, whereas
combined administration of the three drugs completely inhibited tumour development
(Figure 87). Complete tumour resolution took place in 50% of the animals; the
life-spans of others were considerably prolonged.

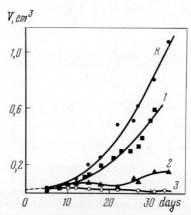

Fig. 87 Effect of prodigiosan (1), cyclophosphamide (2)
and of a combination of cyclophosphamide with prodigiosan
and prednisolone (3) on development of solid sarcoma 37.

9. COMBINED EFFECT OF DRUGS AND IRRADIATION

Methods for selective radiosensitization of tumours, involving the use of drugs, is
important. The problem is considered here in terms of quantitative kinetic and
physico-chemical aspects (Gotlib et al., 1970; Pelevina, 1973; Maksumova et al.,
1972a,b; Krugliakova et al., 1964; Odintsova and Krugliakova, 1976; Voronina et
al., 1972; Smotryaeva et al., 1972).

The search for methods to increase selective radiation damage to DNA by intensification of processes involving free radicals is one approach for increasing the effect
of radiotherapy on tumours. Inhibitors-antioxidants, stable free radicals, and
alkylating agents are compounds capable of damaging the molecular structure of DNA
and inducing changes in the cell's response to irradiation.

The effects of propylgallate (PG), triacetoneamineoxyl (TAN) and MNU on the radiosensitivity of tumour cells were studied because their products of conversion in
the living body are radiomimetic.

The combined effect of irradiation and chemical compounds can be evaluated by the
changes in parameters of the 'dose-effect' dependence described in a general form
by the equation (Puck et al., 1956):

$$S = 1 - (1 - D/D_{37})^n$$

where S is the fraction of surviving cells, D is the radiation dose, D_{37} is the
dose causing an e-times decrease in survival (i.e. up to 37% of controls) and
characteristics of a lethal irradiation, n is obtained by extrapolating the linear

section of the semilogarithmic anamorphosis of the equation to the value $D = 0$ (Figure 88A).

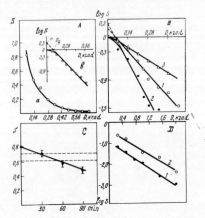

Fig. 88 Effect of propylgallate (PG) and its oxidation products on effectiveness of radiation. (A) Survival of LL-line cells as a function of the γ-irradiation dose; (B) same for irradiation (1) and for combination of irradiation with PG added 18 hours before (2) or 15 minutes before (3) irradiation (Gotlib *et al.*, 1970); (C) changes in radiation reactions of LL-line cells in relation to time of preliminary PG oxidation; (D) survival of ascites NKLy tumour cells after irradiation (1) and on combined irradiation with PG treatment *in vivo* (Pelevina, 1973).

The linear section of the semilogarithmic anamorphosis is described by the function

$$\log S = \log n - 0.434 \; D/D_{37}$$

or after substitution of variables of $\log n = 0.434 \; (D_q/D_{37})$

$$\log S = \frac{0.434}{D_{37}} \; (D - D_q)$$

where D_q is the threshold dose above which the radiation effect is lethal. Since n and D_q are related values, it is more convenient to use D_q which has a certain physical sense (Figure 88A). The lower the D_{37} dose, the greater is the slope of the appropriate straight line and the stronger is the lethal effect.

The influence of PG (at a concentration $2 \cdot 10^{-5}$ M) on the irradiation effectiveness in experiments with LL line cells was found to be greatly dependent on the time of preliminary cell incubation with PG. When PG was added 18 hours before irradiation it exerted a radiosensitizing action and the dose D_{37} decreased by a factor of 1.6, while the administration of PG 15 minutes before irradiation had a protective effect, and the dose D_{37} increased 1.85 times (Figure 88B). The value of D_{37} in controls was 120 rad.

One of the reasons for this phenomenon may be the sensitizing effect of PG oxidation products, in particular, of free radicals of the semiquinone type formed in cells or in culture medium in the course of prolonged incubation. Indeed, the

addition of partly oxidized PG fifteen minutes before irradiation resulted not in a
protective effect, but in cell decay increasing with the PG oxidation extent
(Figure 88C).

Similar results were obtained *in vivo* for NKLy ascites tumours in mice treated with
PG. A single administration of PG directly before irradiation induced a protective
action and increased the fraction of viable cells (Figure 88D). For a solid tumour
the preliminary single administration of PG caused a radiosensitizing effect. The
extent of radiosensitization, i.e. the relation between radiation doses inducing
resolution of 50% tumours (ED$_{50}$) was approximately equal for different irradiation
schedules (Pelevina, 1973).

Type of irradiation	ED$_{50}$, p	Extent of radiosensitization
Single irradiation	1500	
Same with PG	500–600	2.9–3.0
Three irradiations	2700	
Same with PG	900–1000	2.7–3.0

A comparative study of the effects of combined irradiation and PG treatment at
logarithmic and stationary growth stages was carried out for a culture of HeLa
cells (Maksumova *et al.*, 1972a,b). At the stage of stationary growth (8 to 12 days,
Figure 89a), HeLa cells displayed a low mitotic activity. 70% of cells did not
enter the phase of DNA synthesis for 4 days; the mitotic index was 0.6% (at the
logarithmic stage it was 40%). At the same time the reproduction capacity of the
cells was virtually similar for both stages (clone formation was 72-73%). The
radiation doses D_{37} for resting and proliferating cells were approximately similar
(181 and 188 rad, respectively). However, there was a marked decrease in the

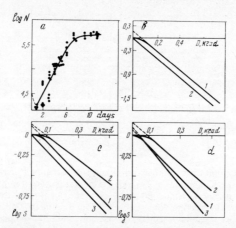

Fig. 89 Effectiveness of irradiation and its combined action
with propylgallate at various stages of tumour growth.
(a) Kinetics of growth of HeLa cell number in culture; (b)
survival of HeLa cells at logarithmic (1) and stationary (2)
growth stages as a function of radiation dose (Maksumova *et
al.*, 1972a); (c) same for irradiation (1) and combined
action of irradiation and PG added 15 minutes (2) or 18 hours
(3) before irradiation at the logarithmic growth stage;
(d) same at the stationary growth stage (Maksumova *et al.*,
1972b).

capacity of resting cells to restore sublethal damage. The combined effect of PG and irradiation was the same for proliferating and resting HeLa cells. Increase in survival was observed for both groups of cells when the contact with PG was short (protective effect), whereas a prolonged action of PG caused stronger irradiation damage (radiosensitization) (Figure 89c,d). This suggests that a combination of PG with irradiation would be highly effective for the treatment of tumours containing many resting cells.

The difference in the effects of PG and its oxidation products was supported also by experiments on a molecular level. Short-term action of PG on isolated DNA was found by Krugliakova et al. (1964) to result in a radio-protective effect caused by interaction of the inhibitor with radicals formed both by water radiolysis and from DNA molecules.

On the other hand, reactive intermediates exerting a radiomimetic effect and causing damage to the DNA structure are known to form from PG in the presence of oxygen in an aqueous medium. The addition of oxidized PG decreases the viscosity of the DNA solution. This effect is a direct function of the extent of PG oxidation (Figure 90A). The number of single and double cleavages of the DNA macromolecules progressively increases with time. With prolonged action (up to 80 hours) this damage is equivalent to that caused by low (up to 20 krad) radiation doses (Figure 90B) (Odintsova and Krugliakova, 1976). The dependences of the protective effect on PG concentration and of the radio-sensitizing effect on the time of interaction with oxidized PG are given in Figure 90C.

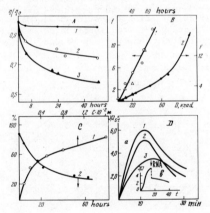

Fig. 90 Protective action of propylgallate for irradiation of DNA. (A) Changes in DNA solution viscosity in the presence of non-oxidized (1) and PG oxidized during 1 (2) and 2 (3) hours; (B) formation of single (1) and double (2) cleavages in DNA molecules as a function of the radiation dose (circles) and in the presence of oxidized PH (triangles, additional x-axis); (C) dependence of the propylgallate protective action on its concentration for isolated DNA (1) and on the time in the presence of oxidized PG (2); (D) change in chemiluminescence in PG oxidation (0.82 · 10⁻² M by O₂ in controls (1) and upon adding 82 μg/ml (2) and 164 μg/ml (3) of DNA to the initial mixture (a) or 600 mkg/ml of DNA at the moment of attaining the luminescence maximum (b) (Odintsova et al., 1976).

Thus, the sensitizing effect of PG seems to be due to the damage it does to DNA during oxidation, and this increases the cell's radiosensitivity. The interaction of DNA with intermediates of a free radical nature is corroborated by the decrease in the intensity of chemiluminescence of PG oxidation after addition of DNA (Figure 90D) (Odintsova and Krugliakova, 1976).

Similar effects would be expected for stable free radicals. The properties and reactions of nitroxyl radicals in chemical systems have been described earlier (Rozantsev, 1980).

Indeed, a number of stable radicals of this class, especially triacetonamide-N-oxyl (TAN)

$$
\begin{array}{c}
O \\
\parallel \\
H_3C \quad CH_3 \\
H_3C \quad N \quad CH_3 \\
\mid \\
O^{\cdot}
\end{array}
$$

have a radiosensitizing effect on cell cultures under anaerobic conditions (Agnew and Skarsgard, 1972; Emmerson, 1967). Up to half the cells in some tumours do not get enough oxygen. For example, the ascite strain NKLy is such a tumour. The low lethal effect of irradiation characterized by a dose value $D_{37} = 400$ r is evidence of an acute NKLy cell hypoxia at certain periods of tumour development (Figure 88D).

Intraperitoneal injections of TAN at a dose of 350 mg/kg 15 minutes before irradiation raised by a factor of 1.5 the number of cells with chromosome aberrations caused by irradiation. When the interval between introduction of the nitroxyl radical and irradiation was increased to 30 minutes and more the radiation effectiveness remained the same (Voronina et al., 1972).

It was found by the EPR technique that after a single injection of TAN the nitroxyl radical content in cells of NKLy ascites tumour rapidly decreased with a rate constant $3.8 \cdot 10^{-1}$ sec $^{-1}$, according to first-order reaction kinetics (Figure 91A). Decay of the TAN free radicals in NKLy cells occurred at approximately the same rate (Figure 91B). Thirty to sixty minutes after injection TAN was virtually

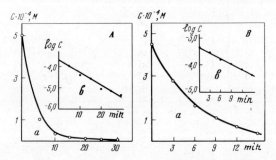

Fig. 91 Kinetics of changes in paramagnetic label concentration in cells of NKLy ascites tumour after single administration of TAN: (A) in vivo; (B) in vitro (Voronina et al., 1972).

absent. When TAN was injected into mice with solid tumours NKLy, the paramagnetic label was distributed uniformly over the bulk of the tumour node. Its maximum concentration was attained 15 minutes after the injection, and after 45 minutes the drug was completely removed from the tumour. Thus the radiosensitizing action of TAN is directly related to its presence in the tumour.

Compounds of such a type are especially suitable for increasing the radiosensitivity of tumours at the terminal stages of their development under conditions of considerable hypoxia (Brustad *et al.*, 1972). The optimum antitumour effect is achieved by irradiating the tumour when it contains the maximum nitrozyl radical.

Pre-administration of MNU also increases the lethal effect of cell irradiation (Maksamova *et al.*, 1972b). This result is natural, since the damaging action of MNU on DNA is known and the lethal damage of a part of the cells might be related to this fact (Smotryaeva *et al.*, 1972; Tseitlin *et al.*, 1975).

The antitumour effect of combined irradiation and chemical treatment is controlled by the ratio of effects of these therapies. Of great importance in this case is the elaboration of tests and programmes providing optimal doses and treatment regimens.

According to Burlakova *et al.* (1965, 1973), the result of combined use of radiation and drugs can be predicted from the specificity of changes in the antioxidative activity (AOA) of the lipid fraction of animal liver in the course of tumour growth and the action of chemotherapeutic drugs. It was found, in particular, that the combined action of radiation and of the inhibitor of radical processes can lead both to a decrease and to an increase in AOA, depending on the dose. It can be seen in Figure 92 that there are four regions of the combined inhibitor and radiation effect: that of radiation protection by the inhibitor both of the tumour and of the body, that of a stronger radiation effect, that of radiation protection of the tumour and of a stronger action on the body, and that of body protection and a stronger radiation effect on the tumour.

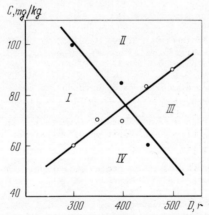

Fig. 92 Regions of various effects of irradiation and of the drug on tumour growth (hepatoma 22) and animal body. (I) Tumour protection and intensification of irradiation action on the body; (II) intensification of the action of irradiation on tumour and body; (III) intensification of irradiation action on tumour and body protection; (IV) protection of tumour and body.

It is important to evaluate the possibility of such an approach to combined therapy of cancer clinically. The general regularities found in the course of experimental and clinical studies give us reason to consider that in this way it would be possible to evaluate the general response of the tumour and the body as a whole to the combined action of radiation and of the radiosensitizing chemical agent.

10. RESPONSE OF PRIMARY TUMOURS AND METASTASES TO CHEMOTHERAPY

The development of many metastatic experimental tumour processes resulted in the death of some animals from early metastases in experiments. This was characteristic of Walker carcinosarcoma and Zaidel ascites hepatoma. Therefore, a two-factor difference criterion permitting quantitative evaluation of the drug's effect on the tumour process and taking into account the death and the irregularities of tumour growth in individual animals, was used in experimental comparative studies on the response of primary and metastatic tumour to thiophosphamide (Thiotepa), cyclo-phosphamide, diazane and methylnitrosourea.

The experimental data were processed with a BESM-6 computer. The calculated drug effectiveness is given in Table 41 with a 95% reliability.

The values of drug effectiveness in Table 41 show a clear-cut difference in the effects of drugs on primary tumours and metastases. This depends both on the properties of the tumours and drugs, and on the chemotherapeutic regimen used. When the treatment of Walker carcinosarcoma is started on the third day, there is a greater effect on metastases, whereas diazane and methylnitrosourea affect preferentially the primary tumours. The greatest effect on metastases is caused by cyclophosphamide, and that on primary tumours by thiophosphamide.

The start of treatment on the seventh day, when the process is generalized in most animals essentially alters this ratio, and the effectiveness of all drugs decreases slightly. However, the inhibition of the growth of metastases is twice that obtained with diazane. When chemotherapy is started later, diazane appears to be the most effective out of the other drugs studied, since along with inhibiting metastases in a way resembling the action of thiophosphamide, it has a stronger inhibiting effect on the primary tumour.

The Zaidel ascites hepatoma is mich more resistant to chemotherapy than the Walker carcinosarcoma. All the drugs studied are more effective in inhibiting the growth of metastases than primary tumours. Diazane is the most active drug for multiple injections. The inhibition of primary tumour growth is virtually independent of the treatment schedule, while the inhibition of metastases increases by 30% on multiple injections of diazane.

Thus, it seems to be possible to evaluate quantitatively the effect of various antitumour drugs on metastasizing tumours.

Examples of kinetic curves demonstrating the action of chemotherapeutic drugs on primary tumours and their metastases are given in Figure 93 plotted using the BESM-6 computer. The curves for survival in controls and experimental animals are also given in this Figure.

TABLE 41 Effectiveness values (ϰ) for action of therapy of primary tumours and their metastases

Drug	From 3rd day multiple injections		From 7th day multiple injections		From 2nd day single injection		From 2nd day multiple injection	
	Primary tumours	Meta- stases	Primary tumours	Meta- stases	Primary tumours	Meta- stases	Primary tumours	Meta- stases
	Walker sarcinosarcoma				Zaidel ascites hepatoma			
Thiophosphamide	6.02± 0.29	7.08± 0.31	2.49± 0.17	4.89± 0.19	-	-	1.72± 0.07	2.42± 0.12
Nitrosomethylurea	2.28± 0.11	1.68± 0.09	1.07± 0.07	1.25± 0.08	-	-	0.92± 0.05	2.14± 0.10
Diazane	4.27± 0.20	2.39± 0.15	3.85± 0.18	4.74± 0.22	1.69± 0.15	1.97± 0.16	1.56± 0.09	2.97± 0.14
Cyclophosphamide	4.72± 0.23	8.28± 0.35	-	-	-	-	-	-

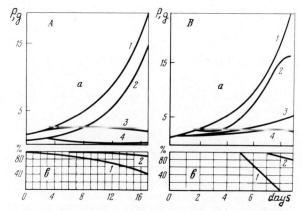

Fig. 93   Response of metastases and primary tumours to
chemotherapy.   (A) Thiotepa for Walker carcinosarcoma;
(B) diazane for Zaidel ascites hepatoma: (a) kinetic curves,
1, 2 — primary tumour and metastases in controls;   3, 4 —
same for chemotherapy;   (b) curves for survival: 1 — controls,
2 — chemotherapy.

11.   SURGERY OF EXPERIMENTAL TUMOURS

Post-operative recurrence and metastasization of malignant tumours represents a
serious clinical problem.   Experimental studies are very rare and are mainly
qualitative.   The data reported in sparse kinetic papers on post-operative
recurrences are rather contradictory and it is difficult to draw any conclusions.

The recurrence of the Guérin carcinoma after combined treatment with benzoteph and
surgical excision of part of the tumour was discussed by Arendarevskii (1977).
The processing of tabular data given in the original paper for controls and experiment showed that tumour growth was described by an exponential function $V = at^b$.
The growth rate of recurring tumours after combined treatment with surgery and
benzoteph ($b_e = 7.7$) was four times higher than in controls ($b_c = 1.9$) and three
times higher than after administration of benzoteph alone ($b_e = 6.2$) (Figure 94a).
These results can be related to both the surgical repair and the immunosuppressive
effect of benzoteph.   It is difficult to evaluate the relative contribution of
each factor since no data on the kinetics of tumour growth recurrence after
surgical operation alone were given.

A somewhat unusual picture of the growth of recurring carcinoma 755 was observed
after surgical excision of the tumour (Chirigos *et al.*, 1962):   in this case
recurrence was observed on the sixth day.   Up to the 40th day the growth rate of
the recurring tumour differed slightly from that of controls (0.5 and 0.6 mm/day,
respectively), then growth stopped for a prolonged time and from the 60th day it
recommenced at a rather higher rate (0.8 mm/day) compared to controls and to the
initial recurrence period (Figure 94c).   The causes of this pattern of growth are
not clear: it might be related to the intensity of secondary immunological
reactions changing with time.   However, it is characteristic that in this case the
growth rate of the tumour recurrence after surgery slightly differed from that for
an intact tumour.

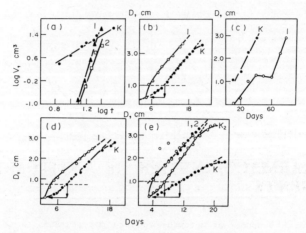

Fig. 94   Developmental kinetics of post-operative recurrence
of experimental tumours: (a) Guérin carcinoma (1 — operation
and benzoteph treatment, 2 — benzoteph) (Arendarevskii, 1971);
(b) Guérin carcinoma (data from Parkanskii and Konovalova,
1973);   (c) adenocarcinoma 755 (Chirigos *et al.*, 1962);
(d) same (from Parkanskii and Konavalova, 1973);   (e)
sarcoma 45 (1 — transplantation with dilution 1:10, 2 — with
dilution 1:1) (Parkanskii and Konavalova, 1973).

A detailed kinetic study of post-operative recurrence for sarcoma 45, Guérin
carcinoma and adenocarcinoma 755 showed that the growth rate of recurring tumours
for the periods of linear growth usually did not exceed the growth rates of the
control tumours (Figure 94b,d,e).   An exception is the sarcoma 45:   the growth rate
of the control tumour transplanted as a tumour cell suspension (dilution 1:10) was
half that for a 1:1 suspension (1.1 and 2.4 mm/day, respectively).   However, in
both cases the rate of post-operative recurrences were the same (1.8 mm/day).   It
will be noted that here the growth rate both in controls and of the recurring
carcinoma 755 was considerably higher (1.6 - 2.1 mm/day) than in the above mentioned
study (0.5 - 0.8 mm/day) (Chirigos *et al.*, 1962) and no periods of no-growth were
observed.

A sharp increase in the growth rate observed for all cases soon after surgery
attracts special attention (Figure 94b,d).   Even in 1-2 days for sarcoma 45 and
Guérin carcinoma and in 3 days for adenocarcinoma 755 the tumours attained the pre-
operative size.   Then their growth rate considerably decreased, approaching that
of controls.   In specific experiments the effect was actually found to consists of
increasing the tumour growth rate, rather than to operative trauma or appearance
of a post-operative hepatoma.   It is possible that in the case of palliative tumour
removal processes similar to those observed in the regenerating liver takes place
in a residual tumour fragment.   Intensive DNA synthesis (Kholms, 1956) is known to
be observed in the liver even 24 hours after partial hepatectomy and 85-90% of
the cells enter mitoses in 26-33 hours (Yokayama *et al.*, 1953).

The results of these investigations provide evidence for the possibility of experimental modelling of post-operative recurrences of transplanted tumours of various
types, and this permits the finding of certain general rules for their development

CHAPTER 1

PHARMACOKINETICS OF ANTITUMOUR AGENTS

The use of quantitative methods in studying experimental and clinical cancer chemotherapy depends on our knowledge of the pharmacokinetics of antitumour drugs.
Along with specificities of the chemical structures of these drugs and their activities on metabolism, the time of their action and their effective concentrations in
tumour and normal tissues are also important. These factors depend on intensity of
supply, distribution, conversion and discharge of the drug and of its active
metabolites in the body. The regularities of these processes are the subject of
pharmacokinetic research. The basic pharmacokinetic concepts have been described
in monographs by Dost (1968) and Wagner (1971).

The general pharmacokinetic regularities are valid for chemical compounds of
different types and varying biological action. For this reason pharmacokinetics
usually classifies biologically active drugs by the types of chemical compounds
they belong to. The antitumour drugs fall into various classes of compounds.
Therefore the pharmacokinetics of antitumour drugs can be considered both as a
part of general pharmacokinetics and as a part of cancer chemotherapy.

A condensed survey of the main models and methods of general pharmacokinetics
devised at the Institute of Chemical Physics, Academy of Science, USSR, the application of these to certain problems of cancer chemotherapy, and the pharmacokinetic
data on a number of new antitumour drugs are discussed in this Chapter.

1. METHODS AND MODELS

Experimental studies on the pharmacokinetics of biologically active compounds
including antitumour drugs involve measurements of the concentration of a compound
and the products of its conversion (metabolites) in various body organs and tissues
at various times after the start of administration. Such problems may be solved by
the conventional methods of chemical kinetics. Pharmacokinetics deal with micro-
concentrations of drugs which have to be detected in very complex, multi-component
systems. Many known physico-chemical techniques such as chromatography, mass-
spectrometry, polarography, and radiospectroscopy, optical and other methods of
analysis, are used for this purpose. For example, gas-liquid chromatography was
used to detect 5-fluorouracil in blood plasma, in the form of its volatile tri-
methylsilyl derivative (Windheuser *et al.*, 1972).

The high sensitivity of radioisotope techniques permits direct sample measuring of the distribution of drugs and of their metabolites inside organs and tissues, even at cellular and subcellular levels. Radioisotope techniques give the most precise results for drugs present in minute concentrations, for example some antimetabolites and antibiotics. When the drug is metabolized in the body, one can tell the concentrations of both the drug and its metabolites. The kinetic curve may be complex and difficult to interpret. Also, labelled drug fragments may become involved in biosynthetic processes. The specificities of the pharmacokinetics of labelled drugs can also be ascribed to the paramagnetic spin-labelled analogues of antitumour compounds.

The spectrophotometric method, based on the capacity of the nucleophilic reactant, 4-γ-(nitrobenzyl)pyridine, to form dyed compounds as a result of alkylation, is widely applied for detection of total concentrations of the drug and its derivatives. The spectrofluorimetry technique is the most precise, sensitive, and selective. It is valid for a wide range of antitumour agents, such as ethylene imines, antimetabolites, compounds of vegetable origin, antibiotics, etc. Its sensitivity is 10^{-15} M (Yudenfrend, 1965).

Good results are obtained by the use of the polarography technique for drugs capable of oxidation or reduction, such as alkylating compounds or phenols. Its sensitivity is 10^{-9} M (Korenman, 1967).

Radiospectroscopy has been used recently for quantitative detection of antitumour drugs. For instance, thiophosphamide was detected by the NMR (Cates, 1973), and its paramagnetic analogue in normal and tumour animal tissues by the EPR technique (Konovalova et al., 1976).

The bactericidal activity of many antitumour drugs permits use of highly-sensitive microbiological methods for detection of these drugs. Part of the sample is placed in a vessel with a microbial culture, and the level of the sample's bactericidal activity is evaluated by the extent of the inhibition of microbial growth. This method makes no distinction between the initial compounds and their active metabolites, and this seems to account for the non-monotonic character of the pharmacokinetic curves for distribution and elimination of 5-fluorouracil and methotrexate (Tugarinov, 1971).

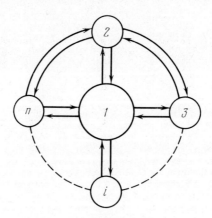

Scheme 2 Multicomponent pharmacokinetic model of a living
body with one central (1) and $n-1$ peripheral (2, 3 ...i...n)
parts.

Administration of antitumour agents before transplantation is also used (Kline *et al.*, 1968). The residual activity of the drug and its active metabolites administered at various times before tumour transplantation are determined.

The experimental data is analyzed in terms of a mathematical model to give quantitative parameters characterizing the pharmacokinetic behaviour of the drug in the body. The so-called multicomponent open linear models representing the body as a set of interlinked components, homogeneous and isotropic for the administered drug, are most widely used in pharmacokinetics (Scheme 2). Individual tissues and organs, their combinations, blood as the general transport system, as well as excretions, the environment, new chemical or physico-chemical states of biologically active compounds (metabolites, complexes) are the system's components.

The mathematical description of such systems is based on premises related to the main processes of the drug in the body.

Transfer or transport of the drug, between and inside the components occurs mainly by diffusion: this is controlled by the concentration gradient. Active transport connected with the selective response of individual cell components is possible for drugs close in structure to natural metabolites, in particular antimetabolites. A simple mathematical description of active transport is given by the equation

$$\frac{dC}{dt} = - \frac{AC}{A + C}$$

similar to the Michaelis equation. Here C is the compound concentration, B is the constant characterizing the affinity of the transport-realizing systems to the compound transported. For low concentrations of the drug ($C \ll B$) this equation reduces to a quasilinear one, for high concentrations ($C \gg B$) to a zero order equation.

The binding of drugs with proteins and other cell components obeys the law of mass action. On condition that the amount of binding agents considerably exceeds the concentration of the administered compound, the process of binding can be considered as a reversible pseudomonomolecular process.

With low drug concentrations metabolism can be considered to be a monomolecular process. Enzymatic conversions are described by the Michaelis equation, which in the case of low substrate concentrations reduces to a first-order equation.

These premises are valid for most antitumour drugs. Indeed, the maximum possible concentrations of many antitumour compounds in the body fall within $10^{-8} - 10^{-5}$ M. The concentration of main binding agents (albumins in plasma) is 10^{-3} M and the known values of the Michaelis constant for enzymatic conversion of the drug in animal and human liver range from 10^{-4} to 10^{-3} M.

Thus the pharmacokinetic behaviour of antitumour compounds in the body can be described by a system of linear differential first-order equation:

$$\frac{dC_i}{dt} - \sum_{\substack{j=1 \\ j \neq i}}^{n} k_{ij} C_i + \sum_{\substack{j=1 \\ j \neq i}}^{n} k_{ji} C_j \tag{1}$$

with reliable solutions of the kind:

$$C_i = \sum_{j=1}^{n} A_{ij} \exp\left(-r_j t\right) \tag{2}$$

Here k_{ij} and k_{ji} are the rate constants, the subscripts i and j denote the components, n is the total number of components, r_j and A_{ij} are constant coefficients representing known algebraic functions of constants k and of the initial conditions i.e. those of concentrations C_i and of the rates of their changes dC_i/dt at time $t = 0$ taken as the reference point. In certain cases (on administering large drug doses) nonlinear differential equations have to be considered as well. Then the solution of system (1) will be obtained by numerical methods, making use of digital or analogue computers.

In practice, the pharmacokinetic curves can, as a rule, be approximated either by one or by the sum of two exponential functions, depending on whether the body is considered as a one- or two-compartment system.

The one-compartment model implies rapid and proportional distribution of the drug over the body directly after administration. Change in the total amount of the drug in the body (P) as well as of its concentration at any site (for example in blood) will be described by a first-order equation:

$$dC/dt = -kC; \quad dP/dt = -kP \tag{3}$$

where $k = k_m + k_e$ is the overall rate constant for decrease in the amount or concentration of the drug owing to metabolism (k_m) and to excretion (k_e). It is assumed that the drug concentration in the body directly after administration attains the value $C_0 = D/V$, where D is the dose, V is the drug distribution volume. Solving equation (3) for initial conditions $t = 0$, $P = D$, $C = C_0$, we obtain:

$$C = C_0 \exp(-kt); \quad P = D \exp(-kt) \tag{4}$$

or in a logarithmic form

$$\log C = \log C_0 - 0.434\, kt; \quad \log P = \log D - 0.434\, kt.$$

Straightening in semilogarithmic co-ordinates is used for evaluation of the model parameters from experimental data.

Loss of the drug in excretions is also a linear process occurring at a rate directl proportional to the drug concentration in blood.

$$dP_e/dt = k_e VC = k_e D \exp(-kt) \tag{5}$$

This expression can be used for evaluation of the pharmacokinetic parameters from the values for drug elimination rates, which is particularly convenient under clinical conditions. The value $\Delta P_e/\Delta t$ is taken as the rate, where ΔP_e is the amount of the drug eliminated within a sufficiently short time interval Δt; the calculated value corresponds to the middle of interval Δt. The logarithmic form of equation (5) is used for evaluation of the parameters

$$\log (\Delta P_e/\Delta t) = \log (k_e 0) - 0.434\, kt.$$

In practice the parameter $t_{\frac{1}{2}} = \ln 2/k$, the half-life of elimination numerically equal to the time during which the concentration or amount of the drug in the body decreases by half, is used along with the numerical values of constant k.

However, in many cases the initial sections of semilogarithmic anamorphoses of pharmacokinetic curves depart from linearity and this can be accounted for by the two-compartment model (Riegelman et al., 1968). This model represents the body as a system consisting of two parts — the central part (blood, extracellular fluid) and the peripheral part (tissues and organs) according to the scheme:

$$\xleftarrow{k_{10}} C_1 \xrightleftharpoons{k_{12}} C_2 \xrightarrow{k_{20}}$$

where C_1 and C_2 are drug concentrations in the compartments, k_{12} and k_{21} are the rate constants for drug exchange between the compartments, k_{10} and k_{20} are rate constants of elimination from the central compartment and of inactivation in the tissues. It is assumed that immediately after administration the drug is rapidly and uniformly distributed over the bulk of the central component and then over the organs and tissues, with simultaneous removal with excretions and by metabolism mainly from the central component. The model is described by a set of differential equations:

$$dC_1/dt = -(k_{10} + k_{12})\, C_1 + k_{21}C_2$$

$$dC_2/dt = -(k_{20} + k_{21})\, C_2 + k_{12}C_1$$

whence for the initial conditions $t = 0$, $C_1 = D/V_1$, $C_2 = 0$, we have

$$C_1 = A_1 \exp(-r_1 t) + A_2 \exp(-r_2 t)$$

$$C_2 = A_3 \exp(-r_2 t) - \exp(-r_1 t)$$

where

$$A_1 = \frac{D}{V_1}\frac{a - r_2}{r_1 - r_2}; \quad A_2 = \frac{D}{V_1}\frac{r_1 - a}{r_1 - r_2}; \quad A = \frac{D}{V_1}\frac{k_{12}}{r_1 - r_2};$$

$$r_{12} = 0.5[(a + b) \pm \sqrt{(a - b)^2 + 4k_{12}k_{21}}];$$

$$a = k_{10} + k_{12}; \quad b = k_{20} + k_{21}.$$

Most often the analysis of experimental curves for drug concentration changes in blood consists in finding the values $A_{1,2}$ and $r_{1,2}$ and then using these values for calculation of the half-life of distribution ($\ln 2/r_1$) and elimination ($\ln 2/r_2$), as well as the volumes of initial and final distribution ($V_1 = D/(A_1 + A_2)$; $V_2 = D/A_2$). One can calculate the administration regimens departing from these parameters, compare the pharmacokinetics of various compounds, evaluate the individual and species differences, characterize quantitatively the effect of various factors on pharmacokinetics, etc. Knowledge of the rate constants k_{ij} permits evaluation of the mean coefficient of distribution over blood and tissues $K_p = k_{12}/k_{21}$ and establishing the contributions from individual paths in the overall process of drug elimination from the body.

Obviously it is impossible to determine all four constants from the values of parameters $A_{1,2}$ and $r_{1,2}$ since they are related by three conditions only

$$k_{10} + k_{12} + k_{21} + k_{20} = r_1 + r_2$$

$$k_{10}k_{21} + k_{10}k_{20} + k_{12}k_{20} = r_1 r_2$$

$$k_{10} + k_{12} = (A_1 r_1 + A_2 r_2)/(A_1 + A_2).$$

In some cases, when the inactivation constant in tissues k_{20} is vanishingly low, or the metabolism constants k_{12} and k_{21} are equal, such a definition becomes possible.

It will be noted that for many lipophilic compounds the values of distribution volume calculated from the model parameters exceed the real volumes of plasma, extracellular fluid, and even of the whole body. The notion of an 'apparent' distribution volume was introduced in this connection. Most probably such an incompatibility stems from the lack of precision of the models.

In this sense the pharmacokinetic models involving specific organs and systems with their volumes, blood flow rates, coefficients of drug distribution in blood and tissue, and elimination parameters, are more promising. Such models were first worked out for the antitumour agents methotrexate and cytosine-arabinoside (Ara-C) (Zaharko, 1972). Obviously these models permit solving the problems of comparative pharmacokinetics dealing with adoption of experimental results clinically.

The problem of a strictly mathematical description of pharmacokinetic data is complex and it is being developed at the present (Fell and Stevens, 1975).

2.   PHARMACOKINETICS IN CANCER CHEMOTHERAPY

The general notions of pharmacokinetics are applicable to the behaviour of compounds exerting various biological effects and the antitumour drugs are no exclusion in this sense. Indeed, analysis of the data reported on the behaviour of more than twenty antitumour drugs of different classes, in the human body and in experimental animals, showed a good consistancy between experimental pharmacokinetic curves and the equations for one- and two-component models (Gorkov, 1971). Certain results of this analysis in generalized co-ordinates $\tau = kt$ and $\eta = C/C_0 = P/D$ (see equation 4) are given in Figure 95. The values of pre-exponential factors and rate constants for individual drugs are given in Table 42.

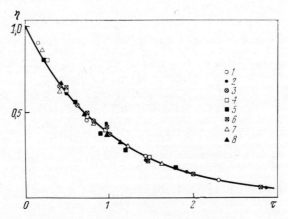

Fig. 95 Generalized kinetic curve for discharge of anti-tumour compounds of different classes from the body in man and experimental animals; the drug corresponding to points 1 - 8 are listed in Table 42.

TABLE 42   Parameters of antitumour drug elimination from the body
in animals and man (Gorkov, 1971)

Number	Drug	Dose, mg/kg	Species	Medium	C_0, mkg/ml	k, hour^{-1}
1	Embichine	3.0	Dog	Blood	0.20	2.90
2	Thiotepa	3.0	Dog	Plasma	1.73	0.96
3	TEPA	3.0	Dog	Plasma	1.80	0.20
4*	5-Fluorouracil	15.0	Man	Serum	27.00	5.50
5	Methotrexate	0.1	Man	Plasma	0.13	0.13
6	Cytosine-arabinoside	250.0	Mouse	Plasma	0.25	2.0
7	Colchicine	400.0	Hamster	Liver	5.50**	0.80
8*	Daunomycin	3.0	Rabbit	Whole body	60.0**	0.14

*Only the linear sections of semil-logarithmic anamorphoses were used.
**Values are given as a percentage of the dose.

One of the most widely encountered problems of general pharmacokinetics is the
evaluation of the rates and extents of intake (absorption) of the drugs from the
sites of their extravascular (subcutaneous, intramuscular, oral) administration.
A direct method for the evaluation of the absorption rate consists of measuring the
amount of drug present at the site of administration at various times. Naturally,
this method is inapplicable clinically. Evaluation of the absorption rate can be
made in this case from the curves for changes in drug content in blood or from its
discharge rate if the site of drug administration is taken into account as an
additional peripheral component in the general model of distribution and elimination of the drug. When the body is considered as a one-compartment model, the
following scheme satisfies this notion:

$$P_a \xrightarrow{\ k_a\ } P \xrightarrow{\ k\ }$$

where P_a and P stand for the amount of drug at the site of administration and in
the body, k_a is the absorption rate constant, k is the rate constant of drug elimination from the body. Owing to the relatively insignificant volume of the initial
site of drug administration one can neglect the reverse transport of the drug and
consider the transfer to be unidirectional. The drug supply to the blood flow is
also assumed to occur by way or ordinary diffusion. Initially $t = 0$, $P = 0$, $P_a = D$
and the drug concentration in the body (in blood) after-administration changes in
accordance with the equation

$$C = \frac{fD}{V} \frac{k_a}{k_a - k} \left[\exp(-kt) - \exp(-k_a t) \right]$$

where f is the bioavailability (the extent of absorption). The value f ($f \le 1$) is
often called the biological assimilation of the drug.

Figure 96 presents the kinetic curves for changes in concentration of oxyurea (A)
and dibunol (B) in blood of cancer patients after oral administration of drugs at
doses of 80 and 50 mg/kg, respectively. Functions of the following form have been
obtained:

$$C_A = 200 \left[\exp(-0.23t) - \exp(-3.50t) \right], \text{ mg/kg}$$

$$C_B = 2 \left[\exp(-0.26t) - \exp(-0.86t) \right], \text{ mg/kg}$$

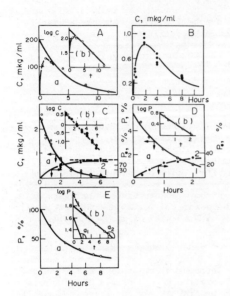

Fig. 96 Pharmacokinetics of antitumour drugs for extravascular administration and elimination from the body. (A), (B) — hydroxyurea (A) and dibunol (B) in blood of man after oral administration (Gorkov *et al.*, 1969); (C) hydroxyurea in rat blood plasma (1) and its elimination (2) (Philips *et al.*, 1967); (D) the colchicine in hamster liver (1) and its elimination (2) (Fleischmann *et al.*, 1968); (E) general contents of daunomycin in the rabbit body.

The elimination rate constants for both drugs are seen to be approximately similar (0.23 and 0.26 hour^{-1}; $t_{\frac{1}{2}} = 3$ hours) but the absorption rate constants and the appropriate absorption half-life differ markedly (3.5 and 0.86 hour^{-1}; 0.2 and 0.8 hour). Apparently dibunol was not completely absorbed from the intestines and this explains the low value of the pre-exponential factor. Assuming that the drug distribution volumes are similar, the absorption extent for hydroxyurea would be twice as high as for dibunol. Indeed, direct measurements of excreted unaltered dibunol showed that about 80% of the dose was not absorbed and was lost from the body within two days (Gorkov *et al.*, 1969).

Since the rate of drug elimination is directly proportional to its concentration in blood, the data on changes in the drug elimination rate can also be used for evaluation of the intake rate constants. The extent of intake can be evaluated from the relation of overall elimination of the drug after intravenous to extravascular administration. When the compound administered is labelled, the extent of uptake can be evaluated from the total amount of labelled compounds eliminated.

Indeed, analysis of the data available shows that the evaluation of pharmacokinetic parameters from the curves for changes on their content in blood and excretions coincide in the case of antitumour drugs as well. For instance, the elimination of hydroxyurea from blood plasma and excretion in the rat are described by expressions with similar exponential indices (Figure 96C):

$$C = 2.5 \exp (-0.6t), \text{ mg/ml}; \quad P_e = 70 \left[1 - \exp (-0.6t)\right], \%$$

70% of the drug is eliminated in an unchanged state, and the remaining 30% is metabolized. Similar indices were obtained also for the elimination curves of colchicine and for changes in its content in hamster liver (Figure 96D):

$$P_e = 40 \left[1 - \exp (-0.8t)\right], \%; \quad P = 5.5 \exp (-0.8t), \%.$$

In this case only 40% of the drug was eliminated in an unchanged state. The pre-exponential factor was close in its value to that for the relative volume of liver

and this is evidence of uniform drug distribution. Graphical analysis of the data
on discharge of daunomycin (3 mg/kg administered intravenously) with the rabbit
bile (Figure 96E) shows that the pharmacokinetics of this antibiotic are consistent
with the two-compartment model possessing the parameters obtained by the equation

$$P = (D - P_e) = 40 \exp(-0.7t) + 60 \exp(-0.14t), \%.$$

Daunomycin is not removed from the rabbit body by other routes.

Pharmacokinetic analysis is important in comparative studies of various drugs,
particularly for investigation of drugs which are structurally similar. Very often
very small changes in chemical structure have an effect not only on the specific
activity of the drug towards certain tumour tissues, but also on the parameters of
its supply, distribution, metabolism and elimination, and this affects the general
activity of the drug. A survey of data on the relation between structures and
pharmacokinetic properties of molecules was given in a monograph by Notari (1971).
An example is given by changes in the concentrations of two close analogues of
ethyleneimine series, such as Tepa and Thiotepa, in dog blood plasma after similar
single intravenous injections of the drugs (3 mg/kg) (Melett and Woods, 1960).

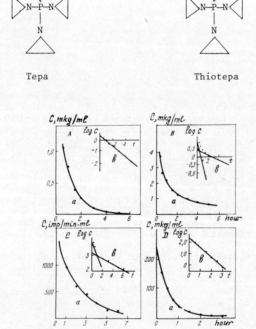

Fig. 97 Pharmacokinetics of drugs as a function of structure
and experimental animal species: Elimination of Thiotepa (A)
and Tepa (B) from dog blood plasma; elimination of cytosine-
arabinoside from dog plasma (C) and mice blood serum (D)
(Dixon and Adamson, 1965; Borsa *et al.*, 1969).

Analysis of experimental curves (Figure 97A,B) shows that a minimal change in structure, such as the substitution of a sulphur atom for an oxygen atom — elements of the same group — results in significant differences in the pharmacokinetics of drugs. Over the whole range of measurements the Thiotepa content changes obey the expression

$$C = 1.73 \exp(-0.96t), \ \mu g/ml$$

The half-life of drug elimination is 43 minutes, and the apparent volume of distribution is $V = D/C_0 = 3/1.73$ 1/kg (or 173%). The change in Tepa concentration over the same range of measurements obeys the bi-exponential relation with a distinct distribution phase (0.0 - 2.0) and with a half-life of elimination of 3.5 hours in the second phase:

$$C = 3.4 \exp(-1.9t) + 1.8 \exp(-0.2t), \ \mu g/ml$$

(Figure 97B). The volume of the central part is 0.59 1/kg, while the apparent volume of distribution is close to the value for Thiotepa (1.67 1/kg). Such a difference in pharmacokinetics can be accounted for in particular by desulphonation of Thiotepa and its conversion to Tepa (Melett and Woods, 1960).

The pharmacokinetic parameters of the drugs serve as quantitative measures of differences in the distribution and elimination of the compounds. Figure 97C,D presents data on changes in concentration of an antimetabolite Ara-C in dog blood plasma (C) and in mouse plasma (D) (Dixon and Adamson, 1965; Borsa *et al.*, 1969). As in the previous case the differences manifest not only in the parameters, but also in the types of models — the elimination curve for dogs is bi-exponential:

$$C = 10^3 \times [7.0 \exp(12.3t) + 1.4 \exp(-0.4t)], \ imp/min/ml;$$

the drug elimination for mice is described by one exponent:

$$C = 250 \exp(-2.0t), \ \mu g/ml$$

The drug distribution and elimination is seen to be slower in dogs than mice ($t_{\frac{1}{2}}$ is 104 and 21 minutes respectively). It is impossible to calculate the distribution volumes because Dixon and Adamson did not state the specific radioactivity of the drug. The distribution volume of Ara-C in mice is 1 1/kg.

Comparative data on methotrexate pharmacokinetics for man and three species of experimental animals are given in Table 43.

TABLE 43 Parameters of distribution and elimination of methotrexate in man, monkeys, dogs and mice (Gorkov, 1971)

Species	Medium	Dose, mg/kg	$t_{\frac{1}{2}}$, hour	V, %
Man	Plasma	0.1 - 10	2.30	75
Monkeys	Plasma	0.3	1.40	187
Dogs	Plasma	0.2	1.50	100
Mice	Serum	5.0	0.50	75
Mice	Serum	50 - 100	0.50	150

Drug elimination was fastest for mice ($t_{1*} = 0.5$ hr) and slowest for man ($t_{\frac{1}{2}} = 2.3$ hr). For monkeys and dogs methotrexate elimination proceeded at approximately the same rate ($t_{\frac{1}{2}} = 1.4 - 1.5$ hr). The values of apparent distribution volumes were different and for mice they changed with the dose. The latter seems to be independent of the non-linear processes in the pharmacokinetics of the drug (Zaharko, 1972).

Chemotherapeutic effectiveness is to a great degree a function of selective drug supply directly to tumours. Tumour resistance to chemotherapy is often due to insufficient supply or a rapid inactivation of the drugs in tumour tissues (Dedrick *et al.*, 1975). For example, the response of Ehrlich carcinoma to alkylating agents is proportional to the capacity of the latter to penetrate into tumour cells (Rutman *et al.*, 1968). The drug penetrates to a lesser extent into cells of Yoshida ascites sarcoma resistant to chlorambucil than it does into cells of a responsive substrain (Still, 1972). The response of a number of mice tumour to daunomycin was determined by the tumour's ability to accumulate and retain the antibiotic (Kessel *et al.*, 1968), and the differences in bromhexitol effectiveness was correlated with the degree of their cumulation in tumour tissues (Institoris *et al.*, 1971).

The problem of selectivity is not yet sufficiently studied. The knowledge of quantitative parameters characterizing the drug's affinity to tissues in different organs is important. The coefficient of compound distribution between blood and tissue is relevant. The differential equation for changes in concentration of the compound in tissue is

$$dC_i/dt = -(k_{i1} + k_{i0})\ C_i + k_1 iC_i \qquad (6)$$

where C_i is the drug content, in tissue, C_1 that in blood, k_{1i}, k_{i1} and k_{i0} are the rate constants of supply, eliminiation and inactivation of the drug. In the equilibrium state $dC_i/dt = 0$ and, consequently,

$$(C_i/C_1)_p = k_{1i}/(k_{i1} + k_{i0})$$

For active transport, the parameters should be considered as quantitative character- istics of the drug's penetration into tissue.

The differential equation (6) with respect to values C_i can be solved if the regul- arities of changes in drug concentration in blood are known. Assuming, for example, that $C_1 = C_0 \exp(-kt)$, we obtain

$$C_i = C_0\ \frac{k_{1i}}{k_i = k} \exp\ (-kt)\ -\exp\ (-k_it) \qquad (7)$$

where $k_i = k_{i1} + k_{i0}$. It follows from equation (7) that the drug content in tissue attains the maximal value in point

$$t_{max} = \frac{\ln(k/k_i)}{k - k_i}$$

The inflection point in the descending branch of the curve corresponds to the value $t = 2t_{max}$. Since values k_{1i} and k_i come into the expression for t_{max} and for the pre-exponential factor in (7), both the maximal content of the drug and the time needed for its attainment can markedly differ for different tissues.

Figure 98 demonstrates data on changes in concentrations of alkylating groups (in light transmission units) in blood and tissues of Guérin carcinoma-bearing rats after intravenous injections of thiophosphamide (27 mg/kg) and of cyclophosphamide (160 mg/kg) and data on changes in Ara-C concentration (100 mg/kg) in blood plasma and spinal fluid of dogs. The following equations were obtained for drug concen- trations in blood (C_1) and in tissues (C_i):

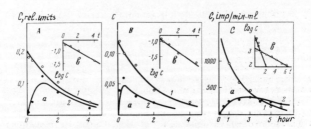

Fig. 98 Changes in the drug content in tumour and normal
animal tissue.
A, B — Alkylating groups in blood (1) and in tumour (2),
Guérin carcinoma in rats after cyclophosphamide (A) and
Thiotepa (B) injections (Mosienko and Pivniuk, 1968).
C — Label content in the blood plasma (1) and in spinal
fluid (2) of a dog after cytosine-arabinoside-H^3 injection
(Dixon and Adamson, 1965).

A. Cyclophosphamide: $C_1 = 0.2 \exp(-0.4t)$; $C_i = 0.18[\exp(-0.4t) - \exp(-2.0t)]$.

B. Thiophosphamide: $C_1 = 0.12 \exp(-0.5t)$; $C_i = 0.60[\exp(-0.5t) - \exp(-4.8t)]$.

C. Ara-C: $C_1 = 1380 \exp(-0.4t)$; $C_i = 339t \exp(-0.4t)$.

The drug distribution coefficients are 0.7 (A), 0.5 (B) and 0.6 (C).

It will be noted that the pharmacokinetic characteristics of drugs for normal and
tumour-bearing animals often do not coincide. This is accounted for by the effect
of the tumour on the body as a whole. This manifests as an increase in the drug
distribution volume in case of a large tumour especially of an ascites tumour, and
in a decrease in the intensity of elimination processes owing to intoxication, etc.

Some specific problems of pharmacokinetics of antitumour compounds can arise in
studying the relations between changes in concentrations of active drug forms in
tumour cells and in the value of the antitumour effect. For instance, it can be
assumed that the number of cells destroyed by the action of the drug on the tumour
is directly proportional to the total number of viable tumour cells $N(t)$, to the
drug concentration $C(t)$ and the time of interaction Δt, i.e.

$$N_e \sim N(t)C(t)\Delta t.$$

In a differential form this expression is

$$dN_1/dt = -aN(t)C(t)$$

where the proportionality coefficient a stands for the specific rate of tumour cell
destruction (or the effectiveness of unit concentration per unit time for the given
cell type). Thus the value a is a quantitative characteristic of the relation
between structure and activity.

The overall rate of change in the number of viable cells is defined as the difference between growth rates and tumour cell destruction

$$dN/dt = N(t)[\phi - aC(t)] \tag{8}$$

where ϕ is the growth rate constant. If at the moment of injection the tumour consists of N_0 cells, integration of equation (8) from 0 to t gives the expression

$$N_e = N_0 \exp\left(\phi t \int_0^t C(t)dt\right) \qquad (9)$$

In order to simplify subsequent calculations the integration limits can be widened from zero to infinity, since the drug is removed from the tumour in a much shorter time than that of tumour development and, consequently, curve $C(t)$ rapidly descends with time. Since according to equation (2) the change in concentration can be described by the sum of the exponents

$$\int_0^\infty C(t)dt = D\int_0^\infty \left[\sum_{j=1}^n A_{ij}\exp(-r_j t)\right]dt = D\sum_{j=1}^n (A_{ij}/r_j) = KD$$

where the constant

$$K = \sum_{j=1}^n (A_{ij}/r_j)$$

is the sum of pharmacokinetic constants. Finally, for a single administration of the drug at a dose D we have

$$N_e = N_0 \exp(\phi t - \alpha D) \qquad (10)$$

where $\alpha = aK$ is a constant value. Assuming that in controls the tumour grows exponentially

$$N_c = N_0 \exp(\phi t)$$

two expressions for the treatment effectiveness can be obtained:

(1) it follows from the definition of the effect as the extent of relative growth inhibition to a fixed time t that

$$E_1 = N_e/N_c = N_0 \exp(\phi t - \alpha D)/N_0 \exp(\phi t) = \exp(-\alpha D); \quad \ln E_1 = -\alpha D;$$

(2) by defining the effect as the shift of the experimental curve relative to the control curve, or, equally, as the difference in the time of attaining similar tumour sizes, from equation

$$N_0 \exp(\phi t_c) = N_0 \exp(\phi t_e - \alpha D)$$

we obtain

$$E_2 = t_e - t_c = \frac{\alpha}{\phi} D.$$

Dose was found to be directly proportional to the effect of drugs of the alkylating type and some antibiotics. It was suggested by Berenbaum (1969) that to introduce a correction for the existence of a minimally effective dose below which the drug has virtually no effect on the tumour would give better consistency:

$$\ln E_1 = -\alpha(D - D_{min})$$

$$E_2 = \frac{\alpha}{\phi}(D - D_{min}).$$

The expressions obtained can be modified for multiple administration assuming that the pharmacokinetic and cytotoxic characteristics (i.e. coefficients K and a) do not change from administration to administration or that their functional dependence on the number of administrations is known. In the first case, for periodic administration of similar doses at similar time intervals, the tumour size τ after n administrations will correspond to the modified expression (10):

$$N_e = N_0 \exp(\phi t - n\alpha D). \tag{11}$$

For sufficiently high n the relation $n = t/\tau$ is roughly fair. Substituting it into (11) we see that in the case of periodic administrations the tumour size changes as follows:

$$N_e = N_0 \exp\left(\phi - \frac{\alpha}{\tau}D\right)t \tag{12}$$

Thus it can be accepted that the exponential nature of the growth persists but the exponential index decreases by a value $\alpha D/\tau$. Substituting the obtained functional expression for ϕ_e in the expression for the activity coefficient $\varkappa^*$ (Chapter 1) we obtain

$$\varkappa^* = 1 - \phi_e/\phi_c = \alpha D/\phi_c\tau.$$

It will be shown later that the linear dependence between effectiveness (value $\varkappa^*$) and the dose for periodic injections was actually confirmed for some new compounds of the alkylating type of action.

It follows from equation (12) that the effect depends on value of the exponential index ϕ, i.e.

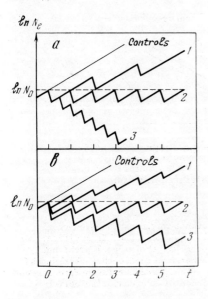

Fig. 99 Hypothetical example of a change in the size of an exponentially growing tumour under various regimens of chemotherapy. (a) $D = $ const, $\tau = 2$ (1), $\tau = 1$ (2), $\tau = 0.5$ (3); (b) $\tau = $ const, $D = 0.5$ (1), $D = 1$ (2), $D = 2$ (3). (Doses and intervals are given in conditional units.)

(1) $(\phi_c - \alpha D/\tau) > 0$ stands for partial inhibition (Figure 99, curves 1);
(2) $(\phi_c - \alpha D/\tau) = 0$ for tumour growth stopping (Figure 99, curves 2);
(3) $(\phi_c - \alpha D/\tau) < 0$ for tumour regression (Figure 99, curves 3).

Generally there exists some function controlling the chemotherapeutic regimens under which the tumour does not grow:

$$\phi_e(D,\tau) = 0. \tag{13}$$

The points above curve (13) in the 'dose-time interval' plot correspond to schedules inducing tumour regression, while those below the curve refer to partial inhibition. There might also be a similar function for normal tissues responsive to the drug. the points lying below the appropriate curve refer to the non-toxic regimens, while the points above the curve characterize treatment regimens under which the drug's toxicity accumulates and becomes lethal. The points lying above the curve $\phi_e(D,\tau) = 0$ for tumour, but lower than for a similar curve for normal tissue, correspond to selective treatment regimens under which the tumour is regressing, while the toxic action on the body is within tolerance limits. Four particular cases reflected in relative positions of the above curves are shown in Figure 100: (a) the region of selective schedules to the left from the point of intersection corresponds to frequent administration at low doses (to continuous infusion at the limit); (b) the same to the right from the point of intersection refers to the infusion of large doses at well-spaced intervals; (c) the region of selective regimens is located between the curves all along the curve lengths — any regimen will be selective in this region; (d) there are no selective regimens (i.e. it is in principle impossible to cause complete tumour regression by this drug).

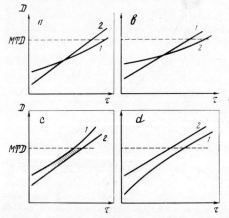

Fig. 100 Regions of selective regimens of antitumour drug administrations (crosshatched sections) as a function of the relative position of the curves $\phi(D,\tau) = 0$ for normal (1) and tumour (2) tissues (MTD is maximum tolerated dose for a single administration).

Such an approach to the search for selective treatment regimens is based on a number of fundamental premises (Berenbaum, 1969). Phenomena such as modifications of the biological properties of tumours in the course of their development and under the action of chemotherapy, the changes in pharmacokinetic characteristics of the drug from administration to administration, etc., are not taken into account. Therefore a practical application of the above method of search for selective regimens requires further development.

Another type of 'dose-effect' exists for compounds having activity proportional to the logarithm of the dose, such as some antimetabolites and antibiotics. Berenbaum expressed this dependence in the form

$$F = (D/D_0)^{-\gamma}; \quad \log E = \gamma \ \lg D_0 - \gamma \ \lg D$$

where E is the fraction of surviving cells, D_0 is the threshold dose, and γ is a constant. Examples of the dependence are given and an attempt is made to provide ground for it in terms of the kinetics of enzymatic processes. A similar dependence can be obtained from a hypothesis of effect saturation at certain concentrations of the drug (Figure 101). If curve $C(t)$ is described by an exponential function, the area under the curve cut off by the straight line parallel to the x-axis will be proportional to the dose logarithm

$$S_{ef} = A + B \ln D$$

where constants A and B are algebraic functions of the value C_{lim} and the pharmacokinetic parameters of the drug (Gorkov, 1971). Substituting the value S_{ef} into equation (9) and making further calculations, we obtain

$$\ln E_1 = A_1 + B_1 \ln D$$
$$E_2 = A_2 + B_2 \ln D$$

where A_1, B_1 and A_2, B_2 are constants.

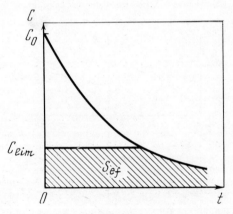

Fig. 101 'Saturation' of the action of some antitumour drugs. Increase in concentration higher C_{lim} does not result in an increase in the effect; S_{ef} is the region of effective action of the drug.

As indicated in Chapter 3, the following drugs recently proposed by the Institute of Chemical Physics, Academy of Science, USSR: dibunol (ionol; 2,6-di-tert.butyl-4-methylphenol), N-methyl-N-nitrosourea (MNU), diazane (1,2-bis-diazoacetylethane) and a paramagnetic analogue of thiophosphamide (PAT) belong to the group of effective antitumour compounds. Preliminary data on the pharmacokinetics of these drugs will be considered.

Dibunol

A generalization of data reported on distribution, metabolism and removal of dibunol from the body of man and experimental animals (Gorkov *et al.*, 1970) reveals a rather complex metabolism of the drug (Scheme 3). The main path of metabolism is a consecutive oxidation of the methyl group in position 4 to alcohol, aldehyde and acid forms, and conjugation of the oxidation products with glycine, sulphuric and glucuronic acids. The dimeric product (see Scheme 3, VI) is formed in the body of rats and rabbits in barely detectable quantities; oxidation of the methyl groups of tert-butyl was observed only in humans. Some metabolites remained unidentified.

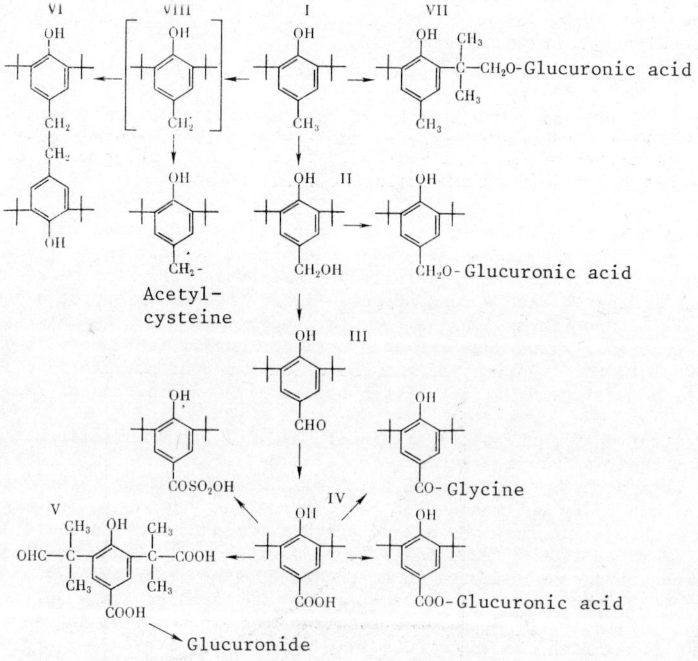

VI   VIII   I   VII

CH_3

$C-CH_2O$-Glucuronic acid

CH_3

CH_2 CH_2 CH_3 CH_3

CH_2

OH

II

CH_2- CH_2OH CH_2O-Glucuronic acid

Acetyl-
cysteine

OH   III

CHO

$COSO_2OH$ IV   CO-Glycine

V CH_3 OH CH_3 OH

OHC$-C-$ $-C-COOH$ COOH   COO-Glucuronic acid

CH_3 CH_3

COOH

Glucuronide

Scheme 3   Route of dibunol metabolism in the body (after Gorkov *et al.*, 1970; Gorkov, 1971).

After single dose of labelled dibunol most of the radioactivity was discharged in the first 2-4 days. Then the rate of elimination decreased considerably; this was ascribed to the drug accumulation in fatty tissue and to enterohepatic circulation of its metabolites. Dibunol was not fully absorbed from the gastrointestinal tract of rabbits and dogs.

Detection of unchanged dibunol in tumour (Walker carcinoma and normal (liver, fat) tissues in rats by gas-liquid chromatography showed that the drug concentration in these tissues was almost double its concentration in blood (Barsel *et al.*, 1976). After a single intraperitoneal injection at doses of 30 or 100 mg/kg the maximum dibunol content in blood (1-2 µg/ml) was observed an hour after injection; afterwards its concentration decreased with a half-life of elimination of about 2.5 hours for both dosages (Figure 102a). The tumour growth had no effect on the distribution and elimination of the drug. It is characteristic that with an

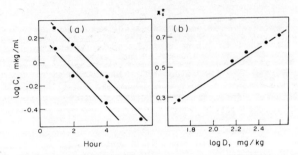

Fig. 102 Kinetics of dibunol elimination from the blood of
rats (a) after single intraperitoneal injection at doses of
30 (1) and 100 (2) mg/kg (Barsel *et al.*, 1976) and the 'dose-
effect' dependence for dibunol (b) for transplanted leukaemia La in mice.

increase in dose from 30 to 100 mg, the drug content increased in a lower proportion in blood, tumour and kidneys, and in a higher proportion in liver and fat
(1.5 - 2.0 and 4 - 6 times, respectively). These facts show the necessity of taking
non-linear processes into account when analyzing the distribution and elimination
of dibunol. A non-linear 'dose-effect' dependence is also characteristic of the
drug. Figure 102b shows that the drug activity coefficient x^* for leukaemia La is
proportional to the logarithm of the dose. Such dependence can be related to the
fact that the antitumour effect of dibunol involves inhibition of redox processes.

The concentrations in the blood of cancer patients after administration of the drug
in various medicinal forms (powder, tablets, pellets) at doses of 3-6 g were close
to those obtained for experimental animals. The elimination rates were also similar: in both cases the mean value of $t_{\frac{1}{2}}$ was about 2.5 hours. However, it is
difficult to conceive that the drug distribution in human tissues is as intense as
in animals, since it was found that a considerable part of the dose (about 80%) was
not absorbed and was eliminated in an unchanged state (Gorkov *et al.*, 1969). Later
on it was found that the dose and the form of the assayed drugs only slightly
affected the kinetics of drug concentration changes in blood, and an equilibrium
count of dibunol in blood (about 0.6 - 1.0 µg/ml) was attained on prolonged administration of the drug (Barsel *et al.*, 1976). It is characteristic that when
prolonged administration was discontinued, the drug level in blood decreased much
more slowly than it did after a single injection. Even in a week the dibunol
concentration was about 0.6 µg/ml, whereas the mean equilibrium level during
administration was 1.0 µg/ml. Possibly this was caused by slow elimination of
the drug from the fatty tissues.

N-Methyl-N-Nitrosourea

This compound is highly reactive and consequently remains in the body in an
unchanged state for a very short time. The distribution of radioactivity in organs
of mice with transplanted hepatoma 22a after injection of MNU labelled at the
methyl or carbonyl group carbon was studied by Lerman *et al.* (1974).

$$CH_3-N-C^{14}-NH_2 \qquad C^{14}H_3-N-C-NH_2$$
$$\quad\ \ |\ \ \|\qquad\qquad\qquad\ \ |\ \ \|$$
$$\quad\ NO\ O\qquad\qquad\qquad NO\ O$$

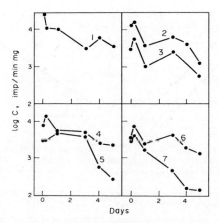

Fig. 103   Changes in label content in the total acid-
insoluble fraction of tissue in hepatoma 22a-bearing mice
after intravenous injection of MNU-C^{14} at a dose of 80 mg/kg.
(1) Blood plasma;   (2) homogenate of brain;   (3) spleen;
(4) liver;   (5) tumour;   (6) kidney;   (7) intestinal mucosa.

Figure 103 shows the measured C^{14} concentrations in the total acid-insoluble
fraction of homogenates of organs and tumour tissue after intravenous injection of
MNU-C^{14} at a dose of 80 mg/kg on the seventh day after tumour transplantation.   The
highest content of labelled meterial is seen to be in the blood plasma.   In 5 days
about 10% of the maximum level observed at the time of first measurement was
present in the plasma.   The content of labelled material in organs attained maximum
values in 5 hours.   The highest concentrations were in brain and liver, whereas in
the spleen, kidneys and intestinal mucosa the concentrations were about 50% lower.
The hepatoma tissues showed a lower level of radioactivity.   A maximum concentration of labelled material in the tumour was attained later than in the organs,
and this difference was ascribed to the lower capacity of tumour tissues for elimination of damaged macromolecules.

On injecting MNU to mice with transplanted leukaemia La, effectiveness of the drug
increased in direct proportion to the dose (Figure 104a).   As already mentioned,
such a dependence is characteristic of drugs of the alkylating type.

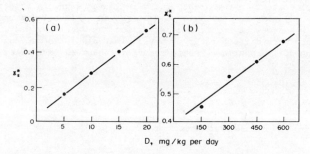

Fig. 104   Dependence of the dose effect for MNU (a) and
diazane (b) for leukaemia La (Gorkov, 1971).

Diazane

The effectiveness of diazane is directly proportional to the dose given for leukaemia La. Preliminary pharmacokinetic data on the drug were obtained by pre-transplantation injections (Konovalova, 1975). Diazane at doses of 150-250 mg/kg was injected intraperitoneally at various time intervals before transplantation of leukaemia La, sarcoma 180 and Ehrlich ascites carcinoma. The residual activity of the drug for leukaemia La was evaluated by the kinetic criteria $\varkappa_S$, and for ascites tumours by the inhibition calculated on the 8th day after tumour transplantation.

In all cases the curves for changes in residual activity had two components: in 1-2 hours the activity diminished to a minimum, then increased, became maximum in 3-4 hours, and then by the 10th hour it gradually decreased to low but measurable values (Figure 105). Such a specific shape for a change in activity may be due to the formation of an active metabolite.

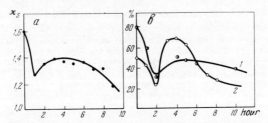

Fig. 105 Changes in residual activity of diazane in experiments with pre-transplantation injections for leukaemia La (a), sarcoma (b1) and Ehrlich ascites carcinoma (b2).

Paramagnetic Analogue of Thiophosphamide

The iminoxyl radical in a PAT molecule is a paramagnetic label which demonstrates the supply, distribution and elimination of the compound and its labelled conversion products. The kinetics of changes in paramagnetic label concentrations in blood and in certain normal and tumour tissues of mice after a single intraperitoneal injection of PAT at a dose of 150 mg/kg have been studied by the ESR technique (Konovalova *et al.*, 1976). The label concentration was determined by the amplitude of the ESR signal in samples of blood and tissues: the signal was a triplet with 15-16 G splitting.

The highest label content in tumour-bearing animals was found in tumour tissue (adenocarcinoma 755) (Figure 106). The concentration of labelled material in blood and liver was somewhat lower, the curves for the label changes were of a compound shape and were different for tumours comparable to normal control animals. The complex shape of the pharmacokinetic curves is observed most often for the labelled metabolites.

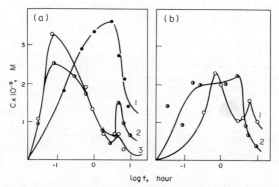

Fig. 106 Changes in spin-labelled concentration in the tissues of mice with adenocarcinoma 755 (a) and intact animals (b) after a single intraperitoneal injection of PAT-1 at a dose of 150 mg/kg (Konovalova *et al.*, 1976). a: tumour (1), blood (2), liver (3); b: liver (1), blood (2).

CHAPTER 5

MOLECULAR MECHANISMS IN CHEMOTHERAPY

Investigation of the action of antitumour drugs at a molecular level is one of the main trends of fundamental studies in current cancer chemotherapy. Problems as important as the rational choice of chemotherapeutic drugs and the development of rules for combined treatment are connected with mechanisms of drug effectiveness.

A number of papers (Larionov, 1962; Ross, 1964; Belousova, 1965; Montgomery and Strack, 1973) deal with the molecular mechanisms of chemotherapy. The alkylation type drugs, the behaviour of which depends on their distinct electrophilic properties, have been studied most extensively. This made possible a complex approach to study of the molecular mechanisms of the action of ethyleneamine and chloroethyl-amine derivatives, based on alkylation reactions of various chemical cell components, in particular of informational biomacromolecules and enzymes.

The success of studies on molecular mechanisms responsible for the effectiveness of antitumour drugs of the antimetabolite group was made possible by the advances in structural and quantum chemistry. The structural analogues of various metabolites act as antagonists of purine and pyrimidine bases, amino acids, vitamins, etc.

The antitumour effect of most antibiotics can also be explained by the above mechanisms. Certain antibiotics (for example, puromycin) are typical anti-metabolites, others may act as alkylating agents (mitomycin C). These problems of cancer chemotherapy will not be discussed in this chapter; instead I shall concentrate on chemical conversions that are or might be responsible for the molecular mechanisms of therapeutic effectiveness of the new types of antitumour drugs proposed at the Institute of Chemical Physics, Academy of Science, USSR.

1. FREE RADICAL MECHANISMS OF THE ACTION OF PHENOL COMPOUNDS

The inhibition of some enzymatic processes is known to be one of the most rational approaches to chemotherapy of various diseases. For cancer chemotherapy this problem could be the finding of possibilities for selective suppression of the redox enzymatic processes in tumour cells. Some 20 years ago inhibitors of free radical reactions were proposed for this purpose. At present this proposal is supported by the current notions about the important role of free radical mechanisms in the vital activity of cells.

In recent years the free radicals were detected directly by the EPR technique at the redox stages of glycolysis, respiration, oxidative phosphorylation, and under the action of various oxidases and dehydrogenases. The principle of interfering with the free radical mechanisms in living cells, by means of compounds binding the free radicals or readily forming new radicals that would disturb the cell metabolism, can obviously be used for chemotherapy.

Since this refers to biochemical and biological experiments, only low-toxicity inhibitors are of practical value. Sich inhibitors are known to be synthesized with the use of phenols (I), aromatic amines (II), quinone (III), etc., as active structures. The elementary reactions of these structures with free radicals $\dot{R}$ resulting both in disappearance of $\dot{R}$ and in the generation of another type radicals from the inhibitor, can be expressed schematically as follows:

$$\text{I.} \quad \rangle\!\!-OH + R^{\cdot} \longrightarrow \rangle\!\!-O^{\cdot} + RH$$

$$\text{II.} \quad \rangle\!\!-NH_2 + R^{\cdot} \longrightarrow \rangle\!\!-\dot{N}H + RH$$

$$\text{III.} \quad \rangle\!\!=O + R^{\cdot} \longrightarrow \rangle\!\!-OR$$

Polyfunctional compounds involving several biological active structural elements can also be used as inhibitors. The virtually unlimited diversity of inhibitor structures is due to the possibility of binding active hydroxyaromatic groups with the structural elements of physiologically active organic compounds of various classes. It will be noted here that certain biologically active compounds involve functional groups typical of inhibitors of free radical reactions. For instance, the B, D, E and P vitamins, the steroid hormones, certain products of amino acid conversions and the alkaloids contain hydroxy groups of the phenol type. The group K vitamins are quinoids.

Certain antibiotics exhibiting antitumour effects, in particular adriamycin, are radical reaction inhibitors. An inhibiting action is displayed by certain anti-tumour compounds of vegetable origin (podophyllin, gossypol), and also by hormonal agents (serotonin, diethylstilboestrol, oestradiol, etc.).

The wide use of antioxidants of the phenol series in chemical research, in various fields of industry and technology, and lately also in experimental biology and medicine, markedly increased the interest in natural phenols and their synthetic analogues often representing biologically active compounds.

The molecular mechanisms of the action of phenol compounds can be due not only to their capacity for inactivating free radical systems; an important part in bio-chemical processes can be played by the phenoxyl (in a general case, by aroxyl) and other intermediate free radicals (for instance, semiquinone radical anions), and also by the intermediates in oxygen reduction — by the superoxide radical $O_2^{\cdot-}$.

In an aqueous solution the $O_2^{\cdot-}$ radicals are in equilibrium with the $HO_2^{\cdot}$ radicals, and the value pK is 4.88 ± 0.10 (Behar et al., 1970)

$$O_2^{\cdot-} + H^+ \rightleftharpoons HO_2^{\cdot}$$

The superoxide radicals are very reactive. Depending on the reactant mixture composition, they can either oxidize to molecular oxygen, or reduce to hydrogen peroxide. At pH 7 the redox potential value E_0 of system $O_2/O_2^{\cdot-}$ is $-0,33 \pm 0.01$ v, and for the system $O_2^{\cdot-}/H_2O_2$ it is $E_0^1 = +0.94 \pm 0.02$ v (Wood, 1974).

Hydroxyl radicals can probably also be formed in this system by reaction of superoxide radicals with hydrogen peroxide (Beauchamp and Fridovich, 1970)

$$O_2^{\cdot-} + H_2O_2 \text{ --- } O_2 + OH^- + OH^{\cdot}$$

Quinones, the oxidation products of phenols, can also oxidize the $O_2^{\cdot-}$ radicals to molecular oxygen

$$X + O_2^{\cdot-} \text{ -- } CX^{\cdot-} + O_2$$

The rate constants of this reaction in an aqueous solution in the presence of isopropyl alcohol (5M) and acetone (1M) are:

Oxidizer	$k\ 10^{-9}\ M^{-1}\ sec^{-1}$
n-benzoquinone	1.0
2-methylbenzoquinone	0.76 ± 0.10
2,3-dimethylbenzoquinone	0.45 ± 0.10
2,5-dimethylbenzoquinone	0.36 ± 0.10
2,6-dimethylbenzoquinone	0.58 ± 0.10
Duroquinone	0.005
Vitamin K	0.0002
2,3-dimethylnaphthaquinone	0.004
Cytochrome C	0.0001

The ability of aroxyl and semiquinone radicals to form complexes with transition metal salts in the active centres of many enzymes will be noted. Such complexes were found to involve copper, iron, cobalt and manganese salts. It is essential that the stability of complexes of metal with radicals varies over wide ranges. For instance, the activation energy for decay of the complex of o-methylphenoxyl with cobalt acetyl acetonate is more than twice that for recombination of o-methylphenoxyl radicals (Figure 107). It can be conceived that such complexes can act as mediators of electron transfer in the chain of biological oxidation. Other possible mechanisms of the contribution of aroxyl radicals to biochemical processes might be due to the reactions of aroxyl isomerization, to their recombination with other free radicals in the system, and to formation of quinolide compounds:

A study of the biological effect of low-toxicity synthetic phenol compounds and of natural polyphenols showed that these are capable of influencing certain biosynthetic processes in living cells, and also exhibit a protective antitumour action. It appeared possible in a number of cases to show that there is a direct relation between the biological effect and the physico-chemical properties of the compounds studied.

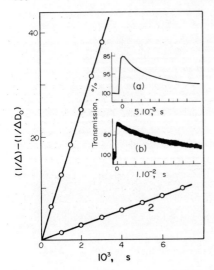

Fig. 107 Oscillograms of spectral changes
at λ = 405 nm caused by decay of o-methylphenoxy radicals (a); complexes of
o-methylphenoxy radicals with cobalt
acetylacetonate (b) in toluene, and their
linear anamorphoses (1, 2).

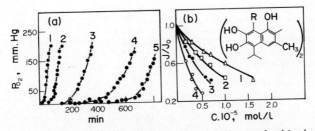

Fig. 108 Kinetic characteristics of the antioxidative and
antiradical activity of hydroxyaromatic compounds (manometric and chemiluminescent methods).
(a) Kinetic curves for oxygen absorption in the oxidation
of methyloleate (1) in the presence of d-oestrone (2), of
$\Delta^{9\,(11)}$-17α-keto-D-homoestradiol (3), of $\Delta^{8\,(9)},^{14\,(15)}$ bis-
dehydro-D-homoestradiol (4) and of $\Delta^{8\,(9)}$-dehydro-D-homoest-
radiol (5); (b) chemiluminescence quenching curves for
ethylbenzene oxidation in the presence of gossypol: (1)
R=-CH=N-CH$_2$-CH$_2$Cl; (2) R=-CH=N-$\langle$ $\rangle$;(3) R=-CHO; (4)
R=-CH=N-$\langle$ $\rangle$-SO$_3$Na.

First of all note the above-mentioned ability of hydroxyaromatic compounds to
interact with free radicals (antiradical effectiveness). A great number of the
phenol compounds series were tested on model systems and the kinetic characteristics of the antiradical effectivity of phenols was evaluated. The results of
these studied are given in the reviews and monographs of Emanuel et al. (1965) and
Denison (1971). Take as examples the data on the antioxidative activity of the
synthetic analogues of steroid hormones (Figure 108a) obtained by the manometric
method, and on the antiradical activity of gossypol and of its derivatives evaluated by the chemiluminescence method (Figure 108b). The relative antiradical
activity of certain natural polyphenols compared to the known inhibitors-antioxidants is:

Compounds and their structural formulae		$\varepsilon_{hl}\ 10^{-4} \cdot$ l/mol at $I/I_0 = 0.5$
	Ionol	3.30
	Propylgallate	62.50
	Kvertsitin	5.80
	Digidrokvertsitin	16.80
	Miritsetin	111.20
	Gossipol	12.0

In order to understand the mechanism of the therapeutic action of phenols it would be essential to find whether exchange interactions of phenols with the free radicals of the biochemical cell components is possible, i.e. to establish the possibility of destroying the biogenic free radicals by the addition of inhibitors. Unfortunately no such direct experiments were made. True, it was found that after an inhibitor (ionol) was added to a system containing free radicals of irradiated protein the EPR spectrum of protein radicals disappeared with simultaneous appearance of a quadruplet due to 2,6-di-tert-butyl-4-methylphenoxyl.

The low-temperature radiolysis method showed that this mechanism was valid for DNA radicals as well: after irradiation of DNA solutions in the presence of propylgallate the EPR spectrum exhibited a signal ($g = 1.0036$, $H = 10e$) characteristic of a semiquinone radical. The summary concentration of free radicals remained the same, but the amplitude of the spectrum component due to DNA became smaller with simultaneous increase in the concentration of radicals from propylgallate (Figure 109). The appearance of EPR signals with a structure corresponding to phenoxyl radicals is evidence of exchange reactions of protein radicals or of DNA with the inhibitors, resembling the inhibition mechanism in chemical radical reactions.

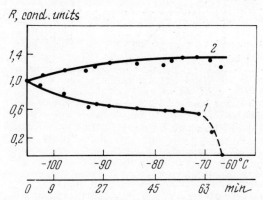

Fig. 109 Changes in DNA (R_{DNA}) and of propylgallate (R_{PG}) radical concentrations on thermal annealing of DNA (2.5 weight %) and propylgallate (0.03 M) aqueous solutions irradiated at $-196°$. $1 = R_{DNA}$; $2 = R_{PG}$.

Certain researchers used phenols and polyphenols as a tool for the study of important biological processes that were assumed to involve free radicals.

Unlike the situation for chemical systems, it had to be expected that not only the inhibitors as such will be active in metabolic processes, but also the radicals formed either from inhibitor molecules by exchange reactions with the radicals of chemical cell components or by inhibitor oxidation in the biological medium.

Thus, it was suggested that incorporation of the inhibitor into the biological system could result both in suppression and in initiation of free radical reactions depending upon the given system conditions and the inhibitor concentration. To find out the regularity of radical formation the oxidation of certain 2,5-di-tert-4-substituted phenols with oxygen in polar media has been studied.

I	R = -H	VII	R = -CH$_2$N(CH$_3$)$_2$
II	R = -C$_2$H$_5$	VIII	R = -CH$_2$N(C$_2$H$_4$OH)$_2$
III	R = -CH$_2$CH(CH$_3$)$_2$	IX	R = -CH$_2$NH$_2$
IV	R = -CH$_2$P	X	R = -CH$_3$CHNH$_2$
V	R = -CH$_2$OCH$_3$	XI	R = -CH(CH$_3$)NH$_2$
VI	R = -CH$_2$OC$_2$H$_5$		

When these phenols were oxidized with molecular oxygen under static conditions in an aqueous-alcohol (1:1) alkali solution, the EPR spectrum exhibited a triplet signal with 1.2 – 1.4 gs splitting and a ratio of intensities 1:2:1 (Figure 110a). In the absence of oxygen the spectrum structure persisted for many minutes.

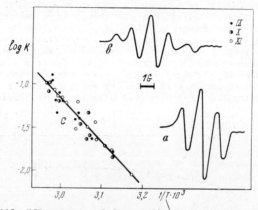

Fig. 110 ESR spectra of free radicals formed in the oxidation of 4-aminealkylphenols with molecular oxygen in an aqueous-alcohol alkali solution (a,b) and the temperature dependence of the decay rate constant for radicals from phenols IX-XI.

At high extents of conversion two additional lines appear to the left and to the right in the original spectrum. They seem to represent a doublet somewhat shifted relative to the main triplet, with a 5.5 gs splitting and a ratio of intensities 1:1 (Figure 110b).

The temperature dependence of the rate constant k for disappearance of radicals exhibiting the triplet before appearance of the doublet has been studied. The temperature dependence for radicals from certain phenols given in co-ordinates log k vs T^{-1}, transformed along axis $1/T$ into the relevant function for phenol (IX) with transformation coefficients close to unity (Figure 110c). The activation energy obtained was 23.0 ± 0.5 kcal/mole.

The correlation of the EPR spectra and of the kinetic regularities for radical consumption suggests that the same radical arises in the oxidation of the phenols studied. The triplet ESR spectrum with a_H = 1.2 – 1.4 gs can be assigned to 2,6-di-tert-butyl-1.4-benzosemiquinone exhibiting, according to the reported data, a triplet with 1.5 gs splitting.

However, the semiquinone radical ion is not the primary product of phenol oxidation in polar media. The oxidation seems to start (both as for oxidation in nonpolar media) by generation of a phenoxy radical which is not always recorded by the EPR method in view of its short half-life. With increase of the conjugation chain and of the size of a substituent in the n-position, the stability of the phenoxy radical increases and in the case, for instance, of a 4-phenyl derivative the phenoxy radical is stable even at room temperature. In the case of 4-(β-hydroxy-ethylamine derivative (VIII) the phenoxy radical could be detected spectrophoto-metrically only by the stopped flow technique. Another evidence of phenoxy radical formation is in certain cases the appearance of methylenequinones — the molecular products of radical disproportionation. The formation of 2,6-di-alkyl-1,4-benzo-semiquinone is accompanied by elimination of the substituent in n-position, and this process is characteristic of the oxidation of 2,4,5-trialkyl substituted phenols in polar media. The following scheme of phenol oxidation with electron donating substituents in n-position was proposed:

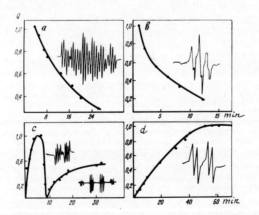

The free radicals formed by alkaline autoxidation of certain polyatomic natural phenols, e.g. caffeic acid, (-)-epicatecholgallate, quercetin, dihydroquercetin, have been studied.

The generation of free radicals in the oxidation of natural phenols is not unexpec-ted, since all these compounds contain pyrocatechol or pyrogallol groups, and the oxidation of such compounds yields free radicals of the semiquinone type. The study of EPR spectra of semiquinone radicals exhibited in the alkaline autoxidation of the compounds studied, and of the kinetic characteristics of radical stability yielded the following results.

Fig. 111   ESR spectra and kinetic curves for semiquinone radicals formed in the oxidation of natural phenols: (a) caffeic acid; (b) epicathecholgallate; (c) dehydro-quercetin; (d) quercetin.

The EPR spectrum of a caffeic acid free radical (Figure 111a) consists of 25 well-resolved lines. The many components of the spectra observed can be ascribed to the great number of nonequivalent protons. The radical concentration decreases exponentially in time with $k = 0.062$ min^{-1}; Q, the intensity of the greatest largest component, as assumed to be unity.

The EPR spectrum of (-)-epicatecholgallate (Figure 111b) represents a triplet (1:2:1). This evidences the splitting of two equivalent protons with a splitting constant 1 gs. Such a triplet with 1 gs splitting was observed for the oxidation of 5-substituted pyrogallols. The radical concentration decreases exponentially in time with $k = 0.1$ min^{-1}.

The quercetin EPR spectrum (Figure 111c) consists of two pairs of well-resolved lines (doublet of doublets) with splitting constants $a_{H_2} = 1.5$ gs and $a_{H_5} = 0.48$ gs. The changes in the signal relative intensity with time have the form of a curve with saturation and are described by a kinetic equation for a first-order reversible reaction

$$Q_t = Q_0 \{1 - \exp [-(k_1 + k_2)t]\}$$

where $k_1 + k_2 = 4.3 \cdot 10^{-2}$ min^{-1}. The stability of the free radicals formed seems to be due to probable dimerization involved in oxidation, i.e. this ensures the persistence of the pyrocatechol group and the reversible conversion

$$\text{semiquinone} \xrightarrow[k_2]{k_1} \text{quinone}$$

becomes possible.

For dihydroquercetin the change in the EPR signal type can be observed in the course of the reaction (Figure 111c). The increase in the several-line signal intensity occurs during the first five minutes.

The hyperfine structure of the EPR signal appearing at the very start of oxidation is very complicated and can be ascribed to the large number of nonequivalent protons. However, a rapid decay of radicals is observed later and in nine minutes from the start of oxidation there appears a new signal in the form of a quartet (1:3:3:1) with each component consisting of two doublets with a splitting constant $a = 4.8$ gs (Figure 111e). Approximately the same splitting is observed in the EPR spectrum of the secondary radicals generated in pyrocatechol oxidation. The part of the curve corresponding to changes in signal intensity with time is similar to the kinetic curve for quercetin and also is described by a kinetic equation for a reversible first order reaction ($k_1 + k_2 = 0.137$ min^{-1}).

It was found that the chemical properties of phenols are responsible for their acting as inhibitors of biochemical free radical processes, primarily of biological oxidation. It is important in this connection that antioxidants suppress the activity of certain redox enzymes playing a leading part in the energy-relations of the tumour cell.

It was found in *in vitro* experiments (Agatova and Emanuel, 1966) that the inactivation of certain enzymes of glycolysis, such as lactic dehydrogenase (LDG), the 3-phosphoglycerin aldehyde dehydrogenase (PGAD) and aldolase by inhibitors is observed only after preincubation of the enzyme with the inhibitor propylgallate (PG) oxidizing in the course of incubation (Figure 112). This suggests that inactivation is caused by free radicals generated in the process of inhibitor oxidation.

The mechanisms of action of the three enzymes are different. LDG and PGAD are known to be redox enzymes, whereas aldolase is a lyase, i.e. a cleaving enzyme.

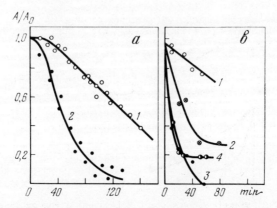

Fig. 112   Kinetic curves for inactivation of glycolytic
enzymes with the oxidized propylgallate. (a) LDG: 1 —
control; 2 — $5 \cdot 10^{-4}$ M of propylgallate. (b) PGAD and
aldolase: 1,2 — control; 3,4 — $5 \cdot 10^{-4}$ M of propylgallate.

A common property of these enzymes is the SH group in the protein molecule. In the
first two enzymes the SH groups enter into the active centre. In aldolase the SH
groups, though not involved in the active centre, are nevertheless important for
sustaining the native structure.

An extensive kinetic study of the effect of phenol compounds on glycolysis enzymes
yielded the activation energies for PG oxidation and LDG inactivation with the
oxidizing inhibitor. The values of these energies coincided (8 ± 0.5 kcal/mole).
In accordance with the data available the activation energy of PG oxidation seems
to be due to the elementary reaction of the propylgallate ion conversion to a
semiquinone radical. The coincidence of the activation energies for PG oxidation
and the protein inactivation shows that the semiquinone radical formation from the
inhibitor is the limiting step of the enzyme inactivation with the inhibitor. The
enzyme inactivation is related to oxidation of the enzyme SH groups with formation
of S-S bonds. The semiquinone radical is reduced to the initial inhibitor, as
seen from the appearance of an induction period in the kinetic curve for PG oxidation in the presence of enzymes (Figure 113). The oxidation of SH groups results
in a disturbance of the native structure of SH containing enzymes. For PGAD and
aldolase this was observed from changes in optical rotation, and for LDG this was
found kinetically from the sharp change in the constant of dissociation of the
LDG-NAD•H_2 complex.

To find out whether the interaction of PG radicals with other protein functional
groups was possible, the effect of PG on the activities of rubonuclease and trypsin
(containing no SH groups) was estimated experimentally. No changes were observed
in the kinetics of PG oxidation and in the activities of these enzymes on combined
incubation (Agatova et al., 1968; Romanovskii et al., 1973). Thus, the low
radical reactivity representing one of the properties of inhibition results in
selective interaction of its radicals with the SH groups of the protein molecule.

The LDG and PGAD enzymes are complex proteins consisting of subunits depending for
enzymatic activity on the state of their quarternary structure. As shown above,
PG has no effect on the specific enzyme activity of the LDG and PGAD dimers, but
markedly increases the dissociation of enzymes, i.e. PG may alter the enzyme
activity of LDG and PGAD by changing the affinity between subunits. PGAD is an

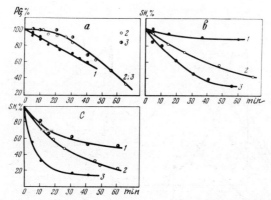

Fig. 113 Kinetic curves for combined oxidation of SH groups
of glycolytic enzymes and PG in a universal buffer pH 9.7 at
30°: (a) PH (1), PG with LDG (2) and aldolase (3); (b)
aldolase (1), LDG (2) and PGAD (3) in the absence of PG;
(c) aldolase (1), LDG (2) and PGAD (3) in the presence of PG.

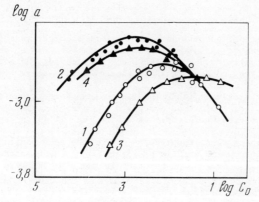

Fig. 114 Effect of PG and cysteine on the enzymatic
activity of PGAD in a glycine buffer pH 8.8 at 10.5°:
(1) native PGAD, (2) PGAD + cysteine; (3) PGAD + PG
$(1 \cdot 10^{-3}$ M); (4) PGAD + PG $(1 \cdot 10^{-3}$ M) + cysteine.

illustrative example in this respect (Figure 114). Comparison of curves 1 and 3
shows that enzyme activation occurs within the concentration range where PG
favours the PGAD tetramer dissociation, and the enzyme activation becomes weaker
within the range where PG contributes to dissociation of the dimer. Such a change
in activity connected with the lower affinity strength between subunits depends on
concentration both of PG and of the enzyme. It appeared that cysteine almost
completely suppresses the action of the molecular PG form by increasing the
affinity between PGAD subunits (Agatova et al., 1968).

Phenol compounds suppress the activity of enzymes in the succinoxidase system of
Ehrlich ascites cells, evaluated quantitatively from the rate of neotetrazolium

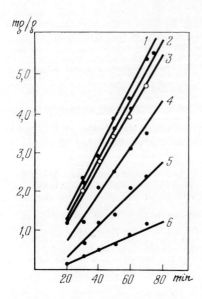

Fig. 115 Kinetics of neotetrazolium
reduction to diformazane with a suspension
of Ehrlich ascites carcinoma cells in the
presence of various inhibitor (ambunol)
concentrations. (1) Control; (2) $3 \cdot 10^{-5}$ M;
(3) $6 \cdot 10^{-5}$ M; (4) $1.5 \cdot 10^{-4}$ M;
(5) $3 \cdot 10^{-4}$ M; (6) $4.5 \cdot 10^{-4}$ M.

reduction to diformazane, as well as by other histochemical methods (Figure 115).
The suppression of enzyme activity occurs at a concentration of phenol compounds
causing no decay of cells; when the inhibitor is removed, the enzyme activity is
to a considerable extent restored. Inhibition of enzyme activity in this system is
observed only in the presence of oxygen. Comparison of enzyme activity suppression
in the succinoxidase system by inhibitors-antioxidants in tumour and normal tissues
shows that the extent of inhibition depends on the level of enzyme activity. The
higher the enzyme activity is in the tissue, the less it is suppressed by inhibitors.

The inhibiting action of PG on respiration and on the accompanying phosphorylation
was studied for isolated mitochondria of liver and of the hepatoma. It was found
that PG suppresses oxidative phosphorylation in the hepatoma mirochondria more
strongly than it does in the liver mitochondria, i.e. there is a certain selectivity in the drug action. There was no marked difference in the PG effect on the
mitochondria in tumour and normal cells, though the effect of respiration
suppression was observed in both cases (Semenova et al., 1965).

The phenol antioxidants were found to suppress other enzyme system as well. The
PG suppresses glycolytic enzymes. The PG, nordihydroguaiaretic acid and α-toco-
pherol are inhibitors of peroxidases, catalase, alcohol dehydrogenase. Phenols
possessing extrogenic activity inhibit the NAD•H$_2$ oxidase, NAD•H$_2$-cytochrome c-
oxyreductase, the cytochrome oxidase; dicoumarol inhibits respiration and phosphorylation and disconnects these processes (Wilson and Merz, 1969); pyrogallol,
sodium gallate and other substituted phenols inhibit the catechol-0-methyltransfer-
ase (Nikodejevic et al., 1970; Baldessarini and Greiner, 1973).

Great possibilities for evaluating the contribution of $O_2^{\cdot-}$ radicals to the mechanism
of the inhibiting effect of phenols on enzymes and other cell components were opene
up by the discovery of a highly specific enzyme, superoxide dismutase, in very
diverse living bodies (McCord and Fridovich, 1969). It catalyzed the dismutation
of superoxide radicals
$$2O_2^{\cdot-} + 2H^+ \rightarrow H_2O_2 + O_2$$

Addition of the superoxide dismutase to the system of autoxidized phenol or amino-
phenol results in sharp inhibition of the autoxidation rate and this is evidence of
the leading role of O_2^- radicals in these processes (Misra and Fridovich, 1969;
Heikkila and Cohen, 1973; Marklund and Marlund, 1974).

To find the possibility of inhibiting enzymatic processes with radical reaction
inhibitors under conditions preventing their autoxidation yielding free radicals,
use was made of xanthinoxidase-catalyzed xanthine oxidation to uric acid. The
latter represents an enzyme with a complex prosthetic group involving, besides
flavin adenine dinucleotide (FAD), also metals (molybdenum and iron). All the
components of the prosthetic group duffer conversions in the course of the reaction:
FAD yields semiquinone, molybdenum and iron change their valence states (Bray *et
al.*, 1965).

Out of the inhibitors tested, only polyphenols appeared to be active. All the
phenols and oxypyridines tested appeared to be ineffective under conditions
excluding the formation of free radicals. The effect of polyphenols on the
xanthine oxidase activity were:

Polyphenol	Coefficient of inactivation of the enzyme
Caffeic acid	4.0
Gallic acid	3.0
Propylgallate	0.9
Resorcin	0.45
Pyrocatechol	0.035

Kinetic analysis of the xanthine oxidase inhibition with polyphenols showed that
it was caused by complexing of polyphenols with the enzyme as such and with the
enzyme-substrate complex.

Model experiments on the complexing of PG with the enzyme prosthetic group components — with flavin and molybdenum — were conducted in order to clear up the
chemical nature of the xanthine oxidase — polyphenol complexes. The stability
constants of PG-flavin complexes on various levels of oxidation-reduction are
(Gonikberg, 1968):

Flavin	K_{st}, M^{-1}	
	pH 6.3	pH 8.1
Oxidized	119	70
Reduced	17	–
Semi-reduced	1550	20

For the FMG-PG complexing at pH 6.3, ΔH^0 = -5000 cal/mole, ΔS^0 = -7.7 cal/mole
grad, ΔF_{298} = 2700 cal/mole. The correlation between stability constants for
complexes of FMN with various donors (including PG) and the energy value of the
highest filled molecular orbit of the donor permit suggesting that charge transfer
contributes to stabilization of such complexes.

Complexing with charge transfer was observed for certain phenols, catechols and
naphthalenediols with various flavins and flavoproteins (Massey and Ghisla, 1974).
For 2,3-naphthalenediol and lumiflavin such a complex was isolated in a crystalline
state and was studied by X-ray-structural analysis. The complex appeared to be of
a 'sandwich' structure, the flavin molecule being located between two molecules of
naphthalenediol.

It was also found that at pH 5.6 PG forms a complex with the molybdate ion in a ratio 2:1 with a stability constant $1.3 \cdot 10^6$ M^{-2}.

The value ΔH^0 of complex formation is -2300 cal/mole; $\Delta F_{298}{}^0 = -8300$ cal/mole, $\Delta S^0 = +20$ cal/mole grad. The complexing kinetics was studied by the stopped flow technique. The first order rate constant for the limiting step of complexing is, according to these data, 6 ± 1 sec^{-1} at 20°. The effective activation energy is about 9 kcal/mole. The enzymatic oxidation of xanthine to uric acid as a model system for study of the mechanism of the biological effect of radical reaction inhibitors is of importance also as a biological source of active O_2^- radicals.

Extensive studies of O_2^- contribution to metabolic processes were started after discovery of the superoxide dismutase. The O_2^- radicals were found to be metabolites in all living bodies utilizing oxygen. The biological sources of O_2^- radicals are, for instance, the autoxidation processes of low-molecular metabolites, of haem-containing proteins, the transfer chains of electrons and mitochondria in microsomes (Fridovich, 1974).

The O_2^- radicals were detected in the enzymatic oxidation of xanthine by the EPR technique. The chemiluminescence arising in the presence of luminol was ascribed to O_2^- recombination. Phenols and oxypyridines act as effective luminescence quenchers (Fridovich, 1977). Quenching seems to be due to capture of O_2^- radicals. These experiments support the hypothesis about the participation of radical reaction inhibitors in direct capture of the active free radicals generated in body in the process of normal metabolism.

The O_2^- radicals are involved in peroxidation of lipids and in the hydroxylation of xenobiotics. PG and other antioxidants were also found to inhibit the metabolism of xenobiotics.

The biological role of the superoxide dismutase is thought to be connected with the body's protection against O_2^- toxicity. The bioantioxidants either present in a cell or administered seem to represent additional protection if the levels of the radical and molecular products of oxygen reduction become elevated (Fridovich, 1974).

As the tumour process (the Ehrlich ascites carcinoma) develops, the enzymatic systems of body protection against toxic lipid peroxidation products become substantially disturbed. In the organs of the tumour-bearing animal the superoxide dismutase activity suffers virtually no change. At the same time the activity of the glutathione reductase and of the glutathione peroxidase (representing utilization enzymes of lipid peroxides) exceeds the activity of these enzymes in norm for certain times of the tumour development (Lankin and Gurevich, 1976). In spite of this, there is still a substantial accumulation of peroxides (Neifakh and Kagan, 1969) contributing to the state of cachexia arising in the body at the terminal stages of tumour growth (Neifakh, 1976).

The glutathione peroxidase activity in the tumour is 2.5 times and that of the superoxide dismutase 12 times higher than in the liver of intact animals. As a result, the rate of peroxide formation in the tumour decreases (due to O_2^- capture by the superoxide dismutase) and the rate of their utilization increases (due to the higher glutathione peroxidase activity). As a result of these processes the tumour tissue contains virtually no peroxides (Lankin and Gurevich, 1976).

The disturbance of phagocytosis in leucocytes of humans suffering from lymphogranulomatosis indicates there is a lower O_2^- concentration in tumour tissue. Normally phagocytosis is accompanied by a higher rate of O_2^- formation (Babir et $al.$, 1973).

The hydroxylation system of xenobiotics during malignant growth and chemical carcinogenesis changes inversely relative to the system of lipid peroxidation (Poliakov et al., 1976), which supports the suggestion that these two systems utilize the same part of the electron transport chain (Wills, 1969; Vladimirov and Archakov, 1972; Levin et al., 1973; Giasuddin et al., 1975).

The above data seem to reflect certain essential details of the molecular mechanism of the biological (including antitumour) effect of phenol compounds capable of regulatory activities in these processes, involving free radicals.

A substantial contribution to these mechanisms can be made by the process of enzyme inactivation due to changes in the number of SS groups. Interesting results were obtained in studying the effects of ionol and sarcolysine on the content of SH and SS groups in Ehrlich ascites carcinoma and in the tissues of the tumour-bearing animal.

The treatment of tumour-bearing animals both with sarcolysine and with ionol inhibits the Ehrlich ascites carcinoma development and prolongs the life-span of these animals: by 2 days with ionol, and 12 days with sarcolysine. This is due to a more prolonged induction period for treated animals and to slower development of the process. Both drugs were administered intraperitoneally at the next day and then again twice in 72 hours after inoculation. Thus in the course of the experiment each animal received three injections, at the 1st, 4th and 7th day of tumour development. Ionol was injected at a dose of 150 mg/kg in a 3% solution of Tween-80, and sarcolysine at a dose of 4 mg/kg in a sodium chloride solution.

The administration both of sarcolysine and ionol to intact animals reduced the amount of sulph-hydryl and disulphide groups and of the protein in blood serum. A decrease in the amount of water-soluble protein in the liver of these animals was observed simultaneously. At the same time sarcolysine induced an increase in the amount of sulph-hydryl groups in liver, whereas ionol has no great effect in this respect. Both sarcolysine and ionol raised the level of SH and SS groups and of the protein in blood serum, as well as the amount of sulph-hydryl groups and protein in the liver of tumour-bearing compared to untreated animals. This increase is observed during the time the drugs are administered. Sarcolysine exhibited a stronger inhibiting effect on tumour growth and also contributed to longer persistence of the elevated level of SH and SS groups in blood serum. As the administration of drugs was stopped and the tumour started growing the amount of SH and SS groups and of protein in the blood serum again decreased.

The increase in SH and SS groups and protein content in blood serum of the animals treated was accompanied by inhibition of their accumulation in the ascitic fluid. Sarcolysine induced a more prolonged inhibition of the SH and SS groups accumulation than did ionol.

The change in the amount of sulph-hydryl groups in tumour cells both of treated tumour-bearing and control animals is of a complicated sinusoidal nature with minima and maxima. The maximum amount of sulph-hydryl groups per cell for treated animals exceeds that observed in controls. The content of protein in water-soluble extracts from tumour cells at the period of drug administration is higher than in controls, though it shows substantial variations. The minima and maxima of protein content in tumour cells coincide in time with those for sulph-hydryl group content.

The changes in the amount of sulph-hydryl and disulphide groups under the action of phenol compounds can be responsible for the changes in many key SH-containing enzymes and in various regulatory factors. These effects can result in substantial disturbances of the biosynthesis of most important macromolecules, and ultimately in inhibition of growth or in regression of the tumour.

It was found in studying the molecular mechanisms of phenol effects (Kukushkina et *al.*, 1966; Gorbacheva *et al.*, 1968; Emanuel *et al.*, 1964, 1976) that phenol compounds hinder RNA and protein synthesis both *in vitro* and *in vivo* (Figure 116). The effects of propylgallate and of ionol on the biosynthesis of protein and of nucleic acids was studied *in vivo* for mice with Ehrlich ascites carcinoma and solid hepatoma 22a.

Ionol in a concentration of 75 mg/kg suppresses by 30%, and in a concentration of 200 mg/kg virtually completely, the incorporation of amino acids.

Moreover, it was found that *in vivo* ionol suppresses to a great extent the incorporation of precursors into nucleic acids. In a concentration 100 mg/kg ionol suppresses by 20%, in 150 mg/kg by 59%, and in 200 mg/kg virtually completely, the incorporation of $8-C^{24}$-adenine.

Thus, the above shows that ionol *in vivo* suppresses the synthesis of protein and of nucleic acid in mice Ehrlich ascites carcinoma. This is also supported by the results in Table 44.

The data in Table 44 show that the nucleic acid fraction is somewhat more responsive to phenol compounds.

It will be noted that in the above an in earlier experiments the inhibiting effect of phenol compounds were observed on direct treatment of the tumour cells.

It was of interest to find out whether the inhibiting action still occurs in the absence of direct contact. Experiments used mice with solid hepatoma transplanted subcutaneously: PG was administered intraperitoneally. The inhibiting effect of PG on cancer cells still occurred; at a 150 mg/kg dose the incorporation of $1-C^{14}$-amino acids into the hepatoma proteins was suppressed by 26%, and at 200 mg/kg by 53% (Kukushkina *et al.*, 1966).

The effect of a water-soluble ionol analogue, of 4-hydroxy-3,5-ditert.butyl-N-N,-di(β-hydroxyethyl)-benzyl amine hydrochloride (ambunol) was also studied (Emanuel *et al.*, 1964). The influence of ambunol on the incorporation of $1-C^{14}$-amino acids into the proteins of Ehrlich ascites carcinoma cells is shown in Figure 116a. Ambunol in a concentration $1.39 \cdot 10^{-4}$ M is seen to suppress by half the incorporation of the label. Virtually complete suppression of biosynthesis is attained at an ambunol concentration of $1.11 \cdot 10^{-3}$ M. The inhibitors of radical reactions were found (Semenova *et al.*, 1965) to suppress the activity of enzymatic redox processes.

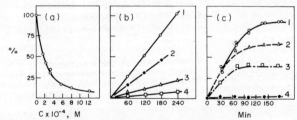

Fig. 116 Effect of phenol series inhibitors on the intensity of $1-C^{14}$-amino acid incorporation into proteins: (a) effect of ambunol (Ehrlich ascites carcinoma); (b) 1 — Hep-2 cells (in the absence of inhibitor), 2–4 — in the presence of propylgallate in concentrations of $0.26 \cdot 10^{-6}$ M, $0.42 \cdot 10^{-6}$ M, and $0.56 \cdot 10^{-6}$ M, respectively; (c) ionol effect *in vivo* (Ehrlich ascites carcinoma), 1 — control, 2–4 — ionol doses of 70, 115 and 200 mg/kg, respectively.

TABLE 44 Suppression of Na C^{14}-formiate incorporation into various fractions of Ehrlich ascites carcinoma cells by ionol and PG 150 minutes after drug administration

Fraction	Ionol (120 mg/kg)			PG (80 mg/kg)		
	Controls imp/min/mg	Experiment imp/min/mg	Suppression %	Controls imp/min/mg	Experiment imp/min/mg	Suppression %
Total acid-insoluble	1173	591	50	641	368	43
	1460	822	44	578	380	55
Nucleic acids	855	345	61	787	363	54
	1677	705	58	–	–	–
Acid-soluble	354	81	77	242	122	50
	786	286	64	–	–	–
Protein	964	672	30	610	347	43
	1696	969	44	–	–	–

An implication of the suppression of these processes can be the disturbance of ATP synthesis, which results in turn in suppression of protein biosynthesis. Indeed, when ATP is added to the incubation medium, protein biosynthesis is increased by some 20%. When ATP is added to the inhibitor-containing system, the decrease in label incorporation is the same as in the absence of ATF. This is evidence that the inhibitor exerts no essential effect on the activation of amino acids, but influences the later stages of protein biosynthesis.

The above is also supported by experiments with the addition of chloramphenicol. Chloramphenicol is known to suppress protein biosynthesis specifically, inhibiting the transfer of RNA-aminoacyl to the ribosomes. When chloramphenicol and ambunol are administered simultaneously, their effect is additive. This might serve as an indication that the protein biosynthesis chain terminates at the same stage under the action both of chloramphenicol and of ambunol.

Similar results were obtained when studying the effect of phenol inhibitors on the biosynthesis processes in a monolayer cell culture of human larynx cancer Hep-2 (Figure 116b). It was found, in particular, that the incorporation of $8-C^{14}$-adenine was suppressed by PG in a concentration $0.14 \cdot 10^{-6}$ M, $0.26 \cdot 10^{-6}$ M and $0.36 \cdot 10^{-6}$ M by 16%, 47% and 60%, respectively. The incorporation of $8-C^{14}$-adenine into nucleic acids appeared to be more sensitive ot PG, than is the incorporation of amino acids into the protein fraction. For instance, at a PG concentration of $0.21 \cdot 10^{-6}$ M the incorporation of $8-C^{14}$-adenine in 180 minutes after the start of the experiment was suppressed by 47%, and that of $1-C^{14}$-amino acids by 30%.

The effect of phenolic inhibitors on incorporation of labelled precursors into proteins and nucleic acids exhibits certain specific features. The suppression of the incorporation of labelled precursors was observed only under anaerobic conditions, supporting the conclusion that only the intermediate forms arising in the course of inhibitor oxidation can act as inhibitors.

Another peculiarity is the existence of threshold (critical) values in the protein biosynthesis suppression as a function of the inhibitor concentration. For instance, up to a 0.05% concentration PG has no effect on C^{14}-glycine incorporation into the Yoshida ascites hepatoma cells. However, at a PG concentration even of 0.1% the protein biosynthesis is suppressed by 60%, and with 0.2% concentration by 95%.

It was also found that the phenol series inhibitors can have an inverse effect on incorporation of labelled precursors. After washing off the Yoshida ascites hepatoma cells their ability to incorporate C^{14}-glycine is restored.

A comparative study of the inhibiting action of phenolic compounds and of an alkylating agent, Thiotepa, widely used clinically, showed that inhibition of protein synthesis *in vitro* requires a concentration of Thiotepa 200 times higher than certain water-soluble phenols. The curves for incorporation of amino acids as a function of the concentrations of phenolic and alkylating compounds markedly differ (Figure 117).

The extent of incorporation (ξ) as a function of the inhibitor concentration (C) can be expressed as

$$\xi = \frac{1}{1 + KC + (KC)^2}$$

whence $$\left(\frac{1}{\xi} - \frac{3}{4}\right)^{\frac{1}{2}} = KC + \frac{1}{2}$$

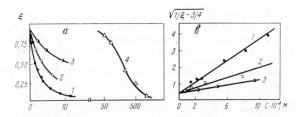

Fig. 117 Effect of phenol series inhibitors and of the alkylating agent on incorporation of $1-C^{14}$-amino acids into protein cells of the Ehrlich ascites carcinoma. (a) Kinetic curves; (b) linear anamorphoses: ambunol (1), di-tert-butyl-4-aminomethylphenol (2), propylgallate (3), Thiotepa (4).

where K is a constant characteristic of the given inhibitor. It will be seen that the value $(1/\xi - 3/4)^{\frac{1}{2}}$ is a linear function of the inhibitor concentration.

Indeed, as seen from Figure 117b, the experimental points for the inhibitor action, expressed in relevant co-ordinates, fall on straight lines. Unlike the situation for most alkylating agents which alkylate first of all the DNA, we have here direct inhibition both of DNA and protein synthesis.

It was found (Gorbacheva et $al.$, 1968) that phenol compounds inhibit transcription processes, acting directly on the enzyme, on the RNA polymerase of the Ehrlich ascites carcinoma cells (Figure 118) which represents an SH-containing enzyme. Consequently, the intermediate forms arising in PG oxidation and acting on the RNA polymerase induce the oxidation of SH groups resulting in inhibition of RNA and of the DNA-like RNA synthesis at the elongation stage (Emanuel et $al.$, 1976). On the basis of the experimental data obtained it can be suggested that disturbance of mRNA synthesis represents the primary 'target' for phenol compounds, resulting further in the inhibition of protein synthesis.

However, it might also be that the intermediate forms of phenol oxidation react with the SH groups of various regulation translation factors, the more so as the

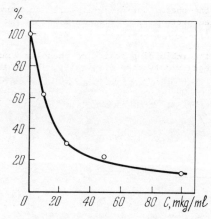

Fig. 118 Effect of propylgallate on RNA polymerase activity.

activities of certain such intermediates are connected with SH groups (Spirin and Gavrilova, 1971).

Such a substantial disturbance of the main biosynthesis processes in tumour tissue treated with phenol compounds induces changes in the duration of individual phases of the cell cycle in tumours (Frankfurt, 1975).

The effect of an inhibitor-antioxidant, ambunol, on the cell cycle in Ehrlich ascites carcinoma has been studied. Mitoses disappeared two hours after administration of the inhibitors for 12 hours. As the duration of the premitotic period was 6 hours, mitotic activity suppression seemed to be caused by the blocking of cell transition from phase G_2 to mitosis. The fraction of cells in the DNA synthesis phase starts decreasing during the first hours after ambunol administration and falls to zero in 9 hours, in a time equal to the S-phase duration. The decrease in cell numbers in the S-phase is the result of the blocking of cell transition from the presynthetic period to the S-phase at a normal rate of cell departure from this phase. Thus, ambunol causes two disturbances in the cell cycle: it blocks transitions $G_2 \rightarrow M$ and $G_1 \rightarrow S$. These disturbances of the cell cycle may be ascribed to the biosynthesis disturbances caused by inhibitors-antioxidants. The blocking of the $G_2 \rightarrow M$ cell transition seems to be due to inactivation of SH groups, since the compounds inactivating SH groups are known to inhibit the transition of cells to the mitotic phase, and the inhibitors-antioxidant interact readily with the SH groups in cells.

It was stated above that inhibition of protein synthesis is a specific property of inhibitors-antioxidants. Various inhibitors are known to inhibit cell transition from the presynthetic period to the DNA synthesis phase. Obviously, complete blocking of the $G_1 \rightarrow S$ transition caused by inhibitors is the result of protein synthesis inhibition. Thus, the action of inhibitors-antioxidants results in biochemical disturbances retarding the passing through the cell cycle and thus suppresses the tumour growth.

2. INTERACTION OF ALKYLNITROSOUREAS WITH NUCLEIC ACIDS

A great deal of attention has been paid lately to study of alkylnitrosoureas as compounds with a wide spectrum of biological action. The representatives of this class of chemical compounds are known to exhibit a strong mutagenic action, as well as specific carcinogenic and antitumour properties, i.e. they are typical radiomimetics of the alkylating series. These effects are due to a great extent to the action of alkylnitrosoureas on protein biosynthesis and to their capacity of modifying nitrogen bases of informational macromolecules.

The chemical specificities of alkylnitrosoureas are their high reactivity and, first of all, their alkylating properties. For instance, the methylnitrosourea readily splits in an alkali medium to form diazomethane which represents an alkylating agent

$$CH_3 - N - C - NH_2 \xrightarrow{\ OH^-\ } CH_2N_2 + 2H_2O + CHO^-$$
$$\underset{NO\ O}{|\ \ \|}$$

$$RH + CH_2N_2 \rightarrow R-CH_3 + N_2$$

Diazomethane methylates various organic compounds containing a mobile hydrogen atom (such as carboxylic acids, amines, phenols, compounds containing NH and SH groups, etc.).

In a neutral medium the methylcarbonium ion formed in the hydrolysis of alkyl-nitrosourea may be responsible for alkylation (Lawley, 1968)

$$CH_3-N-C-NH_2 \xrightarrow{H_2O} [CH_3-N=N-OH + HO-C-NH_2] \longrightarrow CH_3^{\oplus} + N_2 + OH^- + CO_2 + NH_3$$
$$\underset{NO\ O}{|\ \ |} \qquad\qquad\qquad \underset{O}{|}$$

The possibility of modifying DNA nitrogen bases under the action of methylnitroso-urea was demonstrated by Serebrianyi et al. (1969a,b) and Loveles and Hampton (1969). The main alkylation product was 7-methylguanine, although other methylated bases were also observed.

Besides the above alkylation mechanisms, in the case of biologically important macromolecules containing active amino groups, there is also the possibility of formation of urea derivatives:

$$CH_3-N-C-NH_2 + RNH_2 \longrightarrow RNH-C-NH_2 + CH_3OH + N_2$$
$$\underset{NO\ O}{|\ \ |} \qquad\qquad\qquad \underset{O}{|}$$

Indeed, it was found in using methylnitrosourea labelled at the carbonyl carbon atom that the reaction of DNA, i.e. the transfer of the methylnitrosourea carba-moylic $^{14}CO-NH_2$ group to DNA, was possible. The potential sites in DNA are the amino- and hydroxy groups of bases, and also the phosphate groups. A product, N_4-carbamoylcytidine, was detected among other products in a model reaction of methylnitrosourea with cytidine (Smotryaeva et al., 1972; Serebrianyi and Mnatsakanian, 1972).

Summing up the above, the action of alkylnitrosourea can be expressed by the following scheme:

$$R-N-C-NH_2$$
$$\underset{NO\ O}{|\ \ |}$$

Alkylation   Carbamoylation
products   products

Thus, it must be borne in mind when interpreting the biological action of N-alkyl-N-nitrosourea (in particular its antitumour effect) that the structures of bio-logically important macromolecules might be damaged by alkylation and carbamoylation reactions.

The alkylnitrosoureas were found to essentially change the structural properties of DNA, the damage increasing in the order: N-propyl-N-nitrosourea, N-ethyl-N-nitrosourea, N-methyl-N-nitrosourea (Figure 119).

The mechanism of methylnitrosourea action of DNA was studied in detail by Tseitlin et al. (1975) and Wunderlich et al. (1970). The kinetic curves for changes in structural properties of a DNA macromolecule (viscosity, molecular weight) under the action of alkylnitrosoureas are S-shaped (Figure 119) and straighten according to a first order autocatalysis equation. For dimensionless values it is

$$\log \frac{\xi}{1-\xi} = \log \xi' + 0.434\ kt$$

where ξ is the DNA viscosity or molecular weight value normed to the control

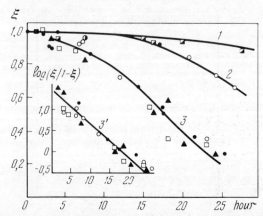

Fig. 119 Kinetic curves for changes in the DNA macromolecule structural properties under the action of N-alkyl-
N-nitrosourea (ANU) derivatives (ratio C_{ANU}/P_{DNA} = 50.1).
(1) N-propyl-N-nitrosourea;   (2) N-ethyl-N-nitrosourea;
(3) N-methyl-N-nitrosourea;   (3') anamorphosis of curve 3
in the autocatalysis equation co-ordinates.

value; ξ' and k are kinetic curve parameters varying with concentrations of the
reactants used.

The observed shapes of kinetic curves are due to that at the initial time (incubation period) the structure damage is slight, but their further accumulation
results in substantial degradation of the macromolecule.

Indeed, during the incubation time only single ruptures appear in the DNA macromolecule, but their accumulation results in double ruptures and this markedly
alters the DNA molecular weight.

Since MNU delay is a first order process with a half-life of 40 minutes, this
suggests that the main effect of MNU on DNA arises during the first hours of the
reaction (caused for instance, by alkylation of the DNA components), and further
on the macromolecule is destroyed by depurinization of alkylated units followed by
the macromolecule degradation (Rosenkranz *et al.*, 1969). This is also supported
by the 'post-effect' observed in the reaction of DNA with methylnitrosourea,
namely by the changes in DNA structural properties for a long time after MNU was
removed from the reaction medium.

It is natural to suggest that the MNU-induced degradation of the DNA molecule is
the result of the accumulation of single (f) and double (F) ruptures which can be
readily calculated from the molecular weight values for double- and single-stranded
molecules.

The kinetic functions for changes in the f and F parameters demonstrate the
consecutive appearance of single ruptures, their statistical accumulation, and the
formation of double ruptures. As seen from Figure 120, the double ruptures in DNA
molecules appear 5 hours after the start of the reaction. This coincides in time
with termination of the incubation period of nitrosomethylurea-induced DNA degradation.

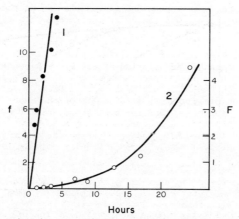

Fig. 120 Kinetic curves for changes in the numbers of
single (1) and double (2) ruptures in reaction of DNA with
N-methyl-N-nitrosourea (ratio C_{MNU}/R_{DNA} = 50:1).

After treatment with methylnitrosourea the DNA IR-spectrum exhibits some changes
in certain absorption bands, but on the whole the spectrum is only slightly
altered.

The changes in intensity of certain IR bands of the DNA spectrum, depending on the
time of interaction with MNU, are shown in Figure 121. The absorption of certain
DNA groups and bonds (of amino groups and conjugate double bonds, and also of
sugar-phosphate bonds) decreases with time. Within the first hour after the start
of the reaction these changes are still indifferent for all bands, except 1580 cm^{-1}.
These results provide evidence that during the first 2-3 hours of the reaction of
MNU wuth DNA there occur deamination and rupture of double bonds in bases, probably

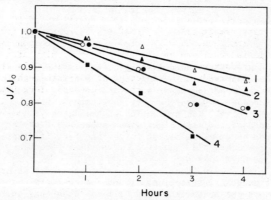

Fig. 121 Relative intensity of certain bands of the IR
spectrum of DNA as a function of the time of interaction
with MNU. (1) 960 cm^{-1} vibrations of sugar-phosphate bonds;
(2) 1605 cm^{-1}; (3) 3350 and 3200 cm^{-1} vibrations of base
aminogroups; (4) 1580 cm^{-1} vibrations of conjugate double
bonds of bases.

as an implication of the methylation and carbamoylation of these bases. The possibility of such processes was found for later reaction stages (Wheeler and Bowdon, 1965).

By conducting the reaction in a medium of low ionic strength it appeared possible to observe carbamoylation and methylation of DNA bases directly from the IR spectra of DNA treated with MNU. The IR spectra exhibited an increase in absorption of the vibrational bands of the amino groups (3350 and 3200 cm^{-1}), of the carbonyl groups (1700 cm^{-1}) and of the methyl groups (2900 cm^{-1}) of the bases. The decrease in ionic strength of the solution seems to lower the stability of the secondary DNA structure and thus to accelerate the MNU action on the bases, thus making possible the detecting of methyl, carbonyl, and amino groups before these intermediates of DNA alkylation start decaying (Gale, 1964; Wheeler $et\ al.$, 1974).

Since the DNA structure in tumours is known to have defects, it is reasonable to suggest that it is more readily damaged by chemical compounds than the DNA in normal tissues. A study of the interaction of MNU with DNA in normal and tumour tissues was conducted by the viscosimetry and the kinetic formaldehyde (KF) methods.

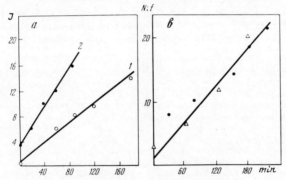

Fig. 122 Increase in defects of the secondary DNA structure
in the reaction with MNU.
(a) liver DNA (1), hepatoma DNA (2);   (b) number of defects
(N) and the number of single ruptures (f).

Defects in the secondary DNA structure against time is shown in Figure 122a: there is a linear dependence on the time of DNA-MNU interaction in all cases. However, the accumulation rate of the secondary structure defects of the DNA samples studied is different. It appeared to be higher with a greater initial concentration of DNA secondary structure defects. The evaluation of the defect accumulation rate constants from the slopes of these straight lines showed that the accumulation rate constant for DNA from hepatoma is almost twice that for an intact mouse liver (C3HA mice): k_{liver} = 4.8 hr^{-1}; $k_{calf\ thymus}$ = 7.5 hr^{-1}; $k_{hepatoma}$ = 9.4 hr^{-1}.

Thus, it was found that despiralization of the DNA secondary structure occurs at the early stages of MNU-DNA interaction. It can be caused either by single ruptures of the DNA sugar-phosphate chains or by local denaturation, since both are recorded as defects by the KF method. The secondary structure defects were compared with the single MNU-induced ruptures of the DNA sugar-phosphate chains of calf thymus (Figure 122b), and the single chain ruptures and the defects of secondary DNA structure are seen to accumulate at the same rate. Calculation shows that a single DNA chain rupture per 10^4 nucleotide pairs corresponds to one defect of the secondary DNA structure, i.e. in the given case each defect represents a single rupture of a DNA macromolecule chain.

The greater susceptibility to damage of tumour DNA, compared to that of normal tissue as determined by the KF method, is consistent with the data obtained by the viscosimetry method. During the first five hours of the reaction of DNA with MNU the viscosity of the solution of DNA extracted from hepatoma decreases much faster than the viscosity of the liver DNA under similar conditions.

Use of the KF method for analysis of the structure damage of DNA extracted from normal and tumour tissues (liver and hepatoma of C3HA mice, respectively) made possible the differentiation of quantitative characteristics for interaction of methylnitrosourea with DNA of normal and tumour tissues. This can be essential in understanding the antitumour action of N-alkyl-N-nitrosourea compounds.

The modification of DNA by alkylnitrosoureas can result further in disturbance of DNA synthesis (replication) and of the informational ribosomal and transport RNA synthesis on the DNA plate realized by an enzyme such as the RNA polymerase (transcription), as well as of protein synthesis on ribosomes (translation) in tumour cells.

It was found in various *in vivo* and *in vitro* experiments using different models that the alkylnitrosoureas inhibit preferentially the synthesis of DNA, and to a lesser extent that of RNA and proteins.

In *in vivo* experiments (solid leukaemia L-1210, Ehrlich ascites carcinoma, hamster plasmocytoma) the administration of 1,3-bis-(2-chloroethyl)-1-nitrosourea (20-100 mg/kg) inhibited DNA and RNA synthesis in tumour cells. At higher doses the inhibition of labelled leucine incorporation into proteins was weak (Vladimirov and Archakov, 1972; Gorbacheva and Kukushkina, 1970).

The propylnitrosourea (PNU) in low doses (10 mg/kg) inhibits *in vivo* DNA synthesis in Ehrlich ascites carcinoma cells (Figure 123, curve 1), but substantially activates the RNA synthesis (curve 2). A dose of 100 mg/kg inhibits RNA synthesis from the first minutes after the drug administration (curve 3).

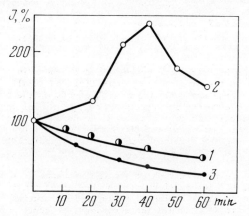

Fig. 123 Effect of propylnitrosourea on incorporation of labelled precursors of nucleic acids in Ehrlich ascites carcinoma cells.

Disturbance of the DNA and RNA synthesis occurs not only in tumour cells, but also in the organs of tumour-bearing and of normal animals (Table 45).

TABLE 45   Effect of PNU on Na C^{14}-formate incorporation into DNA and RNA of
ascites cells, liver and spleen of intact and tumour-bearing mice
(% relative to controls)

Organ	RNA		DNA	
	10 mg/kg, 30 min	200 mg/kg, 120 min	10 mg/kg, 30 min	200 mg/kg, 120 min
Liver: intact	243	31	137	58
tumour-bearing	147	37	133	43
Spleen: intact	74	27	171	53
tumour-bearing	200	32	186	40
Erlich ascites carcinoma cells	160	35	80	30

Separation of the preparations of total RNA of Ehrlich ascites carcinoma cells in the saccharose gradient showed that *in vivo* the propylnitrosourea starts inhibiting the tRNA and rRNA 4 hours after administration of a 200 mg/kg dose.

The nitrosourea has virtually no effect on the transport of fast-labelled RNA from the nucleus to the cytoplasm.

It was found in specific experiments with nuclei of Ehrlich ascites carcinoma cells possessing RNA-polymerase activity and with DNA-dependent RNA synthesis system that, unlike the radical reaction inhibitor, propylgallate, which acts first of all on the transcription elongation stage, the alkylnitrosoureas inhibit RNA synthesis at the stage of enzyme-DNA complexing and initation, acting both on the RNA-polymerase and on the DNA matrix.

This was observed, in particular, when propylgallate was added to a system containing the methylnitrosourea, and this strengthened the inhibiting action on transcription of the rRNA and of the DNA-like RNA.

The alkylnitrosoureas were found to disturb the *de novo* purine synthesis, stimulating the incorporation of formate-C^{14} and serine-C^{14} into the adenine and guanine of the nucleic acids of leukaemia L-1210 and of human leukaemic cells and inhibiting the incorporation of 2-C^{14}-histidine into RNA purines and DNA thymines. Unlike the nitrogen mustard, the alkylnitrosoureas inhibit preferentially the nucleolar RNA synthesis in L-1210 leukaemia cells.

The suggestion that alkylnitrosoureas inhibit at first the DNA synthesis, modifying the nitrogen bases, whereas the disturbances in transcription and translation are of a secondary nature, is widely accepted in literature.

However, experiments *in vivo* and those using an acellular system of protein synthesis showed that inhibition of protein synthesis occurs by direct action of the methylnitrosourea on the translation system (the polyribosomes and the soluble factors of cell fluid).

The administration of MNU to tumour-bearing animals reduces the number of translating ribosomes and results in slower translation (increase in time of the polypeptide chain synthesis). The stage of translation initiation seems to be the most sensitive and this results in accumulation of nontranslating ribosomes.

The system of protein synthesis in liver cells seems to be less susceptible to damage than that in hepatoma cells. The damage is caused by alkylation and carbamoylation of proteins. The difference in damage appearance is probably because most liver polyribosomes are bound with endoplasmic membranes protecting the polyribosomes from damage. It might be, moreover, that certain components of the translation apparatus (tRNA, initiation factors, etc.) are present in limiting concentrations in the hepatoma, and not in the liver.

Naturally such substantial disturbances in the biosynthesis of biologically important macromolecules are reflected also in the cell division specificites due to alkylnitrosoureas. It was found that at the 5th day of leukaemia La development 150 mg/kg of propylnitrosourea causes substantial disturbances in the cell cycle as seen from DNA synthesis suppression, as well as from retardation of transition from the G_2 phase to mitosis. The latter was evident from the fast and deep suppression of the mitotic activity. An important effect of PNU on leukaemic cells is the prolonged disturbance of cell proliferation. For instance, cell proliferation in spleen was retarded for 4 days after drug administration as seen from the marked decrease in the number of cells synthesizing DNA and from inhibition of the label dilution over cells that were in the phase of DNA synthesis at the time of administration. These data are consistent with the substantial and prolonged antitumour effect of PNU administered in a single dose.

3. EFFECT OF DIAZOKETONES ON BIOSYNTHESIS PROCESSES

Diazoketones, i.e. compounds containing the $-C(O)-CHN_2$ group, belong to a little studied class of antitumour drugs. These involve two well-known antibiotics — azaserine (o-diazoacetyl-l-serine) and DON (6-diazo-5-oxo-l-norleucine), and also a near analogue of DON — the antibiotic 1719 (diazomycin) (Ansfield, 1965; Goldberg *et al.*, 1973).

The accepted idea that these drug acts as possible metabolites (glutamine antagonists) is based essentially on structural resemblance:

COOH	COOH	COOH
H—C—NH$_2$	H—C—NH$_2$	H—C—NH$_2$
CH$_2$	CH$_2$	CH$_2$
O	CH$_2$	CH$_2$
C=O	C=O	C=O
CHN$_2$	CHN$_2$	NH$_2$
Azaserine	DON	Glutamine

However, this does not explain the very diverse biological effects of these drugs, in particular the mutagenic effect of azaserine (Iyer and Szybalski, 1958).

Moreover, new supermutagens and effective antitumour compounds have been found in the series of bifunctional diazoketones representing no structural analogues of metabolites. These supermutagens involve diazane (1,2-bis-diazoacetylethane) displaying a wide spectrum of antitumour action (Emanuel *et al.*, 1968).

The high reactivity of diazocarbonyl compounds of the aliphatic series suggests that the general mechanism of their biological effect consists in the participation of diazoketones in selective alkylation of protein molecules. In a weakly acid medium the diazoketones are known to be decomposed by water to form α-ketones:

$$R-\underset{\underset{O}{\|}}{C}-CHN_2 + H_2O \xrightarrow{H^+} R-\underset{\underset{O}{\|}}{C}-CH_2OH + N_2$$

In the same manner carboxylic acids interact with diazoketones to form esters:

$$R-\underset{\underset{O}{\|}}{C}-CHN_2 + HO-\underset{\underset{O}{\|}}{C}-R^\bullet \longrightarrow R-\underset{\underset{O}{\|}}{C}-CH_2O-\underset{\underset{O}{\|}}{C}-R^\bullet + N_2$$

The rates of such reactions accompanied by emission of nitrogen are dependent on the medium acidity and this might be the reason for the selective effect of diazoketones.

The diazoketone ability to form C-substutited pyrrol derivatives is also known:

$$\underset{\underset{H}{|}}{\overset{}{\boxed{N}}} + N_2CH-\underset{\underset{O}{\|}}{C}-R \rightarrow \underset{\underset{H}{|}}{\overset{}{\boxed{N}}}-CH_2-\underset{\underset{O}{\|}}{C}-R + N_2.$$

Such reactions involving diazoketones can probably occur in biological systems. It was found, for instance, that in the presence of copper ions the diazocarbonyl compounds can esterify the carboxyl group in a pepsin active centre, causing complete inactivation of the enzyme (Kozlov et al., 1967). Azaserine and DON interact with the glutamine-transaminase forming selective bonds with the enzyme, the DON selectivity being higher (Hartmann, 1962). It is of interest to note that diazane binds perferentially with proteins and virtually does not interact with DNA, as found by the equilibrium dialysis method (Plugina et al., 1971).

Other possible molecular mechanisms of the diazoketone effects were studied *in vivo* and *in vitro* using bacterial and animal cells.

For instance, azaserine blocks the incorporation of labelled formiate and glycine into the components of normal and tumour cells. DON and azaserine suppress the biosynthesis of inosinic acid and also effectively block the synthesis of purines *de novo* (Levenberg et al., 1957).

Diazane *in vitro* was found to substantially inhibit DNA synthesis in Ehrlich ascites carcinoma cells (Plugina et al., 1969). As seen from Figure 123, equivalent doses of diazane have a lesser effect on biosynthesis of RNA and proteins. For instance, at a 12 mM concentration the incorporation of a labelled precursor into DNA decreases over 6 hours approximately by 50%, the RNA and protein synthesis decreasing by only 10-15%. The effect of diazane on biosynthesis of macromolecules *in vitro* is characterized by reversibility of the cytotoxic effect: after the drug is washed off, DNA synthesis becomes completely restored. The DNA synthesis *in vivo* (hepatoma 22a, leukaemia La) also appeared to be more sensitive to the diazane action. In certain cases, synthesis of DNA was completely suppressed, but that of RNA and proteins was observed. The effect of diazoketones is suggested to involve the inactivation of the enzymes of the DNA synthesizing system, since protein synthesis is needed for restoration of DNA synthesis after the drug has been remove

It was found that diazoketones suppress the ribonucleotide reductase activity
(Plugina *et al.*, 1972), thus inhibiting the synthesis of deoxyribonucleotides.
Such a mechanism can represent the primary effect of diazoketones on the matrix
synthesis. However, the action of diazoketones on other enzyme systems also
cannot be disregarded.

The effect of diazane on the synthesis and processing of RNA was studied *in vivo*
and *in vitro* by incorporation of labelled C^{14}-cytidylmonophosphate (CMP) into
L-1210 leukaemic cells. As seen from the results given below, a low diazane
concentration (25 µg/ml) causes only a slight activation of RNA synthesis. A
higher diazane concentration inhibits RNA synthesis.

The effect of diazane on the RNA polymerase activity *in vitro* is characterized by
the following:

Sample	C^{14} CMP incorporation mole per 1 mg of protein	% relative to controls
Whole sample with native DNA	215	100
Same + diazane 25 µg/ml	260	121
50	204	95
100	183	85
200	112	52

The effect of diazane on the synthesis of RNA precursors *in vivo* is more distinct,
as can be seen from comparison of the following data:

Drug dose, mg/kg	Incorporation of C^{14}-uridine pre-mRNA	% relative to controls pre-rRNA
10	17	26
50	112	158
100	51	62

Administration of 100 mg/kg of diazane results in strong inhibition of the synthesis
of m- and rRNA precursors (49% and 38%, respectively), whereas *in vitro* the same
dose causes a 15% inhibition. Strong inhibition of RNA synthesis with a very low
dose of 10 mg/kg can also be seen.

The difference in the *in vivo* and *in vitro* effects can be due to several reasons:
either to diazane metabolism *in vivo* and/or to the action of diazane on the regulatory protein factors absent in the *in vitro* system. It will also be remembered
that DNA in eukaryote cells is bound with proteins that might affect its matrix
activity. The use of pure DNA in the *in vitro* system is not representative of
physiological conditions because of the different accessibility of DNA to drugs and
the possible effect of diazane on the chromatin proteins.

When C^{14}-uridine was administered for 120 minutes, the incorporation of labelled
diazane (50 mg/kg and 100 mg/kg) into mature r- and mRNA forms was the same as that
mentioned above. This suggests that diazane has no effect on RNA processing. It
is supported also by the different extent of synthesis of the RNA precursors at
various times of the drug action. For instance, when diazane (100 mg/kg) is administered 10 minutes before incorporation of the label, the pre-mRNA synthesis is
inhibited by 49%, and the synthesis of pre-rRNA by 38%, whereas for a time of 45
minutes it is 22% and 20%, respecitvely. If the drug was to impede RNA maturing,
an increase in the time of its action would result in accumulation of high-molecular

precursors. The increase in the inhibiting diazane action with time supports once
more the suggestion that diazane has an effect on the synthesis of RNA precursors,
but not on their processing.

As consistent with the results obtained in studying the molecular mechanisms of the
action of diazoketones as inhibitors of the synthesis of DNA precusors, autoradiographic studies revealed a blocking of the $G_1 \rightarrow S$ transition when L-1210 leukaemia
cells were treated with diazane (Goncharova *et al.*, 1976). This was found in
experimenta with repeated administration of H^3-thymidine. As seen from Figure 124,
the administration of a labelled precursor in the absence of diazane results in a
linear increase in the fraction of labelled cells (a larger number of cells enter
the S-phase within a longer time interval). With a single injection of diazane the
fraction of labelled cells remains the same after four subsequent administrations
of H^3-thymidine. It follows that diazane blocks the transition from the presynthetic phase to DNA synthesis and its effect persists for 8 hours.

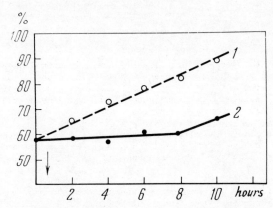

Fig. 124   Change in fraction of labelled cells upon multiple
administration of ^{3}H-thymidine in controls (1) and after
administration of diazane (2).

An autoradiographic study of the cells present in the S-phase at the time of
diazane administration showed that the mean number of granules over the labelled
cells remains constant for more than 30 hours, i.e. division is blocked during this
time. Within the following 40 hours the label dilution is doubled, whereas in
controls a double decrease in the number of granules is observed even in 10 hours.
This is evidence that the intensity of the restored cell division is considerably
lower compared to controls. At the same time the label index throughout the
experiment differed only slightly, which is an indication of the absence of
selective cell dstruction in the S-phase.

Comparison of the mitotic index changes during 40 hours after diazane administratio
with the dynamics of changes in the fraction of labelled mitoses within all control
mitoses suggested that there is no blocking of the $G \rightarrow M$ cell transition and that
there is inhibition of DNA synthesis with cell damage to the end of the S-phase
(Goncharova *et al.*, 1976).

CHAPTER 6

FREE RADICALS AND TUMOUR GROWTH

Very extensive studies of the role of free radicals in normal physiology and various pathological processes have been conducted in recent years. Extensive investigations were facilitated by the use of electron paramagnetic resonance (EPR) techniques making possible detection, identification and quantitative determination of free radicals in various specimens (Ingram, 1972; Pryor, 1976).

The EPR technique can be used in most chemical studies of structures and properties of free radicals. The use of this technique in biological and medical research is difficult. However, with further development of the EPR technique the difficulties are being resolved.

EPR studies of biological substances were first conducted in the middle nineteen-fifties and comprehensive information in this field has been accumulated. Not only the contribution of free radicals to most important processes of cellular vital activity (which was once questioned), but also the role of other paramagnetic centres (mainly metal complexes) have been established. The studies on the mechanisms of most redox enzymatic reactions underlying glycolysis, respiration, phosphorylation, etc. might be mentioned here.

Great attention was paid, especially in the last 15 years, to the role and behaviour of free radicals in various pathological processes, in particular in malignant tumour growth (Emanuel, 1973, 1974a, 1976; Gordy, 1958; Petyaev, 1972; Kozlov, 1973).

Interest in this problem was generated by research into the chemistry of various carcinogenic agents, first of all on their capacity to enter reactions accompanied by transfer of one electron. For instance, some carcinogenic agents were found to possess high electron donor and acceptor properties and to convert readily to free radical states in the course of biological oxidation. The formation of such reactive species naturally has a great effect on many biochemical processes including those responsible for transformation of a normal into a malignant cell (Swartz, 1972).

1. NATURE OF PARMAGNETIC CENTRES IN NORMAL AND TUMOUR TISSUES

Convincing evidence for a quantitative correlation between the changes in intensity of EPR signals and the level of metabolic activity has been obtained.

Paramagnetic centres representing various metal complexes or free radicals of the semiquinone type have been detected in active metabolizing systems. Most centres are localized, as iron and copper complexes and also as free radicals of flavins, uniquinones, and other co-factors of redox enzymes, in the mitochondrial respiration chain (Orme-Johnson et $al.$, 1974a,b).

The EPR signals from haem and nonhaem iron in mitochondria could be recorded only at 100 K and lower, because of the strong spin-lattice coupling characteristic of these paramagnetic centres.

The active centres of proteins containing non-haem iron represent polynuclear iron complexes containing protein RS-groups and sulphur atoms (Sands and Dunham, 1974).

The majority of these complexes are diamagnetic in the oxidized state, and pass to the paramagnetic state by reduction. Signals from non-haem ferroproteins have complex shapes with absorption localized mainly in the 1.94 g-factor region. For example, the EPR spectrum of adrenoxine exhibits an axial symmetry of the paramagnetic centre (g_I = 2.025), (g_{II} = 1.932). The EPR spectrum of the Rieske protein from the third Green complex in mitochondria is still more complex and corresponds to rhombic symmetry (g_1 = 2.026; g_2 = 1.887; g_3 = 1.81). The low-temperature liquid-helium technique of recording EPR spectra exhibited by biological substances permits detection of many non-haem ferroproteins functioning in mitochondria (Orme-Johnson, 1974a,b). At the temperature of liquid nitrogen boiling only an insignificant part of these centres was detected by the EPR technique.

Active centres of both haemoproteins and copper-containing proteins in mitochondria are paramagnetic in the oxidized state only (Orme-Johnson, 1974a,b). In living tissues most metal complexes of enzymatic systems are in the reduced state. Therefore mostly signals from proteins containing non-haem iron are observed in the EPR spectra of these substances.

Free radical states of pathological tissues were the main subject of early research carried out in the USSR and abroad by the EPR technique in the middle of the nineteen-sixties. At that time the EPR technique could not be used for wet samples, since the presence of water markedly decreased the sensitivity of EPR spectrometers. Most investigations made use of lyophilic samples exhibiting the EPR signal from free radicals at g = 2.0057 with $\Delta H \sim 8$ gs. Later on it was suggested that this signal was due to free radicals appearing due to the contact of wet air with the lyophilically dried tissue preparation (Ruuge et $al.$, 1976).

The free radical centres exhibiting EPR signals at g = 2.00 in native tissue are localized mostly in the mitochondria. The major contribution to the EPR signal from free radicals seems to be that from flavins in the semi-oxidized state and from the semiquinone form of ubiquinones.

These free radicals exhibit a slightly asymmetrical EPR signal at $g = 2.0015$ with a halfwidth $\Delta H = 14-15$ gs. The signal is recorded in frozen and in wet native tissue preparations at room temperature. The signal intensity is $10^{14} - 10^{16}$ spin/g. It follows that *in vivo* only an insignificant part of the flavins and ubiquinones in tissues are in the paramagnetic state.

Thus, depending on the technique of sample preparation and conditions of the EPR spectrum recording at $g = 2.00$ at least two different signals are observed: one with $\Delta H = 14-15$ gs (free radical form of organic co-enzymes) and another with $\Delta H = 8$, due to the ascorbic acid anion radical which is absorbed by the proteins

$$O=C-C=C-CH-CH-CH_2$$

The first signal is characteristic of wet (and also of frozen) tissue preparations, the second is observed for lyophilically dried samples.

The intensity of the signal with $\Delta H = 8$ gs is 100% higher than that of the wet tissue free radicals. When there is no contact between the lyophilically dried preparations and air, the recorded signal is identical in its parameters ($\Delta H = 14-15$ gs) to that from a wet tissue radical. Contact of the sample with oxygen of the air induces the appearance of a signal with $\Delta H = 8$ gs. This results in narrowing of the signal to 8-10 gs and in an increase in its intensity.

When studying free radical centres, the technique of sample prearation and the conditions of EPR spectrum recording must always be stipulated. Unfortunately many authors give no precise details of the signals and this makes it difficult to decide to which of the two radical types they belong.

Besides the EPR signals from mitochondria, signals due to the oxidized form of cytochrome P-450 (functioning in the electron transport microsomal chain) and to metal complexes of manganese and molybdenum were also observed for frozen tissues. The signal of cytochrome P-450 is characterized by the g-factor values: $g_1 = 2.42$, $g_2 = 225$, $g_3 = 1.91$. The signal exhibited by manganese complexes has a six-component hyperfine structure, three components falling within the range of $g = 2.17$ to 2.00. Molybdenum complexes representing active centres of xanthine oxidase and sulphite reductase (functioning in liver cell cytoplasm) exhibit an EPR signal at $g = 1.97$.

The EPR spectrum of frozen mouse liver tissue, which is characterized by several signals different in intensity and in g-factors, is presented in Figure 125. By

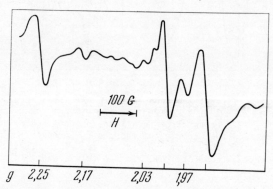

Fig. 125   The EPR spectrum of frozen liver tissue from C3H mice.

assigning these signals to complexes involving non-haem iron, cytochrome P-450, molybdenum and manganese, as well as to free radicals at $g = 2.004$, it is possible to correlate the intensities of individual signals with a specific metabolic process.

The most complete data on the EPR spectra of frozen tissues of various normal animals are given by Ruuge and Kornienko (1969).

Additionally, other signals not inherent in normal tissues are often observed in the EPR spectra of tumour tissues. Their appearance over a wide range of magnetic field strength was shown by Nebert and Mason (1963). However, these signals were not identified. EPR signals at $g = 2.01$-2.016 assigned to metal ions have been observed by Mallard and Kent (1964). Signals with a width of about 34 gs with triplet hyperfine structure exhibited by certain tumours were ascribed to inter-action of an unpaired electron with the ^{14}N nucleus (Brennan *et al.*, 1966). A certain regularity in the variation of the g-factor of a single signal from tumour tissue was found in research conducted clinically (Wallace *et al.*, 1970).

A signal at $g = 2.035$ in the early stages of development of malignancy was reported by Vithayathil *et al.* (1965). It was exhibited by rat liver long before the appearance of a tumour. However, in subsequent studies of the carcinogenic action of diethylnitrosoamine and dimethylaminoazobenzene no signals at $g = 2.035$ came from the liver. The same signal was recorded in the livers of rats fed with oxidized fish oil. The signal intensity ($g = 2.03$) changed during the course of the experi-ment and a characteristic maximum was observed on the 20th day (Figure 126a). The signal at $g = 2.03$ can also appear in rat liver due to the action of agents possess-ing no carcinogenic activity such as acetone, ether, ethanol, decylxanthogenate, and phenol (Figure 126b) (Emanuel *et al.*, 1973). The above agents were admin-istered in maximum tolerated doses, so that the signal appearance seems to be related to the cytotoxic action of chemical compounds damaging or blocking the electron carriers in mitochondria containing non-haem iron.

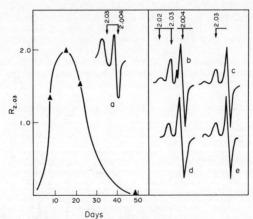

Fig. 126 Nitrosyl iron complexes in rat liver after various
treatments.
(a) The EPR spectrum from the livers of rats fed oxidized
fish oil and the kinetics of changes in intensity of the
signal at $g = 2.03$; (b) the EPR spectra of rat liver treated
with decylxanthogenate (b), acetone (c), ethanol (d) and
phenol (e).

It was found later that non-toxic doses of a compound can induce the signal at
$g = 2.03$. This signal is exhibited by the liver and kidney of rabbits under the
action of certain non-inhalation narcotics. The histological changes observed
indicate development of moderate hypoxia and the absence of toxic action. The
signal at $g = 2.03$ appeared only at the time of most acute action of narcotics and
persisted for only a short time in the post-narcosis period.

The unspecificity of the signal at $g = 2.03$ for early stages of the development of
malignant growth was corroborated by its presence in necrotic tissues (Brennan *et
al.*, 1966) and in isolated tissues under various conditions of storage (Azhipa *et
al.*, 1966).

A later investigation of the nature of the signal showed (Azhipa *et al.*, 1969;
Woolum and Commoner, 1970) that dinitrosyl complexes of non-haem iron bound with
two closely located RS-groups of protein were responsible for this signal:

$$\begin{array}{c} \text{S} \diagdown \quad \diagup \text{NO} \\ \quad \text{Fe}^+ \\ \text{S} \diagup \quad \diagdown \text{NO} \end{array}$$

EPR triplet signals unusual for biological objects were obtained for many experimental tumours frozen whilst in the stage of active metabolism (Saprin *et al.*, 1966;
Mil *et al.*, 1971). These signals with a half-width about 75 gs are characterized
by the values $g_1 = 1.98$, $g_2 = 2.03$, $g_3 = 2.07$, and also by the presence of hyperfine
triplet structure with $g_m = 2.007$ and splitting $H = 15$ gs. For instance, such signals
were found in the tissue of sarcoma 45, Walker carcinosarcoma, hepatoma 22a, etc.
(Figure 127a,b). The signals are very stable: their shape and intensity persist
for many days after thawing and keeping in an open ampoule at room temperature.
Comparative studies of triplet signals in the EPR spectra of tumour tissues and
model nitrosyl complexes of haem-containing proteins (catalases, cytochromes, haemoglobin) under different treatments, such as heating, oxidizing or reducing agents,
showed their complete identity. Thus, the triplet is due to nitrosyl complexes of
various haemoproteins.

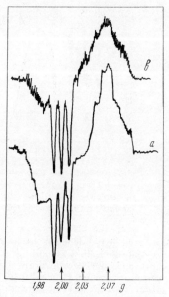

Fig. 127   The EPR spectra of nitrosyl
           iron complexes in tumours.

           (a) Walker carcinosarcoma;
           (b) hepatoma 22a.

It was suggested in the course of fractionation of tumour cells to subcellular components, that the triplet signals could be due to metal complexes, localized in mitochondria and microsomes (Borukaeva *et al.*, 1969). The functional activity of the latter was disturbed, but not completely suppressed. Signals of a similar kind can appear under the action of carcinogens on nitrosyl complexes of microsomal haemoproteins as well as in tissues in the course of other processes not related to malignant growth. It will be noted here that not all tumour tissues exhibited triplet signals. Ascites tumours, for example, exhibited an ordinary single signal, at a g-factor close to that for a free electron. For ascites sarcoma 180 the signal was markedly asymmetric.

It can be concluded from the above that it is still difficult to use the signal type and its radiospectroscopic characteristics for cancer diagnosis. On the whole the only reliable difference between normal and tumour tissues lies in the intensities of their EPR signals, and this could be taken as the basis for studying the rules for changes in the paramagnetic properties of the organs and tissues in the course of carcinogenesis and of tumour growth.

2. CHANGES IN PARAMAGNETIC PROPERTIES OF TISSUES DURING CARCINOGENESIS

Changes in the tissue's free radical content represent a specific phenomenon accompanying carcinogenesis. Certain kinetic regularities for changes in signal intensity in frozen tissues were found for various types of viral and chemical carcinogenesis. An increase in free radical content in the process of cell infection with various adenoviruses was observed for cultures of embryo fibroblasts of hamsters and rats. As seen in Figure 128a, a distinct increase in the intensity of the signal at g = 2.004, becoming maximum on the 4th day, was observed even on the next day. Of interest was the sharp simultaneous intensification of aerobic glycolysis in cells of the infected culture (Figure 128b) (Saprin *et al.*, 1971).

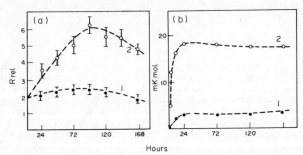

Fig. 128 Free radicals and aerobic glycolysis in hamster fibroblast culture: (a) relative intensity of the signal at g = 2.004 in the EPR spectra of cells in normal (1) and under the action of adenovirus type 12 (2); (b) intensification of aerobic glycolysis in cells of infected culture (2) compared to normal (1).

More complex regular dependences were observed for changes in paramagnetic properties of tissues of animals during carcinogenesis. In the case of diethylnitrosourea administration a 40% decrease in the free radical content of liver compared to normal was observed until the 10th day. Soon after there was an increase in the free radical content rising to a maximum on the 22nd day (50% above normal), with

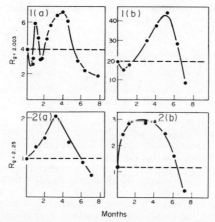

Months

Fig. 129   Content of free radicals (curves 1a,b) and of
cytochrome P-450 (curves 2a,b) in rat liver during carcinogenesis induced by diethylnitrosoamine (a) and dimethylaminoazobenzene (b).

a subsequent gradual decrease to normal (Figure 129a) (Wallace *et al.*, 1970).   A
period of decrease in the free radical concentration at the initial period of
carcinogenesis was also observed with other carcinogens used.   Similar data were
obtained for the tissues of liver, muscle and lungs in rats treated with 3,4-benzo-
apyrene, dimethylbenzanthracene and 20-methylcholanthrene (Abdurasulov *et al.*, 1967).
A decrease in the EPR signal intensity (g = 2.003) was observed in the first 15 days
of the experiment, which corresponds to the initial section of curves 1a,b in
Figure 129.   This section is similar to the curves for the effects of toxic doses
of DDT and benzene, and also of strongly oxidized sunflower oil.   This seems to be
evidence of the toxic action of the carcinogenic agents, rather than of their
specific action.

As seen in Figure 129a, a prolonged period of increase in the EPR signal intensity
was noted after 40-50 days of carcinogen action, when the free radical concentration became close to normal values.   To the 90-110th day the free radical
concentration became maximum, exceeding the norm by 75%.   This phenomenon can be
conceived to be specific for the action of different carcinogenic agents.   For
instance, 2-acetylaminofluorene caused a considerable increase in free radical
content in liver of experimental animals to the 90-110th day.

This period is characterized histologically as the stage of diffusive and focal
hyperplasia.   With further development of hepatocarcinogenesis, when in 130-150 days
tumours arise in most animals, the free radical concentration decreased;   in
developed tumours it appeared to be half the normal concentration.

Similar changes were also observed in the course of hepatocarcinogenesis under the
action of dimethylaminoazobenzene: at early stages of carcinogen action the free
radical content decreased by 30%;   at the stage of diffusion-focal hyperplasia
(2-5 months) the free radical processes became more intense and in growing tumours
the free radical content again decreased to half normal values (Figure 129b).

These regularities are in agreement with the data reported by other authors.   For
example, a decrease in free radical content compared with normal was observed both
at the early stages of carcinogenesis caused by dimethylaminoazobenzene (DAAB) or

acetylaminofluorene (AAF) and in the tumours induced by these agents (Sidorik, 1964).

Tissue	Time of experiment	Relative amplitude of EPR signals at g = 2.004
Liver of intact rats	–	1.0
Liver of rats treated with DAAB	8-30 days	0.7
Hepatoma (DAAB)	5-10 months	0.25
Liver of rats treated with AAF	8-30 days	0.6-0.7
Hepatoma (AAF)	6-10 months	0.3

Along with changes in the intensity of the signal at g = 2.004 in the course of carcinogenesis changes were observed also in the cytochrome P-450 signal at g = 2.25, connected with the cytochrome P-450, the terminal oxidase of the microsomal system of multipurpose oxidases. The intensity of this signal was so high that it was readily recorded not only in isolated microsomes, but in the whole liver tissue.

Such changes in signals, exhibited by other paramagnetic centres as well, are characteristic of even the early stages of chemical carcinogenesis. For instance, a marked suppression of the microsomal detoxic system and a five-fold increase in the intensity of the signal at g = 2.05 under the action of aminoazofluorene were observed in two months.

Changes in the cytochrome P-450 content and its considerable decrease in tumours evaluated by the amplitude of the signal at g = 2.25 (curves 2a,b in Figure 129) were observed in the course of carcinogenesis induced by diethylnitrosoamine and dimethylaminoazobenzene. For example, the cytochrome P-450 content in developed tumours was reduced 4-5 fold as compared to normal liver. This phenomenon might be related, in particular, to the reduced capacity of tumour cells for conversion of the hepatocarcinogenic agent. At the same time activation of the microsomal system of multipurpose oxidases by means of the so-called inductors is known to be possible. Various chemical compounds including the inhibitors of free radical processes, proposed as antitumour drugs, can be inductive.

It is interesting to compare experimental data on the increase in cytochrome P-450 concentration upon administration of an inhibitor of free radical reactions (ionol) and on its anticarcinogenic effect during chemical carcinogenesis induced with dimethylaminoazobenzene, 3,4-benzoapyrene and dimethylbenzanthracene.

In 1967 the effect of ionol on hepatocarcinogenesis caused by n-dimethyl-aminoazo-benzene was studied under the assumption that free radical reactions were intensified (stimulated) in the course of malignant growth. The experimental animals (rats) received for 150 days a food containing n-dimethylaminoazobenzene (0.6%) and ionol (0.3%) dissolved in corn oil. Tumours arose neither in the thirty Wistar rats, nor in the fourteen August rats in the course of the whole experiment (12-15 months). No pre-tumour changes were observed after various terms of combined feeding of rats with the carcinogen and ionol (Figure 130a).

The anticarcinogenic effect of inhibitors-antioxidants of the phenol series was later confirmed by other researchers (Wattenberg, 1972, 1973). It was found that such an effect was exerted by ionol and butylhydroxyanisole in the chemical carcino-genesis induced by polycyclic hydrocarbons. These phenolic antioxidants inhibit development of mouse pre-stomach and rat mammary tumours (reducing the number of tumour-bearing animals and the number of tumours in an animal). A similar effect of butylhydrocyanisole was observed for lung cancer arising in mice after DMBA, benzoapyrene, urethane and diethylnitrosoamine were added to their food.

A water-soluble analogue of ionol (4-hydroxy-3,5-di-tert-butyl-α-methylbenzylamine hydrochloride) was also found to be an anticarcinogenic agent for subcutaneous

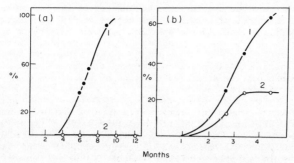

Fig. 130   Kinetic curves for changes in the frequency of
appearance of tumours induced by dimethylaminoazobenzene
(1a) and 3,4-benzopyrene (1b).   Anti-carcinogenic action
of ionol (2a) and 4-hydroxy-3,5-di-tert.butyl-α-methyl-
benzylamine hydrochloride (2b).

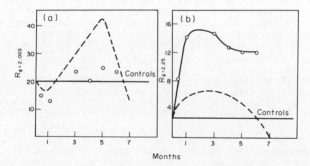

Fig. 131   Concentration of free radicals (a) and cytochrome
P-450 (b) in rat liver under combined action of dimethylaminoazobenzene and ionol.   The dotted curves refer to
changes during carcinogenesis induced by dimethylaminoazobenzene.

sarcoma induced in rats with 3,4-benzopyrene (Figure 130b) (Burlakova and
Molochkina, 1974).

As to the changes in the EPR spectra of liver tissue induced by a diet including
carcinogen and ionol, it can be seen in Figure 131a that the free radical concentration first decreases, and then (at the stage of diffusive and focal hyperplasia)
slightly increases, remaining however at a normal level.

The cytochrome P-450 content increases approximately 2.5-fold under the action of
dimethylaminoazobenzene, whereas with a diet involving the carcinogen and ionol the
intensity of signal at g = 2.25 is almost six times higher, with subsequent persistence of this level for a long time (Figure 131b).   This provides evidence that
ionol is capable of acting as an inducer of the enzymatic system of multipurpose
oxidases in liver microsomes.

Though the mechanism of the anticarcinogenic action of radical process inhibitors
is not yet clear, it can be conceived to be based on the antiradical properties of
antioxidants and their capacity to inactivate radicals (see Chapter 5, section 1).

In connection with the above regularities in changes of the tissue's paramagnetic properties under the action of chemical carcinogens it is expedient to state here also the possibilities of the kinetic approach to investigation of mechanisms of action of various factors of the environment on living bodies.

Such an approach was first realized when studying the paramagnetic properties of rat liver and brain under the action of DDT (one of the most widely used insecticides), benzene, and oxidized fats.

Figure 132a demonstrates the peculiarities of action of the above compounds causing alteration of the stationary level of free radicals in rat liver. When use was made of DDT and benzene, the stationary concentration of free radicals considerably deviated from normal, even at the end of the experiment. A sharp suppression of free radicals in brain was observed (Figure 132b).

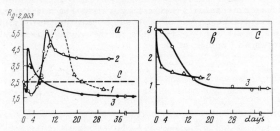

Fig. 132   Changes in free radical concentration in liver (a)
and brain of rats fed with oxidized sunflower oil (1),
benzene (2) and DDT (3).

Thus it is evident now that free radical centres and paramagnetic metal complexes suffer various changes in the course of tumour growth. Study of these changes can be of importance for the problems of early diagnostics of malignant diseases, the elucidation of methods for prophylaxis and therapeutic treatment of cancer, and studies concerning mechanisms of the action of environment factors on living bodies

3.   KINETIC REGULARITIES FOR CHANGES IN THE RADICAL CONTENT IN THE COURSE OF TUMOUR GROWTH

Inhibitors of free radical processes were worth investigating as antitumour drugs, especially as it was also assumed that the free radical reactions were intensified during rapid tumour growth and, as a consequence, the free radical concentrations increased. For a long time this point of view received no experimental confirmation; the data reported were very contradictory. For instance, an increased content of free radicals (compared to normal) was found in four transplanted tumours in rats (rhabdomyosarcoma, lymphosarcoma, sarcomas M-1 and SSK) (Petyaev, 1972):

Tissue	Number of cases studied	10^{16} spin/g
Sarcoma M-1	20	10.1 ± 2.0
Sarcoma SSK	20	6.8 ± 1.0
Rhabdomyosarcoma	20	4.5 ± 0.5
Muscle (normal)	20	2.54 ± 0.2
Heart (normal)	10	2.8 ± 0.02
Lymphosarcoma	20	7.6 ± 1.0
Thymus (normal)	4	1.02 ± 1.33

A similar effect was also reported for blood leucocytes of patients with leukaemia (Pavlova and Livenson, 1965).

At the same time the free radical content in tissues of certain liver tumours (Commoner *et al.*, 1954; Truby and Goldzieher, 1958), of sarcoma (Saprin *et al.*, 1971) and of other experimental tumours was found to be lower than in appropriate normal tissues.

However, the kinetic approach to studying of the changes in free radical content in malignant growth was not used in all these projects. Yet it is just the know-ledge of kinetic regularities for changes in free radical concentrations during tumour processes that opens up new possibilities for investigation of the nature of malignant growth, for working out rational principles of cancer chemotherapy and for finding new antitumour drugs.

Experimental analysis of regular kinetic changes in free radical states in the process of tumour growth completely corroborated this point of view. The regul-arities established permitted interpretation of the contradictory data on free radical content variation during malignant growth.

A considerable increase in free radical content was always found in tumour tissues at the inital latent stage of development. A decrease in the free radical level always corresponded to the terminal phase of tumour growth (Saprin *et al.*, 1967).

The EPR spectra of tumour tissue, blood and organs of tumour-bearing animals were obtained for lyophilically dried sampled with moisture no higher than 1.4 - 1.6%. The samples were prepared in argon with subsequent evacuation of the ampoules. The signal halfwidth was 8-10 gs.

Statistical treatment of the results obtained made use of the weighted average of the EPR signal amplitude, of the dispersion values and reliable intervals for each run of experiments. The kinetic curves for changes in free radical content in the course of tumour development were plotted on the basis of these calculations (Figure 133).

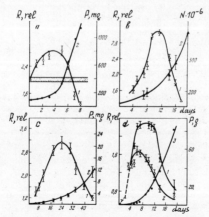

Fig. 133 Kinetic curves for tumour development and changes in the free radical content in the lyophilized samples of tumour tissues: (a) transplanted leukaemia La; (b) ascites form of sarcoma 37; (c) solid sarcoma 37; (d) Walker carcinosarcoma (curves 1 and 2 refer to peripheral and central parts of the tumour).

As seen from Figure 133a, the free radical concentration in spleen, the most damaged organ, increased at the initial stages of experimental leukaemia La and attained maximum values on the 4th - 5th day. It will be emphasized that the free radical concentration suffered changes earlier than did any other known symptom of the leukaemia process, such as the increase in spleen weight, leucocyte count and haemocytoblast number in peripheral blood and marrow. To the time of the animal's death the free radical content in spleen was considerably lower than normal. Thus, it is evident from this curve that for samples taken at the terminal stages of malignant growth the free radical concentration would be much lower than normal, and this was actually observed also by the authors who did not conduct kinetic studies.

Similar regularities of changes in free radical concentrations were observed for development of ascites and solid tumours. The kinetic curve for changes in free radical content in tumour tissue during sarcoma 37 growth is given in Figure 133c. A regularity of this kind is characteristic also of the ascites sarcoma 37 (Figure 133b).

It will be noted that a rather long phase of exponential growth is specific of the above tumours: it permits evaluation of the effective time of tumour weight (or volume) doubling ($T = \ln 2/\phi$) and the characterization of each stage of tumour growth by the doubling number ($n = t/T = \phi t/\ln 2$). By norming the x-axis in such a way and by plotting the EPR signal amplitude referred to its maximum value along the y-axis, it is possible to generalize these experimental results.

TABLE 46   Kinetics of changes in free radical concentration for transplanted tumours of various types

	Leukaemia La			Sarcoma 37 (ascites)			Sarcoma 37 (solid)	
Days	Relative signal	Doubling number	Days	Relative signal	Doubling number	Days	Relative signal	Doubling number
1	0.867	0.97	4	0.56	1.72	6	0.446	0.96
2	0.895	1.94	5	0.64	2.16	8	0.49	1.28
3	0.947	2.91	7	0.685	3.02	11	0.63	1.76
4	1.000	3.88	8	0.75	3.45	18	0.905	2.89
5	1.000	4.85	9	0.974	3.88	24	1.00	3.86
6	0.845	5.82	11	1.00	4.75	30	0.94	4.81
7	0.537	6.79	14	0.826	6.04	34	0.70	5.46
			16	0.611	6.9	40	0.505	6.41
8	0.450	7.76	18	0.453	7.76	46	0.385	7.37

$\phi = 0.67$ day^{-1}	$\phi = 0.297$ day^{-1}	$\phi = 0.111$ day^{-1}
$T = 1.03$ days	$T = 2.32$ days	$T = 6.23$ days

The data given in Table 46 show the maximum concentration of free radicals was attained by the time corresponding to 4-5 doublings of the tumour. Such a small number for transplanted tumours can be easily explained by the great number of transplanted cells: the leukaemia La inoculum consisted of 10^7 cells, that of ascites sarcoma 37 of 6×10^6 cells.

The transformation of these data for a tumour arising from one cell suggests that about 20 doublings would be needed here to attain the size of the effective inoculum representing approximately one-third of the total number of transplanted cells. It is very important that the time of attaining the maximum which corresponds to 24-25 tumour doublings falls in the initial phase of tumour growth, and in principle this could be taken as a basis in the working out of methods for early diagnosis of tumour processes.

The vital activity of cells is known to be different for various parts of the tumour. The central cells have less blood supply and rapidly decay, forming foci of necrosis. For this reason it was expected that cells of different layers would have different free radical contents.

It was found experimentally that the free radical contents in peripheral and central parts of the Walker carcinosarcoma were different: it was considerably higher for the peripheral zone of the tumour than for the central parts (Figure 133d). The maximum level of free radical content in the peripheral tumour layers persisted for 6-7 days whereas the level in the central sections decreased immediately after attaining the maximum.

In comparing the kinetic parameters for the decrease in free radical content and for tumour growth over a certain time interval it can be seen that there is a direct relationship between these parameters. The results given in Table 47 demonstrate that the experimental data on the increase in tumour size and free radical content can be described by linear functions $\log P/P_1 = \log R/R_1 = 0.4343\tau$, where $\tau = (t - t_1)\phi_R = (t - t_1)\phi_t$ (Figure 134).

TABLE 47   Kinetic parameters of changes in free radical concentration and tumour growth

Tumour	$(t-t_1)$, day	ϕt, day^{-1}	ϕ_R, day^{-1}
Solid sarcoma 37	25–40	0.08	−0.06
Ascites sarcoma 37	14–20	0.14	−0.15
Walker carcinosarcoma	11–19	0.16	−0.12

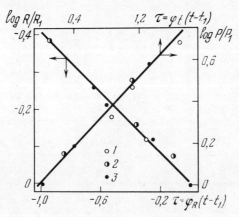

Fig. 134 Linear semilogarithmic anamorphoses of segments of kinetic curve segments of steady fall of free radical concentration (R/R_1) and tumour growth (P/P_1). (1) Ascites sarcoma 37; (2) solid sarcoma 37; (3) Walker carcinosarcoma.

TABLE 48 Summarized data on kinetic studies of free radicals in experimental tumours

	Type of tumour	Method of determining free radical concentration	Strain of animals	References
1.	Leukaemia La	EPR (lyophilized samples)	C57Bl mice	
2.	Sarcoma 37 (ascites)	" " "	Non-inbred mice	
3.	Sarcoma 37 (solid)	" " "	" "	
4.	Walker carcinosarcoma	" " "	Non-inbred rats	Saprin et al. (1967)
5.	" "	EPR (frozen samples)	" "	Driscoll et al. (1967)
6.	Melanoma B-16	" "	C57Bl mice	Wallace et al. (1970)
7.	Gardner lymphosarcoma	" "	C3H mice	Driscoll et al. (1967)
8.	Sarcoma 180 (solid)	Graft co-polymerization (tumour globulins)	Non-inbred mice	
9.	Sarcoma 45	Graft co-polymerization (tumour lipids)	Non-inbred rats	
10.	Ehrlich ascites carcinoma	Graft co-polymerization (tumour protein and lipids)	Non-inbred rats	Goloshchapov et al. (1973)
11.	Harding-Passey melanoma	Graft co-polymerization (tumour protein and lipids)	C3HA mice	Goloshchapov et al. (1973)
12.	Hepatoma 22a	EPR (frozen samples)	" "	
13.	" "	" "	" "	Varfalomeev et al. (1976)
14.	Leukaemia	" "	AKR mice	Dodd and Giron-Conland (1975); Swartz et al. (1973)
15.	Leukaemia LZ	" "	C57Bl mice	Khistianovich et al. (1977)
16.	Leukaemia P-388	" "	BDF$_1$ mice	
17.	Leukaemia L-1210	" "	" "	
18.	Mammary gland cancer	" "	C3H mice	
19.	Cloudman melanoma	" "	DBA/2 mice	
20.	Melanoma B-16	" "	BDF$_1$ mice	

Rows 15–20 (braced): Studies conducted in the laboratories of the Institute of Chemical Physics, Academy of Science, USSR

Further development of the kinetic method for the study of free radicals in biological systems made it possible to analyze a large number of animal and human
tumours, and to extend the method also to techniques other than EPR for detecting
free radicals. By now about 20 types of tumours have been studied kinetically
(Table 48).

Kinetics of changes in the free radical content in the course of tumour development
was also studied by Wallace and his groups (USA) (Wallace *et al.*, 1970; Driscoll
et al., 1967). The curves for changes in the free radical content in the peripheral actively-growing part of the Walker carcinosarcoma were obtained in three
independent experiments. The curves are similar in general shape, the points of
maximum amplitude of the EPR signals refer to similar values. However, these
curves are shifted by one day relative to each other. Unfortunately, the absence
of kinetic follow-up of the tumour growth rate does not allow us to transform along
the time axis and to present the curves in co-ordinates 'amplitude *vs* doubling time'.

On the whole the authors found a complete analogy between their results and the
data obtained earlier by Soviet researchers. For instance, a study of the fast-
growing melanoma B-16 showed that the maximum free radical content appeared at an
early time in the phase of fastest growth.

Similar changes in the free radical content in tumours were demonstrated by the
method of graft co-polymerization (Kozlov, 1973).

This method is based on the capacity of biogenic free radicals to initiate polymer-
ization of a radioactive monomer (for example the ^{14}C-amide of acrylic acid)
incorporated into the living body. By measuring the radioactivity of a chosen
tissue and the individual chemical components of cells one can judge the amount of
grafted monomer in biological substances.

According to data obtained by Bogdanov and Goloshchapov, the extent of labelled
acrylamide in the organs and tissues of non-inbred mice correlated with the radical
content determined for lyophilically-dried samples by the EPR technique (Figure 135).

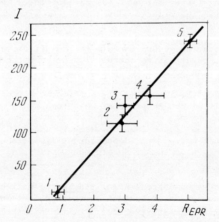

Fig. 135 Correlation between the free radical content
determined by the EPR technique (R) and the specific activity
of ^{14}C-acrylamide (I) introduced into the muscle tissue (1),
kidney (2), liver (3), lungs (4) and spleen (5).

It was shown by the method of graft co-polymerization that the changes in free radical content in cells of sarcoma 180 were described by an extreme function with the maximum falling at an early stage in the highest tumour growth rate. If the factor of exponential growth ($\phi = 0.23$ day^{-1}) and the time of tumour doubling ($T = 3.0$ days) are calculated from the data given above, the maximum will be attained after 4 doublings. The changes in free radical content in tumour lipids and in the liver of tumour-bearing animals with sarcoma 45 are of a similar nature.

The kinetic curves for changes in specific radioactivity of the grafted monomer in proteins and lipids of the Ehrlich ascites carcinoma cells (EAC) and of the Harding-Passey melanoma cells exhibit a maximum at the phase of highest tumour growth rate (Figure 136): the maximum free radical concentration in lipids and proteins of EAC falls for 3 days, and for the Harding-Passey pigment melanoma the concentration falls over the first 16 days (Goloshchapov et $al.$, 1973).

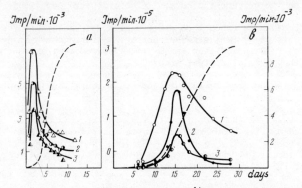

Fig. 136 Changes in the activity of ^{14}C-acrylamide introduced into proteins (1), free (2) and bound (3) lipids of
tumour tissues in the course of Ehrlich ascites tumour (a)
and Harding-Passey melanoma (b) development. The dotted
line denotes the kinetic curves for tumour growth.

It seemed to be important to generalize all the quantitative data available and to find on this bases the quantitative correlation between the kinetic parameters of tumour growth and the changes in free radical content (Emanuel, 1974).

The exponential dependent $N = N_0 \exp(\phi_t)$ is sufficiently general to permit description of the initial growth phase of most tumours.

The experimental points in Figure 137 for various tumours up to five doublings are close to the theoretical curve $\eta = 2^n$. Subsequent deviations from the exponential dependence at later stages of tumour development correspond to a transition to the linear phase of tumour growth, where $N = N_1 + bt$.

The region of tumour development characterized by the maximum growth rate value can be obtained from the condition of contact of the exponent and the straight line corresponding to equality of functions and their derivatives

$$N_1 + bt = N \exp(\phi t)$$

$$b = N \exp(\phi t).$$

Thus, the time of attaining the maximum growth rate:

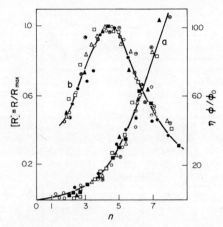

Fig. 137   Generalized kinetic growth curves for transplanted
tumour (1) and changes in free radical content in tumour
tissues (2).

$$t_{w_{max}} = \frac{1}{\phi} - \frac{N_1}{b}$$

As an example of such an analysis of tumour growth kinetics, consider the regularities of transplanted Harding-Passey melanoma development (Goloshchapov *et al.*,
1973). These data are best described by the autocatalysis equation which gives the
time of attaining the maximum tumour growth rate at the inflection point. The time
of tumour doubling in the exponential phase can be found by the least squares
procedure from the linear section of the semilogarithmic anamorphosis. Up to the
20th day tumour growth can be satisfactorily described by the exponential dependence
with the growth factor $\phi = 0.29$ day^{-1}. Thus the time of tumour doubling is
$T = \ln 2/\phi = 0.693/0.22 = 3.1$ days. The parameters of the melanoma linear growth
stage found by the least squares procedure are: $N_1 = -4.4$, $b = 0.30$ day^{-1}.

Substituting these values into the expression

$$t_{w_{max}} = \frac{1}{\phi} - \frac{N_1}{b}$$

we obtain $t_{w_{max}}$ = 18.9 days. It would be worth mentioning for comparison that
$t_{w_{max}}$ found in approximating the data by the autocatalysis equation was 18.2
days for changes in the mean tumour diameter, and 19.0 days for changes in
the melanoma weight.

Knowing the doubling time T for every experimental tumour, we find $n = t/T$, i.e. the
number of doublings at which the tumour attains the highest tumour growth rate.
The results in Table 49 show that n varies within close limits (5.0 - 6.9 doublings)
for the cases considered and the average value is 5.6 ± 0.3. This conclusion holds
for various ways of expressing tumour growth parameters and is independent of the
chosen characteristic of tumour development (weight or volume of tumour, volume of
ascitic fluid or number of tumour cells).

Analysis of the data on changes in free radical content as a function of the
doubling number was carried out for relative values R/R_{max} standardized to the

TABLE 49 Kinetic parameters characterizing the changes in free radical contents in experimental tumours

Tumour	ϕ, day^{-1}	$t_{W\max}$, day	$n_{W\max}$	$n_{R\max}$	$\Delta = n_{W\max} - n_{R\max}$	$\dfrac{n_{R\max}}{n_{W\max}}$
Leukaemia La	0.690	5.5	5.5	4.4	1.1	0.80
Sarcoma 37 (ascites)	0.232	13.4	4.6	3.5	1.1	0.76
Sarcoma 37 (solid	0.104	33.2	5.0	3.5	1.5	0.70
Walker carcinosarcoma	0.261	13.1	5.0	3.5	1.5	0.70
Melanoma B-16	0.263	16.1	6.2	5.0	1.2	0.81
Sarcoma 180 (solid)	0.332	14.4	6.9	5.7	1.2	0.83
Ehrlich carcinoma (ascites)	0.84	4.1	5.1	3.7	1.4	0.73
Harding-Passey melanoma	0.22	18.9	6.3	5.3	1.0	0.84
Average values			5.6±0.29	4.3±0.32	1.3±0.07	0.77

highest free radical concentration in the given tumour. The data on free radical content in lyophilized samples of tumour tissues determined by the EPR technique, and the data on the extent of labelled acrylamide incorporation into chemical components of the cells obtained by the graft co-polymerization method were used for this purpose.

Graphical analysis in co-ordinates $n \log R/R_{max}$ showed that both branches of the extreme curve for changes in free radical content can in all cases be described by exponential dependences with positive and negative values of the exponentials. The number of doublings $n_{R_{max}}$ corresponding to maximum free radical content was determined at the crossing point of appropriate anamorphoses. As seen in Table 49, the value $n_{R_{max}}$ changes within two doublings (from 3.5 to 5.7 doublings) and the average value is 4.3 ± 0.3.

The general character of changes in free radical content during tumour development is clearly seen in Figure 137 presenting the data on various experimental tumours averaged to the value $n_{R_{max}}$.

It will be readily seen by using average values of $n_{W_{max}}$ and $n_{R_{max}}$ that $n_{W_{max}} - n_{R_{max}} = 1.3$, i.e. the maximum free radical content is attained approximately at the point preceding by one doubling that of the highest tumour growth rate.

This conclusion seems to be of a general character. Besides the above examples it is supported also by the results obtained for the kinetics of changes in specific content of free radicals in frozen samples of hepatoma 22a and transplanted melanomas with various extents of pigmentation in the course of tumour development. The relative intensities of the signals of semiquinone radicals and other paramagnetic centres in tumours and in host liver in the course of transplanted heptoma 22a growth (Varfalomeev *et al.*, 1976) were found to change in the same sense. The maxima in kinetic curves were observed at the point preceding by one doubling that of the highest tumour growth rate (Figure 138). For transplanted melanomas a similar dependence characterizes the change in intensity of signal at $g = 2.004$ due to radical anions of the indolequinoid fragment of melanin (Bogdanov *et al.*, 1977).

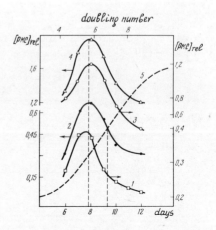

Fig. 138 Changes in paramangetic centre concentrations during the growth of hepatoma 22a: g = 2.003, tumour (1); g = 1.94, liver (2); g = 2.25, liver (3); g = 2.003, liver (4); curve for tumour growth (5).

An EPR study of wet samples of the spleen of AKR/j mice revealed that the content of ascorbic acid radicals increased during the induction period of leukaemia (Dodd and Giron-Conland, 1975). This is in agreement with the general regularity mentioned above for changes in free radical content during tumour growth.

At the same time investigation of the paramagnetic properties of frozen liver and spleen samples for AKR/j mice leukaemia (Swartz et al., 1973) showed an increase in free radical concentration (signal with $\Delta H = 14$ gs) in spleen and a decrease in liver almost throughout the whole leukaemia disease duration.

Similar data were obtained when studying free radical concentrations in frozen samples of mouse liver for various generalized forms and ascites forms of experimental leukaemias (Figure 139) (Khistianovich et al., 1977).

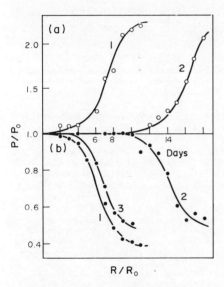

Fig. 139 Changes in free radical content (b) and in liver weight (a) for experimental leukaemias: (1) leukaemia LZ; (2) the first generation of spontaneous leukaemia; (3) leukaemia P-388 (weight of the liver unchanged).

A steady decrease in free radical content was observed in all cases studied (Table 50). The decrease in free radical concentrations (R/R_0) to the moment of attaining the maximum growth rate ($t_{W_{max}}$) was reported to be greater for the generalized forms of leukaemias, compared to the ascites variants. At the terminal stage of various leukaemia forms the free radical content became less than half of the initial value.

TABLE 50 Free radical content in the liver of mice
in the course of experimental leukaemias

Strain of tumour	Strain of mice	$t_{W_{max}}$, day	(R/R_0)
Leukaemia La	C57B1	4.0	0.7
Leukaemia LZ	C3H	7.0	0.6
First generation of spontaneous leukaemia	AKR	15.0	0.6
Leukaemia L-1210	BDF$_1$	4.5	0.9
Leukaemia P-388	BDF$_1$	5.5	0.9
Lymphatic leukaemia L-5178	DBA$_2$	8.5	0.9

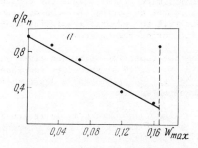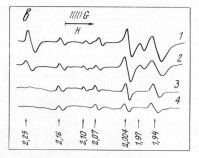

Fig. 140 Paramagnetic centres in the tissues of normal liver
and transplanted hepatomas: (a) relative content of free
radicals in normal ($R/R_0 = 1.0$) and regenerating liver, and
also in hepatomas with various growth rates; (b) stands for
EPR spectra of frozen tissue samples of normal liver (1),
minimally deviated hepatoma 46 (2) and rapidly growing
hepatomas 60 and 22a (3,4).

For transplanted hepatomas with various degrees of differentiation (Figure 140)
the relative free radical content, evaluated by the signal intensity ($g = 2.004$) in
the EPR spectrum of frozen tissue samples, regularly decreased with increase in
maximum tumour growth (Varfalomeev *et al.*, 1976; Bogdanov *et al.*, 1976). This is
supported also by the results of qualitative studies (Commoner *et al.*, 1954; Truby
and Goldzieher, 1958) in which the decrease in free radical content of hepatomas
was compared with that in liver. At the same time the free radical content in
regenerating liver (maximal regeneration rate $(dx/dt)_{max} = 0.164$ day^{-1}) did not
substantially differ from normal.

All these pecularities of changes in specific free radical content in homologous
tissues seem to be controlled by the extent of differentiation, rather than by the
proliferating activity of radicals. The dysfunction of certain enzymatic systems,
specific of hepatomas, is reflected in the decrease in intensity of most EPR
signals. A number of signals ($g = 1.97, 2.10, 2.25$) are absent for frozen samples
of rapidly growing hepatomas 22a and 60 (as compared to normal liver or to
minimally-deviated hepatoma 46) (Figure 140a,b).

A study of liver mitochondria and three transplanted Morris hepatomas (Onishi *et
al.*, 1973) showed that the intensity of the EPR signal from the (Fe–S) complex was
somewhat reduced in the slow-growing hepatoma 16, compared to normal. At the same
time a considerable decrease in the intensity of this signal was reported for the
rapidly growing hepatoma 7777. However, the absence of marked differences in the
spectrum of mitochondria of hepatoma 7800 growing at a medium rate suggested that
there is no correlation between the above data and the hepatoma growth rates.

It is very important to study the physico-chemical characteristics not only of
tumours, but also of host organs.

The data (Goloshchapov *et al.*, 1973) on changes in free radical content in proteins
and lipids of mouse liver in the case of Ehrlich ascites tumour and Harding-
Passey melanoma are given in Figure 141. The curves are seen to be of an extreme
character. The specific amount of grafted monomer in liver lipids is minimal in
the phase of highest tumour growth rate.

An increase in the specific amount of grafted monomer in liver proteins was

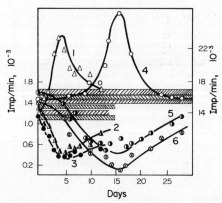

Fig. 141   Changes in introduced monomer activity in liver
proteins and lipids for Ehrlich ascites carcinoma and
Harding-Passey melanoma: (1) proteins; (2) free lipids;
(3) bound lipids; (4) proteins; (5) free lipids; (6)
bound lipids.

observed simultaneously. The maximum free radical content in proteins was found
on the 5th-6th day of EAC development and on the 15th-16th day for melanomas.

The correlation of data on the amount of grafted acrylamide in proteins and lipids
of tumour tissue (Figure 137) and in host liver (Figure 141) leads to an important
conclusion. The extent of acrylamide grafting in proteins and lipids is seen to
change in parallel for the cells of Ehrlich ascites tumour and the Harding-Passey
melanoma. Conversely, the amount of grafted monomer in the bound lipid fraction
of host liver increases with decreasing grafting level in proteins and vice versa.
A similar dependence characterizes the ratio of free radical content in proteins
to that in lipids of host liver under the action of a radical process inhibitor
(Goloshchapov and Burlakova, 1973). Such differences between the changes in free
radical states in proteins and lipids of tumours and tissues of host organs might
depend on the regulating mechanism specificity related to the membrane systems of
normal and tumour cells.

The reaction of host blood and organs to changes in the concentration of free
radicals in tumours is essential for early diagnosis and therapeutic control.

For example, EPR studies showed similar changes in the free radical contents in
host blood in the cases of solid and ascites forms of sarcoma 37 (Figure 142a,b)
and Walker carcinosarcoma (Figure 142c), corresponding moreover to regular changes
in the leucocyte count (Saprin et al., 1967). Of a slightly different nature are
the regularities of changes in free radical concentration in the blood of animals
with transplanted leukaemia La (Figure 142d). The level of free radicals in the
first four days was lower than normal. However, a marked increase in the free
radical content in blood was observed afterwards along with leucocytosis growth
and an increase in the number of tumour cells in the blood.

The main signal at g = 2.05 due to a copper-containing protein, ceruloplasmin, was
recorded in frozen blood plasma, and was different from the lyophilized samples.
However, the increase in intensity of this signal is not a specific feature of the
tumour process, since a similar effect was observed for other pathological states
as well (Mailer et al., 1974).

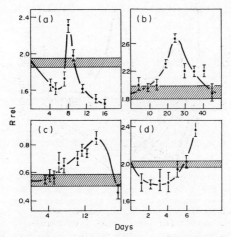

Fig. 142 Kinetics of changes in free radical concentration
in the peripheral blood of animals with solid (a) and the
ascitic (b) forms of sarcoma 37, Walker carcinosarcoma (c)
and leukaemia La (d).

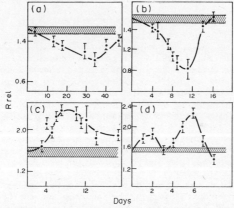

Fig. 143 Free radical content in host liver for ascitic (a)
and solid (b) forms of sarcoma 37, Walker carcinosarcoma (c)
and leukaemia La (d).

The content of free radicals in the viscera of tumour-bearing animals as a rule
decreases, while in the tumour it increases. An example is the change in the
amount of free radicals in liver during ascites and solid sarcoma 37 development
(Figure 143a,b).

Similar results were obtained making use of the graft co-polymerization method:
the extent of labelled acrylamide grafting in the liver tissues was minimal for
solid sarcoma 180. The content of semiquinone radicals in the livers of rats with
sarcoma 45 was below normal (Kozlov, 1973). Similar changes were observed in the
adrenal glands of animals bearing Walker carcinosarcoma. However, the curve for

changes in free radical content in the liver of animals with Walker carcinosarcoma has the opposite shape (Figure 143c). For leukaemia La this relation is even more complex (Figure 143d). Of a similarly complex type are the regularities for changes in the free radical concentrations in lungs for leukaemia La and in spleen for sarcoma 37 and Walker carcinosarcoma. These deviations unmistakably indicate the complex nature of the interrelationship between tumour and host in terms of the free radical processes.

Complex changes in the free radical content of host organs have been known for some time. The curves with two maxima for changes in the free radical content were obtained for spleen and liver of rats with Walker carcinosarcoma. Extreme changes in the content of free radical states with a maximum on the 6th day after transplantation were observed in liver and spleen of C3H mice with Gardner lymphosarcoma.

With melanoma B-16 (Wallace *et al.*, 1970) the maximum free radical content in liver, spleen and lungs fell within a period of 15 to 16 days. This virtually coincides with the time of attaining the highest growth rate and the maximum free radical content in the tumour. The concentration of free radicals considerably increased when metastases appeared in the above organs.

The above-mentioned data on the specificity of changes in free radical content in different organs and tissues of tumour-bearing animals showed that although much empirical information has been obtained, the data reported are rather disconnected and this prevents a strictly quantitative generalization.

4.   EFFECT OF ANTITUMOUR AGENTS ON FREE RADICAL
      CONTENT

The essential changes in intensity of free radical reactions in the course of transplanted tumour development made it possible to study the relevant effects of various antitumour drugs belonging to inhibitors of free radical processes, anti-metabolites and alkylating agents.

Russian researchers carried out such experiments on lyophilized tissue samples.

5-Fluorouracil (5-FU) is an antimetabolite which has been assayed and is now widely used clinically. The experiments were conducted for transplanted leukaemia La, and 5-FU was administered from the 4th day after transplantation (maximum content of free radicals in spleen) (Emanuel, 1974b; Bogdanov *et al.*, 1976, 1977; Onishi *et al.*, 1973; Goloshchapov and Burlakova, 1973; Mailer *et al.*, 1974).

At a dose of 25 mg/kg 5-FU hardly affected either the leukaemia or the level of free radicals in spleen.

Substantial inhibition of leukaemia development accompanied by complex changes in free radical content in spleen and liver were observed at a dose of 60 mg/kg (Figure 144a). Unlike the inhibitors of free radical reactions, 5-FU markedly changes the pattern of free radical states in normal animals and increases the free radical content in the above organs. It will also be noted that 5-FU does not induce an irreversible decrease in radical content and a maximum in the kinetic curve for free radical content in the spleen of animals with leukaemia precedes the repeated increase in spleen weight.

The effect of alkylating drugs (sarcolysine, Thiotepa, propylnitrosourea) is very similar to that of 5-FU. For example, sarcolysine at a dose of 4 mg/kg consider-ably inhibits the leukaemia process ($\varkappa^* = 0.32$). The free radical concentration first decreases and then rises, attaining by the 7th day the same value as in

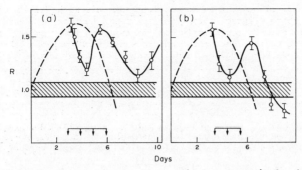

Fig. 144 Changes in the free radical content in lyophilized
samples of the spleen for leukaemia La (dashed line) and for
the treatment with 5-fluorouracil (a) and sarcolysine (b).

controls (Figure 144b). Just as in controls, this is the time at which vigorous
leukaemia development begins. Such regularities were also observed in the livers
of animals with leukaemia.

Thus, as with 5-FU, sarcolysine does not prevent pathological deviations from the
normal free radical level, but merely reschedules it.

Propylnitrosourea (PNU) administered on the first day after transplantation of
leukaemia La considerably inhibits leukaemia development ($x^* = 0.53$) with simultaneous reduction of the free radical content in the spleen. At the same time the
level of radicals in blood virtually returns to normal and the leucocyte count also
remains normal. This suggests a relationship between free radical concentration
and the leucocyte count in the peripheral blood of animals with transplanted
leukaemia. When PNU was administered starting from the 5th day, the antileukaemic
action was stronger ($x^* = 0.62$) and the changes in the free radical level in spleen
resembled those caused by sarcolysine or 5-FU. With the given schedule of PNU
administration the leucocyte count and the free radical content were within normal
limits.

The effect of PNU on the ascites form of sarcoma 37 consisted in a marked inhibition of the accumulation of ascitic fluid and tumour cells with a simultaneous
considerable decrease in the free radical content. However, the action of PNU on
tumour cells of ascites sarcoma 37 seems to be less specific than that on leukaemic
cells since the concentration of free radicals decreased to a lesser extent than
for leukaemia and the life-span of animals was not significantly prolonged.

The action of Thiotepa was studied for the Walker carcinosarcoma. Kinetic curves
for changes in the free radical concentration in the peripheral and central parts
of the tumour are shown in Figure 145a,b.

Under the action of the drug the tumour growth rate becomes half that of controls
($x^* = 0.5$). After Thiotepa administration the free radical content in the peripheral parts of the tumour at first slightly decreases, but later, despite continuing drug administration, it increases attaining the level in controls with shift
in time of 6 days. Then it decreases again, and subsequently increases with
renewal of tumour growth.

A similar picture was observed for the central part of the tumour (Figure 145b),
the only difference being that the maximum shift in time was 2 days. This might
be due to weaker action of the drug on the central part of the tumour, compared to

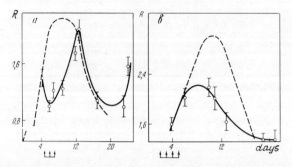

Fig. 145 Kinetic curves for changes in free radical
concentration in the central (a) and peripheral (b) parts
of Walker carcinosarcoma under the action of Thiotepa.

the peripheral regions. The administration of Thiotepa does not affect the type
of changes in the total leucocyte count and in the free radical content. Only
their maxima shift in time, but the curve shapes remain the same in both cases.
Attention will be drawn to the fact that the values of these shifts correspond to
the period of tumour inhibition under the action of Thiotepa.

Marked changes were observed in the free radical level in spleen, liver, adrenal
glands. These changes always represented a decrease in the free radical content
with subsequent restoration to the level in controls.

Resolution of the tumour with complete normalization of the free radical content
in blood and in all organs under the drug action was observed in 10% of the animals.

The capacity of inhibitors of free radical processes to reduce the free radical
content in Ehrlich ascites carcinoma cells was discovered in 1960. Under the
action of propylgallate it decreased approximately 6-fold.

A similar effect of propylgallate was observed for solid hepatoma 22a.

More detailed information about the effect of inhibitors on the free radical content
in tumours was obtained in kinetic studies of one of the most widely used antioxidants, ionol (2,6-di-tert.butyl-4-methyl-phenol). The drug was injected in a
dose of 150 mg/kg at 24-hour intervals starting from the first day after leukaemia
La transplantation (Figure 146a) and at doses of 100, 150, 200 mg/kg at times
corresponding to maximum free radical content in the spleen of animals bearing
leukaemia La (Figure 146b).

The level of free radicals markedly falls under the action of ionol. The kinetic
curves for changes in free radical concentrations at the sites of drug injection
are exponential, as seen from the respective semilogarithmic anamorphoses (Figure
146d). The calculated kinetic rate constants (k) of the decrease in free radical
content and the increase in spleen weight compared to controls are shown in the
table opposite.

On the basis of these data a conclusion can be reached on the correlation between
the antiradical and antileukaemic effects of ionol.

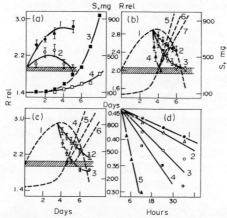

Fig. 146   Changes in the free radical content of the spleen
during leukaemia under the action of inhibitors of radical
reactions: (a) changes in free radical content in controls
(1) and in experimental animals (2) with ionol administration
at 24-hour intervals;   (3) and (4) are corresponding curves
for changes in spleen weight;   (b) effect of ionol on free
radical content (2-4) and on the leukaemia development rate
(5-7);   (c) 'diphenyl' effect on changes in free radical
concentration (2,3) and leukaemia development rate (5,6);
(d) semi-logarithmic anamorphoses of curves for steady fall
of free radical concentration under the action of ionol (1,
3,5) and 'diphenyl' (2,4).

Dose, mg/kg	Rate of increase in spleen weight compared to controls	$k \ 10^{-3}$, hour
	Ionol	
100	0.91	3.5
150	0.73	6.9
200	0.55	34.0
	'Diphenyl'	
125	0.67	4.4
175	0.62	10.4

Similar regularities were found for another inhibitor of radical reactions —
4-hydroxy-3,5-di-tert.butyl-4[1]-methyl-diphenyl ('diphenyl') administered against
leukaemia at doses of 125 and 175 mg/kg, equivalent to ionol doses of 100 and 150
mg/kg (Figure 146c). It was reported earlier that substituted hydroxydiphenyls in
equimolar doses exert a high antileukaemic effect. The above results also show a
more marked decrease in the free radical content, since the relevant constants
appear to be higher for diphenyl than ionol.

After drug administration was discontinued the shapes of kinetic curves became
somewhat different. Probably the inhibitor has a finite effect in the living body
and subsequently the free radical concentration in spleen increases again. The
free radical content always decreased to less than normal before the animal's

death. This phenomenon was observed repeatedly and seems to be specific of changes in the free radical content in the terminal stages of tumour growth.

This reduction in the free radical content for leukaemia La probably also applies to other types of experimental tumours. In any case ionol administered orally caused inhibition of the ascites sarcoma 37 and a decrease in free radical content in the ascitic fluid.

It follows that the inhibitors of free radical reactions are capable of reducing the free radical content in animal organs in the case of transplanted leukaemia and in ascitic fluid for sarcoma 37. The strongest effect is achieved by administering the drug within the period of maximum free radical content in malignant cells.

The rate constant for the steady fall of free radical concentration is seen to depend on the dose and to correlate with the antitumour activity value.

5.   CERTAIN REGULARITIES OF CHANGE IN THE FREE RADICAL CONTENT OF HUMAN TUMOURS

The results obtained when studying the kinetic regularities of changes in free radical content undoubtedly warrant wide use of the EPR technique in oncological practice, most of all for early diagnosis of malignant tumours and for control of the effectiveness of therapy.

This is evident from the first results obtained for human tumours by the EPR technique. An increase in the intensity of the EPR signal from leucocytes of patients with chronic lymphatic leukaemia (Pavlova and Livenson, 1965) and from the liver of leukaemic patients has been reported earlier. It was found in studies of the paramagnetic properties of tissues of 80 patients with stomach cancer that the free radical content in the peripheral part of the tumour was twice, and in the central part 1.5 times higher than in unchanged stomach mucosa. Metastases in regional nodules exhibited signals 3.5-fold more intense than those from unchanged mucosa.

A five-fold increase in free radical content was observed in cancer of the cervix uteri and pulmonary cancer, but Commoner and Ternberg reported in 1961 that the pulmonary metastases of a patient with cancer of the large intestine gave no EPR signal. No EPR signals were exhibited by tissues of the glioblastoma, neurinoma, meningioma, etc.

These early qualitative clinical investigations of free radical states were followed by details studies of the kinetic regularities of changes in the free radical content in leucocytes of patients with chronic forms of myeloid leukaemia and lymphatic leukaemia in the USSR between 1967 and 1970.

The regularities of changes in free radical content in the course of experimental leukaemia, and their relation to the stage of leukaemia process development attracted attention primarily because these changes were observed ahead of other macroscopic symptoms of leukaemia. Therefore it appeared to be important to find out whether similar regularities would hold for tumour cells in the case of human leukaemia, and what metabolic processes could be responsible for it.

Free radical concentration in leucocytes of 160 patients with chronic myeloid leukaemia and of 170 patients with chronic lymphatic leukaemia have been measured when studying the kinetic regularities of changes in the free radical content in leucocytes of leukaemic patients (Kassirskii *et al.*, 1967).

The free radical concentrations in leucocytes were measured at the time the patient arrived at the hospital, and during treatment. The kinetic curves for changes in free radical content in leukaemic cells were plotted taking into account the haematological pattern of leukaemia and various methods of therapy. The free radical content in leucocytes of 50 patients was measured and compared with normal.

The extraction of leucocytes was carried out by the usual technique. Lyophilized and wet samples were used for determining the free radical content.

The EPR signal for all cases observed was asymmetric and single with a half-width 10 15 gs and g-factor 2.003 typical for biological tissue. The EPR spectrum of 'leukaemic' leucocytes differed neither in shape nor in the g-factor from the EPR spectrum of donor leucocytes both for lyophilized and wet samples. Only in individual cases of chronic lymphatic leukaemia an additional signal at $g = 2.09$ was observed in wet leucocyte samples. Its nature is not yet clear. Moreover, the EPR intensity recalculated in terms of an equivalent number of leucocytes (20 mg of dry weight of 1 ml of $2×10^8$ cell suspension) was lower for wet samples than for the lyophilized ones.

The free radical content in leucocytes of patients with chronic myeloid leukaemia was on the average twice the normal level, and four times that in leucocytes of patients with chronic lymphoid leukaemia. The changes in free radical concentrations in the leucocytes of peripheral blood during the development of chronic forms of myeloid and lymphoid leukaemias were sufficiently well described by exponential kinetic curves with close constant values: 0.19 and 0.20 $week^{-1}$ respectively.

A kinetic study of the behaviour of free radicals during leukaemia shows that the progress of the disease is characterized by an increase in the free radical content in leucocytes up to a certain time after which the body undergoes rapid degeneration. In this period the level of free radicals in leucocytes sharply decreases (Figure 147). The kinetic curve shape is similar to that for changes in free radical content in animal organs in the course of experimental leukaemia (Figure 133a).

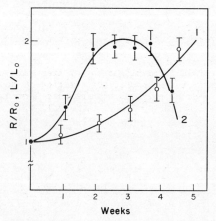

Fig. 147 Leucocytes count in blood (1) and the relative content of free radicals (2) in patients with chronic lymphatic leukaemia.

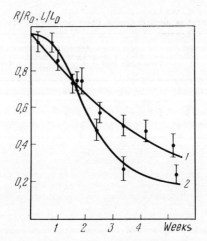

Fig. 148   Changes in leucocyte count (2) and the relative
content of free radicals in leucocytes (1) in the course of
treatment of patients with chronic lymphatic leukaemia.

The kinetics of changes in leucocyte free radical concentration under successful
chemotherapy shows that the free radical level in leucocytes regularly decreased
with clinical remission (Figure 148). These results were obtained when treating
chronic myeloid leukaemia with myelosane and 6-mercaptopurine, and chronic
lymphatic leukaemia with prednisolone, leukeran, and dipin.

However, despite the clinical remission of patients, the free radical content in
leucocytes remained elevated in most cases, without returning to normal. This
elevated concentration of free radicals in leucocytes of patients during remission
might be evidence of a minority of leukaemically modified cells in peripheral
blood.

The follow-up of 6 patients discharged from hospital in a state of remission, but
with an elevated free radical content in peripheral blood leucocytes, revealed
that the remission period tended to be shorter for these patients.

Comparison of the kinetic curves for changes in the free radical content in leucocytes of leukaemic patients and for leucocyte counts in peripheral blood under
successful therapy shows that the decrease in free radical content in leucocytes
proceeds faster than the leucocyte count in peripheral blood. This phenomenon
might indicate an earlier alteration of leucocytes at the molecular level, as a
reaction to therapy.

Analysis of the changes observed in free radical content in tumour cells and the
results of comparative studies of the EPR spectra of model systems make it
reasonable to consider that the EPR signal from biological tissue is due to active
centres of the enzymes responsible for electron transport in redox enzymatic
systems. The system of oxidative phosphorylation also contributes to the EPR
signal.

The intensity of respiration (by oxygen consumption) and glycolysis (by increase in
lactic acid content) as well as the ATP content in leucocytes of donors and patient
with myeloid and lymphatic leukaemias are shown in Table 51. Incubation of leuco-

TABLE 51 Respiration, glycolysis, ATP content and free radical concentration in leucocytes under the action of metabolic poisons

	O_2 consumption	Increment of lactic acid content	ATP content	Free radical concentration %
Donors (normal)				
Leucocytes + Gl	1120	7.1	154	100
" + Gl + BA	1070	0	49	60
" + Gl + SF	1000	0	90	100
" + Gl + DNP	1150	12.0	160	80
" + Gl + Ol	1130	8.0	150	95
Chronic lymphatic leukaemia				
Leucocytes + Gl	1104	8.7	112	100
" + Gl + BA	1275	0	25	50
" + Gl + SF	1300	0	75	95
" + Gl + DNP	1320	13.0	100	50
" + Gl + Ol	1150	8.0	98	90
Chronic myeloid leukaemia				
Leucocytes + Gl	112	0	133	100
" + Gl + BA	25	0	0	60
" + Gl + SF	75	0	80	90
" + Gl + DNP	100	9.0	122	40
" + Gl + Ol	98	7.0	110	90

Note: The data are given for 10^9 cells. Values averaged over 60 experiments. Error $\pm 10\%$. Gl is glucose; BA is monobromacetate, 8×10^{-4} M; SF is sodium fluoride, 2×10^{-2} M; DNP is 2,4-dinitrophenol, 8×10^{-4} M; Ol is oligomycin, 2×10^{-4} M.

cytes from leukaemic blood containing various metabolic poisons reveals that the free radical concentration reduces considerably only under the action of 2,4-dinitrophenol, separating oxidative phosphorylation at the initial stages. The free radical concentration reduces in this case by 50 per cent. The use of oligomycin, which separates oxidative phosphorylation processes at a later stage, has no marked effect on the free radical content in 'leukaemic' leucocytes.

Incubation of leucocytes from donor blood containing 2,4-dinitrophenol and oligomycin revealed no great effect of these metabolic poisons on free radical concentration.

The free radical content in leucocytes remained unchanged both on glycolysis suppression by sodium fluoride and on stimulation of glycolytic processes under anaerobic conditions. Monobromine acetate markedly affected the concentration of free radicals. However, the changes in free radical concentration can be assumed to be caused by damage of the oxidative phosphorylation system.

These results are evidence of certain shifts in the oxidative phosphorylation in leucocytes in patients with myeloid and lymphatic leukaemia and are thus an additional indication that leukaemic transformation of haemopoiesis is accompanied by certain changes in the leukaemic cell metabolism seemingly involving free radical stages.

Another example of the possible use of EPR technique in clinical practice was
reported by Wallace *et al.* (1970). He gave the characteristics of 152 clinical
cases of mammary gland tumour, 63 being histologically diagnosed as cancer, and
89 as various benign tumours.

The large amount of experimental data permits the finding of a correlation between
the g-factor value and the probability of detecting a malignant tumour: the higher
the probability, the larger is the g-factor.

The width of signals from the peripheral tumour part was 10.6 ± 0.35 gs, while for
a normal tissue or for a benign tumour it was 12.5 ± 0.45 gs.

In tumours 1 to 4 cm in diameter the relative concentration of free radicals was
much higher than in the adjoining tissue. This relation indicated changes in free
radical content in peripheral parts of the tumour. Tumours of about 4 mm in
diameter were reported to exhibit the same level of free radicals, as did normal
tissues. This was thought to be a direct consequence of extreme regularities for
changes in free radical content, for example, in the development of transplanted
tumours.

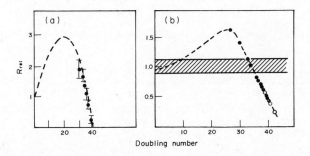

Fig. 149 Changes in free radical content in tumours (a)
and blood (b) of patients as a function of the doubling
number (Wallace *et al.*, 1970).

The extreme dependence obtained experimentally (Figure 149a) was used when describing the results of changes in free radical content under clinical conditions. The
curves for changes in free radical content as a function of the doubling number
can be plotted under the assumption that a tumour of 1 mm diameter corresponds to
20 doublings, and a tumour of 1 cm corresponds to 30 doublings (Gerstenberg, 1965).
Wallace *et al.* (1970) considered only the descending section, since only this could
be obtained in the clinical period of investigation. The satisfactory approximation of these data and also of those on changes in free radical content in the
blood of patients will be noted (Figure 149b). A reliable increase in the signal
amplitude (at $g = 2.003$) was obtained in studying free radicals in the blood
coming from cancerous stomach in the late stages of the process.

Thus, the study of free radical mechanisms and of changes in paramagnetic properties of tissues in the course of tumour development has become one of the most
important trends of investigation in experimental and clinical oncology.

CHAPTER 7

KINETIC BIOCHEMISTRY OF TUMOURS

A study of the kinetics of biochemical shifts displayed by tumour tissues can be of great importance in the choice of certain parameters that characterize the extent of tumour growth and are valid for setting up criteria of the effectiveness of therapy (Emanuel, 1965).

Certain biochemical differences between tumour and normal tissues, the extraordinary metabolism of the tumour, and the activity of enzymes limiting the rates of the most important metabolic processes have been established by now. Many reviews and monographs deal with these problems (Weber, 1961; Belousova, 1965; Manailov, 1971; Salyamov, 1974; Weber and Lea, 1966; Webber, 1974; Shapot, 1975).

This chapter is concerned mainly with changes in certain biochemical or biophysical characteristics of tumour tissues relative to the kinetics of tumour growth. Such studies were conducted using various types of spontaneous, induced and transplanted tumours. The best results were obtained for hepatomas with different growth rates, making possible correlation of certain biochemical values with rates of tumour growth.

From these results Weber developed a semi-quantitative molecular-correlational concept for assessing at a molecular level specific features of growth rate.

From the diverse biochemical shifts observed both in tumour tissue as such and in other tissues of the tumour-bearing animal, those connected with growth and division of cells are the most important.

A study of the life cycle of normal cells in the process of carcinogenesis showed that disturbances of the relation between proliferation and differentiation of cells are characteristic of the development of the malignant state. For tumours arising from renovating populations (for instance, for planocellular carcinoma) the fraction of differentiated cells diminishes, thus showing the extent of equilibrium disturbance between cell proliferation and differentiation.

For tumour arising from non-renovated populations (spontaneous tumours of mammary glands), the main disturbance in the cell life cycle consists of the transition of cells from the rest phase to the presynthetic period in the absence of stimulation (Frankfurt, 1975).

Models of cell proliferation have been proposed in this connection. However, the actual molecular mechanisms of regulation disturbance are not yet clear.

239

Consequently it is essential to find out the changes in metabolic processes that provide a biochemical interpretation of disturbances in cell proliferation and differentiation.

1.   CARBOHYDRATE METABOLISM

The study of the difference between energy metabolism of normal and tumour tissues has been directed towards the relationship between the respiration and glycolysis processes. These studies were based on the well-known intensification of glycolysis in tumours.

Glycolysis accounts for about half the energy required by the tumour cell and results in the formation of low-molecular precursors for biosynthesis of amino acids and nucleotides. The intensity of the glycolytic process was repeatedly confirmed both experimentally (Aisenberg, 1961; Woods and Vlahakis, 1973) and clinically (Shapot, 1973), and it represents the most critical difference between tumour and normal metabolism.

But not all tumours exhibit intense glycolysis and thus this feature cannot be considered as a characteristic of cancer cell energetics. For instance, it was found in studying minimally deviated slow-growing hepatomas that the aerobic or anaerobic glycolysis in hepatoma 5123 is very slow (Aisenberg and Morris, 1961). This hepatoma exhibits a moderate respiration intensity which increases four to five times after the addition of succinate, and it does not exhibit the Crabtree effect, i.e. respiration is not suppressed by glycolysis. On the whole the main characteristics of respiration and glycolysis processes for these hepatomas and for normal cells are not substantially different.

A study of carbohydrate metabolism in fast-growing hepatomas revealed an intense aerobic glycolysis common for tumours. Hepatomas with various extents of differentiation showed a good correlation between glycolysis level and rate of tumour growth (Weber, 1974).

The gluconeogenesis process involving certain enzyme systems is characteristic of normal liver cells.

A number of cell enzymes can be distinguished at the basic stages of glycolysis and gluconeogenesis. The general regularities of changes in enzyme properties and their relation to tumour growth were established for tumour tissues. These regularities are connected with activation of the key enzymes of glycolysis (hexokinase, phosphofructokinase and pyruvate kinase) and with retardation of the basic gluconeogenesis stages involving glucose-6-phosphatase, fructose-1,6-diphosphatase and pyruvate carboxylase. The above regularities of the carbohydrate metabolism are shown in Scheme 4. Moreover, differences were noted in the isoenzyme spectra of certain enzymes and in the Michaelis rate constant values.

For instance, considerable changes were observed in the activity of hexokinase, an enzyme responsible for the rate of the initial stage of biological glucose oxidation. Indeed, under the action of 3-methyl-N,N-dimethyl aminoazobenzene hepato-carcinogenesis was accompanied, even at early stages, by a five-fold increase in hexokinase activity (Sharma et al., 1965). A similar increase in hexokinase activity was observed for benzopyrene-induced skin cancer, and it was suggested that this factor might be used for early diagnosis of malignant processes (Adachi et al., 1969). For a number of transplanted tumours the histological differentiation and the changes in hexokinase activity were found to be related to the tumour growth rate $G = 0.02 + 0.042$ (Knox et al., 1970). In particular, such a linear correlation was observed for five hepatomas with different growth rates (Figure 150a).

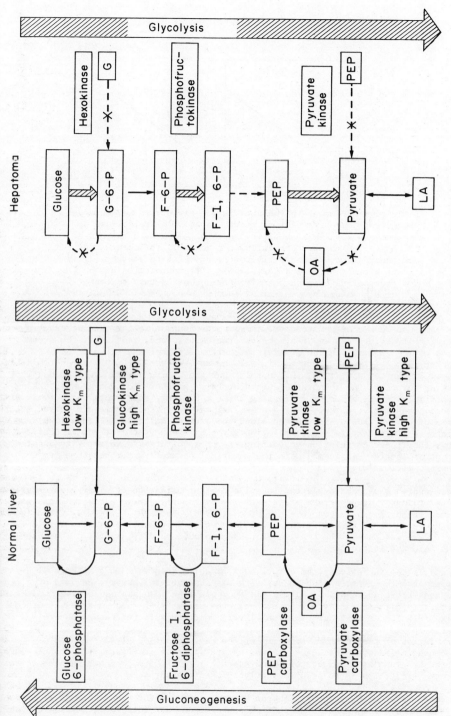

Scheme 4 Main glycolysis and gluconeogenesis stages in normal liver and hepatoma (Weber, 1974)

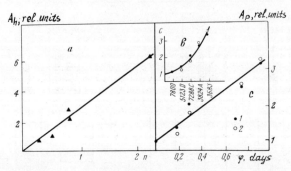

Fig. 150 Change in the activity of glycolysis key enzymes
in hepatoma with various growth rates: (a) relationship
between hexokinase activity and hepatoma growth rate (n =
number of tumour generations per month); (b) changes in
phosphofructokinase activity (1) and lactate content (2) in
hepatomas (Weber and Lea, 1966); (c) correlation of the
phosphofructokinase activity (1) and of lactate content (2)
with hepatoma growth rate (Weber and Lea, 1966; Weber, 1974).

The same dependence of hepatoma growth rate was found also for the increase in
activity of another key enzymes, phosphofructokinase and, judging by the accumulation of lactic acid, in the general intensity of glycolysis (Figure 150b)
(Sweeney et al., 1963). In the original papers (Weber, 1961, 1974; Weber and Lea,
1966; Sweeney et al., 1963) the correlations are semi-quantitative, because in
drawing the plots the authors used an arbitrary scope of hepatoma growth, taking
them simply in the order of increasing rates. However, such plots can be made of
a more quantitative nature, if the numerical values of the parameters characteristic of tumour growth are plotted along the growth rate axis. Figure 150b demonstrates a semi-quantitative correlation given by Sweeney et al., and Figure 150c
shows the linear correlation connecting the phosphofructokinase activity and the
amount of lactic acid formed with the numerical parameters for hepatoma growth
(Knox et al., 1970).

The elevated lactic acid content is evidence that oxidation of glucose in experimental tumour tissues occurs preferentially by the glycolytic pathway. This was
found for Novikov hepatoma (Ashmore et al., 1958), Ehrlich ascites carcinoma (Wu
and Packer, 1959), mammary gland carcinoma, etc. When Ehrlich ascites carcinoma
cells were incubated with C^{14}-glucose under aerobic conditions, 95% of the label
went into the lactic acid.

Alongside the increase in the activity of glycolysis enzymes in hepatomas with
various growth rates, a drop in activity was observed for the key enzymes of gluconeogenesis: glucose-6-phosphatase and fructose-1,6-diphosphatase (Weber and
Morris, 1963). In fast-growing hepatomas the activity of these enzymes is minimal
(Figure 151). In contrast to normal liver, most transplanted hepatomas are
incapable of inducing these enzymes under the action of glucocorticoids. The
correlation of the relative activity of the key enzymes of glycolysis and of
gluconeogenesis with the hepatoma growth rate is shown in Figure 152 (Shapot, 1975)
The authors use as a measure of tumour growth rate the times of attaining a certain
tumour size, which is an insufficiently scientific approach.

No correlation with the hepatoma growth rate was found for other enzymes of carbohydrate metabolism, such as glucose phosphate isomerase, aldolase, glyceraldehyde-
3-phosphate dehydrogenase, phosphoglycerate kinase and lactate dehydrogenase.

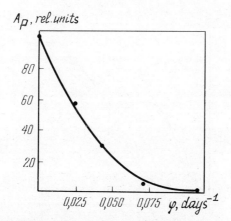

Fig. 151   Relationship between fructose-1,6-diphosphatase activity and tumour growth rate (Weber and Lea, 1966;   Knox *et al.*, 1970).

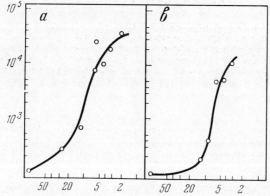

Fig. 152   Imbalance of glycogenolysis and gluconeogenesis processes in hepatomas with various growth rates.   (a) Changes of the ratio of hexokinase to glucose-6-phosphatase activities;   (b) same, of phosphofructokinase to fructose-1,6-diphosphatase.

At the same time it was noted that a certain change in the enzymatic activity of lactate dehydrogenase in the blood serum of tumour-bearing mice occurs with development of certain transplanted tumours.   There is a close connection between the nature of these changes and various stages of tumour growth (Agatova and Treshchenkova, 1972).

For instance, the induction period for Ehrlich ascites carcinoma development is characterized by a sharp increase in the lactate dehydrogenase activity (Figure 153).   The phase of intense tumour growth is accompanied by a decrease in the activity of lactate dehydrogenase, which remains higher than normal.   At the terminal stage of tumour growth, enzyme activity increases.   The change in enzyme activity during tumour growth was thought to be caused by a change in its

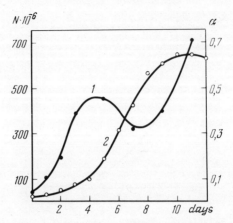

Fig. 153 Changes in lactate dehydrogenase activity (1) in
the course of Ehrlich ascites carcinoma development (2)

isoenzyme content. However, no direct connection between these phenomena was
found.

Besides other specific features of carbohydrate metabolism in tumour tissues it
will also be noted that in the ascites and solid form of Ehrlich carcinoma a
considerable part of the glucose is oxidized via glucose-1-phosphate (Wenner *et al.*,
1958). The growth of transplanted tumours is accompanied by activation of
glucose-6-phosphate dehydrogenase (Weber *et al.*, 1961) and by formation of lactic
acid from glucose-1-phosphate.

The Crabtree effect is also connected with activation of the hexose monophosphate
path of glucose oxidation in tumours, compared to normal tissues. A correlation
was found between tumour growth rate and the oxidation of glucose C_1/C_6 atoms to
CO_2 (Weber and Morris, 1963).

The glucose content in the tumour and adjacent tissues is considerably lower than
normal. For instance, with development of the Ehrlich ascites carcinoma the
glucose concentration in ascitic fluid is less than 8×10^{-5} g/l. The content of
glycogen in transplanted hepatomas and in the livers of tumour-bearing animals
markedly decreases (Misheneva and Goriukhina, 1973). There is a correlation
between tumour growth rate and low glycogen content in liver (Tagi-Zade and Shapot,
1970).

The elevated glucose affinity of cells transformed by the sarcoma virus (MSV) will
be noted in this connection. The Michaelis constant for glucose — a value inverse
to substrate affinity — decreases after transformation (Martin *et al.*, 1971).

Shapot suggested that the tumour acts as a glucose trap (Shapot, 1972). This
functional peculiarity of the tumour, and its systemic action as a nitrogen trap
(Greenstein, 1954), are characteristic of the tumour's relationship to the host.

The tumour cells retain the capacity for tissue respiration. This path of glucose
oxidation *in vivo* does not represent an important energy source in the tumour.
For instance in the Ehrlich carcinoma the glycolytic coefficient is higher than the
respiration coefficient (Kit and Gross, 1959). The latter is also very reduced in
the liver of tumour-bearing rats. At the same time it was found that the level of

respiration remains constant in induced heptoma, in normal and regenerating liver and in the metastases of a chemically-induced tumour (Aisenberg, 1961). Under *in vitro* conditions the ascites cells (ovary Ehrlich carcinoma, Zaidel hepatoma and hepatoma 22) retain a respiration level sufficient for ensuring the energy needed for protein biosynthesis (Ettsiva, 1965).

In discussing the problem of tissue respiration in tumours attention must be given first of all to the decrease in partial oxygen pressures in tumour tissues established for a number of tumours both experimentally and clinically. A reduced oxygen pressure was found for sarcoma 45 cells. For Ehrlich ascites the pO_2 decreased during malignant process development (Figure 154a) (Efimov and Bernshtein, 1968). Figure 154 shows the decrease in oxygen pressure against increasing cell number: this suggests that reduced respiration in tumour tissues is due to local hypoxia, which is corroborated by the Pasteur effect (suppression of glycolysis by respiration) in Ehrlich ascites carcinoma cells under conditions of elevated partial oxygen pressure. When oxygen is introduced into the peritoneal cavity the content of lactic acid in tumour cells decreases with a simultaneous increase in the glucose concentration (Figure 154b). Though the tumour cells retain their potential capacity for respiration, possible disturbances in the functioning of individual enzymes of energy metabolism cannot be excluded.

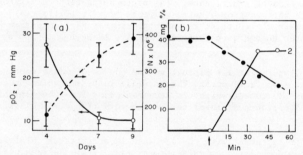

Fig. 154 Partial oxygen pressure and the Pasteur effect in tumour cells: (a) curves for changes in cell number and oxygen pressure in the course of Ehrlich ascites carcinoma development (Efimov and Bernshtein, 1968); (b) changes in glucose (2) and lactic acid (1) concentrations in Ehrlich ascites carcinoma cells.

For instance, besides data on normal functioning of the Krebs cycle in hepatomas (Aisenberg, 1961) there are other data demonstrating its disturbance in Ehrlich ascites carcinoma cells. An increase in the activity of enzymes that split citric acid and a decrease in serine dehydrogenase activity were observed in the course of hepatocarcinogenesis by Wu and Homberger (1969).

As the tumour developed, changes were observed in the activity of other redox enzymes and in its relation to the tumour growth rate (Houglum *et al.*, 1974; Raikhlin and Smirnova, 1967). Ketoreductase activity reduced with faster growth of hepatomas (Houglum *et al.*, 1974). The flavine content in hepatomas was also markedly lowered. The activities of cytochrome oxidase and of succinate dehydrogenase also changed in the course of tumour development. These changes were at first reversible, but later on enzyme inactivation became irreversible (Raikhlin and Smirnova, 1967). Such phenomena might be due to changes in the structure and properties of the membranes in tumour cell mitochondria. For instance, the mitochondrial membranes of tumours are known to display elevated permeability.

Since iron is present in many enzymes of the respiration chain, certain regular
changes in the metabolism of iron-containing proteins will be noted. For instance,
as the growth-rate of certain transplanted hepatomas becomes higher, their capacity
to incorporate iron becomes lower and the ratio of iron to protein in the tumour
ferritin becomes smaller (Figure 155a) (Edwards *et al.*, 1971).

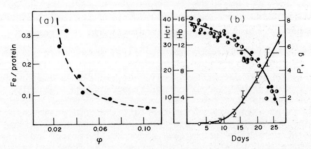

Fig. 155 Changes in iron-containing tumour components as a
function of growth rate: (a) ratio Fe/protein in hepatomas
with various growth rates (Edwards *et al.*, 1971); (b)
haematocrit (Hct, %) and haemoglobin Hb, g%) contents; P
is the tumour weight (Linder *et al.*, 1970).

The changes in lymphoreticular tissues in the course of mouse carcinoma growth are
quite consistent with these data. The increase in plasma volume occurring parallel
with the increase in tumour weight is accompanied by lower haemoglobin and haematocrit counts in the iron-containing cell components (Figure 155b) (Linder *et al.*,
1970).

These data are in agreement with the decrease in activity of catalase in hepatomas
and livers of tumour-bearing animals (Greenstein, 1954; Jeffree, 1958). It was
found, for instance, that even a day after inoculation of sarcoma 180, catalase
activity reduced by half. A regular drop in catalase activity in liver was observed
throughout the growth of transplanted tumours (Figure 156) up to the animal's death.
Such results were obtained for Pliss lymphosarcoma and Zaidel hepatoma.

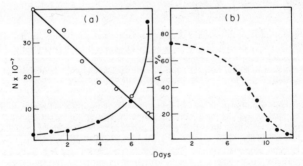

Fig. 156 Changes in catalase activity (%) in the course of
tumour growth: (a) Zaidel ascites hepatoma; (b) Pliss
lymphosarcoma.

Hepatomas with low catalase activity grow faster than those with high catalase activity (Rechcigl *et al.*, 1962). Incorporation of radioactive iron into the liver catalase of tumour-bearing animals was insignificant, or did not occur at all (Ceriotti *et al.*, 1960).

The relationship of energy metabolism to changes in catalase activity and tumour growth kinetics has been established. Tumour development was found to be accompanied by a lower intensity of phosphorylation in liver and spleen of tumour-bearing animals. Catalase activity also decreased.

This is evidence that the tumour growth process is accompanied by regular changes in the intensity of different energy metabolism stages, both in the tumour as such, and in the host body. The kinetic approach allows investigation of quantitative regularities of biochemical shifts and their relationships.

2. NUCLEIC ACIDS

There is no universal standpoint for the molecular mechanisms of carcinogenesis. Cancer is thought to be caused both by gene mutations, and by epigenetic shifts. This can be accompanied by disturbance of replication (DNA synthesis), transcription (RNA synthesis) and translation (protein synthesis).

The data on changes in nucleic acid content in hepatomas with different extents of differentiation and different growth rates demonstrate that a higher DNA content is inherent in tumours (Lea *et al.*, 1966; Bogdanov and Shmonina, 1975). This characteristic should correlate with the growth rates of experimental liver tumours. For instance, the DNA content in slowly growing rat hepatomas is within normal limits, in hepatomas with a high growth rate it is somewhat elevated, and in low-differentiated tumours that have lost their tissue specificity it is very high (Lea *et al.*, 1966):

Hepatoma	DNA content (mg/g) (from Lea *et al.*, 1966)	Mean number of tumour generations per month (from Weber and Lea, 1966)
7800	2.28 ± 0.07	0.3
5123	3.32 ± 0.31	0.4
7288c	3.82 ± 0.14	0.6
3924A	6.66 ± 0.42	1.8
3683	5.58 ± 0.28	2.1
Regenerating liver	2.21 ± 0.10	–

Similar results were obtained for a number of hepatomas in C3HA mice (Bogdanov and Shmonina, 1975).

Comparison of the amount of DNA in normal and regenerating liver showed that despite the high growth rate characteristic of liver tissue after partial hepatectomy, its DNA content remained at a normal level.

The correlation between DNA content and tumour growth rate is observed against a substantially changing RNA content. For several hepatomas the total RNA content was found not to correlate with the growth rate (Weber *et al.*, 1964). This is due to the multiplicity of specific RNA forms and their functions.

The change in the specific content of nucleic cells in tumours is reflected in the

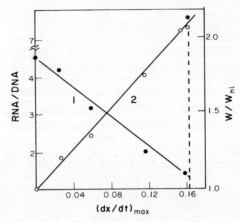

Fig. 157   The RNA/DNA ratio (1) and the initial rate of
thymidine incorporation (2) in hepatomas with various growth
rates relative to normal liver (W_{nl}) (Bogdanov and Shmonina,
1975).

ratio of RNA to DNA.   It will be seen from Figure 157 that the RNA/DNA ratio and
the maximum growth rate of transplanted hepatomas are connected by an inverse
linear dependence (Bogdanov and Shmonina, 1975).   The regenerating liver exhibits
the highest growth rate and thus the highest RNA/DNA value.   For hepatomas 60 and
22a this ratio appeared to be substantially lower than for the liver.   On the whole
the RNA/DNA value is connected with the maximum growth rate of hepatomas by the
equation

$$RNA/DNA = 4.4 - 1.92 \ (dx/dt)_{max}$$

The decrease in the RNA/DNA ratio in hepatomas can be due to the lack of differentiation inherent in tumours.   One of its signs is the retardation or complete
suppression of the synthesis of certain specific proteins.   A similar decrease in
RNA/DNA has also been reported by Mizuno *et al.* (1968).   For instance, for 15 forms
of rat hepatomas the RNA/DNA ratio changed within 1.2 - 2.4, whereas for normal
liver this value was about 3.5.

The differences in metabolism of nucleic acids in normal and tumour tissues are
implicit in the experimental data on changes in DNA and RNA synthesis rates in the
course of tumour growth.   An example of such data can be found in Figure 158.   The
synthesis rate both of DNA (incorporation of C^{14}-thymidine) and of RNA (incorporation of C^{14}-uridine) is seen to reduce with development of the transplanted
leukaemia L-1210.   Most probably the decrease in the synthesis rate of macromolecules is connected with a longer cell cycle in leukaemia development (Goncharova
et al., 1973).

A more intense incorporation of labelled precursors into nucleic acids has been
reported.   For instance, the incorporation of C^{14}-thymidine and deoxyuridine into
the DNA of hepatoma was found to be more intense compared to normal liver, and
there was a correlation between thymidine incorporation and tumour growth rate
(Figure 159).   This correlation permitted the authors to recommend labelled
thymidine as a characteristic of transplanted hepatoma growth rate (Lea *et al.*,
1966).

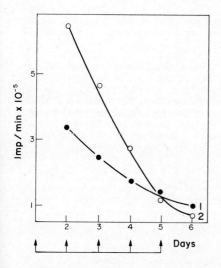

Fig. 158   Incorporation of labelled RNA
(2) and DNA (1) precursors into leukaemia
L-1210 ascites cells in the course of
growth.

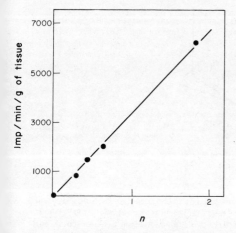

Fig. 159   Incorporation of C^{14}-thymidine
into cells of hepatoma with different
growth rates (n = mean number of tumour
generations per month) (Weber and Lea,
1966).

A more intense RNA synthesis was observed for tumour lymphocytes in humans
(Kogarko *et al.*, 1970). The incorporation of labelled RNA into leukaemia cells
was four times higher than incorporation of H^3-uridine into normal lymphocytes.
With further development of the tumour virtually all leukaemia cells (99%)
intensely incorporate the labelled precursor, i.e. synthesize RNA.

A method of two-stage autoradiography and cytophotometry of one individual cell
was used for quantitative assessing of the combined synthesis of nucleic acids (of
DNA and RNA) in leukaemia lymphocytes. It was found that in tumour lymphocytes
intense RNA synthesis was accompanied by only a small change in DNA synthesis,
whereas in normal cells intense RNA synthesis occurred together with substantial
DNA synthesis. The two processes occur in parallel and are interrelated, whereas
during tumour growth this relationship is disturbed.

A kinetic approach to the metabolism of nucleic acids in transplanted liver tumours with different growth rates and extents of differentiation was used in studying hepatomas in C3HA mice (Bogdanov and Shmonina, 1975; Bogdanov et $al.$, 1973, 1976).

C^{14}-Thymidine incorporation demonstrates the rate of DNA biosynthesis and shows a correlation between the extent of tumour differentiation and DNA synthesis. Hepatoma 46 was closest to normal liver in the initial rate and limiting amount of label incorporation. These characteristics were also close for hepatoma 22a and the regenerating liver. On the whole there is a linear relationship between the initial rate of label incorporation into DNA and the growth rates (Figure 157).

$$W/W_{nl} = 1 + 6.54 \ (dx/dt)_{max}$$

No correlation between the rates of DNA and RNA catabolism and hepatoma growth rates was found in studying the catabolism of nucleic acids in hepatomas, in regenerating liver, and in other organs and tissues of normal animals.

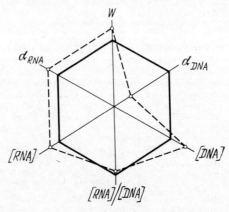

Scheme 5   Main characteristics of nucleic acid metabolism
in normal liver and in minimally deviated hepatoma.

Scheme 5 represents coincidences and differences in the elements of nucleic acid metabolism in normal liver and in minimally deviated mouse hepatoma. It shows the relationship between characteristics of nucleic acid metabolism in hepatoma and normal liver. The regular hexagon represents data obtained for normal liver tissue. In plotting this contour the values of all characteristics: the initial rate of C^{14}-thymidine incorporation into DNA, the extent of DNA and RNA decay during 5 hours of homogenate autolysis, the RNA and DNA contents, the ratio of RNA to DNA, were arbitrary. The relevant characteristics of nucleic acid metabolism for the hepatoma were plotted along every axis.

It will be seen from Scheme 5 that almost all characteristics of nucleic acid metabolism in hepatomas reproduce essentially the pattern inherent in normal liver. An exception is the extent of DNA decay, and this may be evidence of the substantial difference between the minimally altered hepatoma and normal liver.

A relation was found between the extent of spleen infiltration with leukaemic cells and the kinetics of nucleic acid decay at various times of leukaemia development. A regular decrease in the extent of DNA decay in the course of leukaemia development

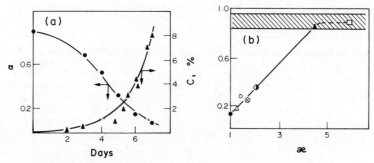

Fig. 160 Catabolism of nucleic acids during leukaemia La:
(a) changes in the specific content of leukaemic cells (C, %)
in spleen and the extent of DNA decay (α) (Bogdanov *et al.*,
1971); (b) extent of RNA decay as a function of antileukaemic drug activities.

was observed for spleen homogenates, accompanied by an exponential rise of leukaemic cell percentage in these homogenates (Figure 160a) (Bogdanov *et al.*, 1971).

It will be noted that at the initial stage of leukaemia development (the 1st to the
4th day), when the percentage of leukaemic cells in spleen does not exceed 10%, the
extent of DNA decay is reduced by half. Further decrease occurs against a substantial increase in the leukaemic cell content at the terminal stage of the process
(at the 5th to 7th day).

The inhibition phenomenon of nucleic acid catabolism was used as a biochemical
characteristic of certain antileukaemic drugs and for kinetic study of their effect
on the decay of nucleic acids in spleen homogenates of mice with transplanted leukaemia La. As the effectiveness of antileukaemic treatment increases, both DNA and
RNA decay accelerates approaching normal under the action of nitrosopropylurea and
diazane. It will be noted that with less active drugs the extent of RNA decay has
a linear relationship to the inhibition coefficient of the leukaemic process
(Figure 160b). The authors suggest that the observed effect can be due both to
the indirect action of antitumour drugs on catabolism and to changes in physico-
chemical properties of nucleic acids induced by these drugs sensitizing the nucleic
acids to the nuclease action.

A study of the metabolic pathways of thymidine conversion in normal, regenerating
and neoplastic liver tissues showed that the rates of C^{14}-thymidine incorporation
into DNA and its decay to CO_2 correlated with the growth rates of certain transplanted hepatomas (Ferdinandus *et al.*, 1971). Table 52 lists the results obtained
for these processes using tissue sections *in vitro*. It is seen that as the rate
of thymidine incorporation becomes higher, the rate of its catabolism decreases.

The activity of one of the enzymes limiting the uracil catabolism rate, of the
dihydrouracil dehydrogenase, decreases in parallel with the rising growth rate of
transplanted hepatomas (Queener *et al.*, 1971). Figure 161 shows the relative value
of thymidine catabolism to CO_2 decreases with the changes in enzyme activity.

The above kinetic regularities of nucleic acid metabolism in tumours reveal certain
characteristic features which are connected with synthesis and inhibition of
nucleic acid catabolism. This can apparently be considered as evidence of the
disturbance of equilibrium between proliferation and differentiation inherent in
tumour growth.

TABLE 52   Thymidine metabolism in hepatomas with various growth rates
(Ferdinandus *et al.*, 1971)

Tissue	Time of attainment of a tumour diameter of 1.5 cm, in months	Relative value of thymidine incorporation into DNA	Relative value of thymidine catabolism to CO_2	Synthesis / Catabolism
Liver	–	1	1	1
9618A	5.8	2.8	0.49	6.15
9618B	4.5	2.92	0.36	8.10
7800	3.0	3.7	0.069	57.5
5123	2.5	7.06	0.065	135.0
3924A	1.0	18.9	0.00094	22100
7288c	0.8	23.6	0.00050	56200
7777	0.7	45.2	0.00064	87000
3683	0.5	39.0	0.00045	115000
9618A₂	0.4	31.8	0.00041	139000

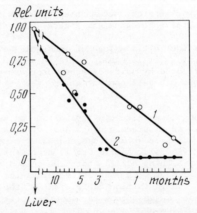

Fig. 161   Relative intensity of thymidine catabolism to CO_2
(2) and the dihydrouracil dehydrogenase activity (1) as a
function of hepatoma growth rate (Queener *et al.*, 1971).

3.   LIPIDS

Lipids are constituents of membranes and are important in the energy relationships
of the cell, so a study of lipid metabolism during the development of various
pathological states, including malignant neoplasms, is rewarding.

The possible role of biological membranes in the regulation of cell metabolism
stimulated studies on the structure, function, chemical and physico-chemical
properties of lipids (Burlakova *et al.*, 1975;   Vladimirov and Archakov, 1972;
Dyatlovitskaya, 1970).   The pecularities of lipid metabolism in the biochemistry
of tumours still remains insufficiently studied.

The relationship of lipid metabolism to carcinogenesis and malignant growth, and
the substantial shifts in quantitative ratios of certain lipid components in the

course of the transplanted tumour's growth stimulated the search for specific 'cancer' lipids. However, the presence of lipids, such as carcinolipin or malignolipin, in tumours was disproved by Bergelson et $al.$ (1967).

At the same time a chemical study of lipid components revealed structural differences in phospholipids of normal and tumour tissues. For instance, hepatoma cells exhibit marked amounts of lecithins with unsaturated fatty acid in position 1, which makes these lecithins different from normal:

$$H_2C\text{--}OCOC_nH_{2n+1}$$
$$|$$
$$HC\text{--}OCOC_mH_{2m-1}$$

$$\overset{O}{\overset{\|}{H_2C\text{--}O\text{--}P\text{--}OCH_2CH_2N(CH_3)_3OH}}$$
$$|$$
$$OH$$

$$H_2C\text{--}OCOC_mH_{2m-1}$$
$$|$$
$$HC\text{--}OCOC_nH_{2n+1}$$

$$\overset{O}{\overset{\|}{H_2C\text{--}O\text{--}P\text{--}OCH_2CH_2N(CH_3)_3OH}}$$
$$|$$
$$OH$$

Liver lecithins   Hepatoma lecithins

An exception is oleic acid: it is uniformly distributed in normal liver lecithins over positions 1 and 2.

The selective nature of the distribution of fatty acids in tumour tissue lecithins was observed also for nephroma RA and Jensen sarcoma. The composition of fatty acids in tumour glycerophospholipids differs from normal in the elevated content of oleic acid and in the low content of arachidonic acid. The presence of lecithins with unsaturated acids in positions 1 and 2 is also characteristic of tumours. This might be the reason why tumour lecithins are less capable of cholesterol solubilization, compared to liver lecithins, and this is reflected in the shift of the cholesterol to lecithin ratio; for instance for hepatomas this ratio is ~1.1, whereas in liver it is ~1.8.

Substantial differences were also observed in the distribution of individual phospholipids in normal and tumour cells.

The regenerating liver cells, just as normal tissues, contain sphingomyelins only in microsomes and cardiolipin in mitochondria.

Unlike normal tissues, sphingomyelin and cardiolipin are present in tumours in microsomes and mitochondria in equal amounts. This can be considered evidence of lack of differentiation because the content of various phospholipids in cells becomes equal (Dyatlovitskaya, 1970). In the minimally deviated hepatoma 48 the lack of differentiation is so indistinct that on the whole the pattern seems to be similar to normal, though cardiolipin is found in microsomes.

Experimental data show a relationship between malignant tumour growth and lipid metabolism. For instance, the lipid content in host liver is higher than in hepatomas (Morris et $al.$, 1964). A considerably smaller incorporation was also observed in hepatomas (Ashmore, 1958; Weber et $al.$, 1961).

These results provide evidence for a lower level of lipid synthesis in hepatomas. As the hepatoma growth rate increases, the intensity of oxidation of fatty acid chains to CO_2 and acetylacetate reduces (Bloch-Frankenthal et $al.$, 1965). The decrease in activity of α-glycerophosphate dehydrogenase occurring in parallel with increasing tumour growth also reveals changes in lipid metabolism (Shonk et $al.$, 1965).

Regular changes in the total contents of lipids and of their individual components, in the composition of fatty acids, and in the physico-chemical properties of the lipid fraction of tumour cells and tissues of hosts are observed in the couse of transplanted tumour growth.

Changes of this kind were observed when studying lipid metabolism in experimental tumours such as Ehrlich ascites carcinoma, the Walker carcinosarcoma, the Sveč erythroleukaemia, etc. (Lankin and Neifakh, 1968). The total amount of lipids in Ehrlich ascites carcinoma cells were sharply diminished on the first day, and from the 5th day reached a constant level which was retained to the terminal stage. A similar course of changes in total lipid content was also observed for Walker carcinosarcoma (Lankin and Neifakh, 1968) and Sveč erythroleukaemia in rats. Some transplanted hepatomas also have a lowered lipid content (Morris *et al.*, 1964).

This effect is similar to that of hypoglycaemia accompanying malignant growth. It seems that a decrease in total lipid content at the initial period of tumour growth is characteristic of most transplanted tumours.

Intensification of lipolysis might be due indirectly to changes in the carbohydrate metabolism of the tumour tissue: there is a definite relationship between the concentrations of carbohydrates and non-esterified fatty acids in the blood.

The content of phospholipids, triglycerides and cholesterol in lipids of Ehrlich ascites carcinoma change mostly during the early stages of tumour growth. Starting from the 5th day after transplantation the concentrations of these fractions in tumour lipids remain virtually constant. The content of free fatty acids in the lipids of Ehrlich ascites carcinoma was reduced by half within the period of 3 to 14 days of tumour growth (Figure 162, curve 2), while the content in the lipids of ascites plasma increased more than 2.5 times between the 7th and 14th day (Figure 162, curve 2).

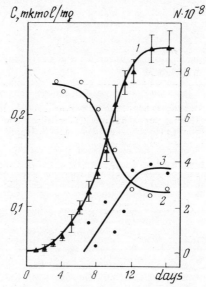

Fig. 162 Changes in lipid content for Ehrlich ascites carcinoma: (1) increase in the number of ascites cells; (2) changes in the content of free fatty acids in tumour cells; (3) increase in fatty acid content in plasma.

The changes in the percentage of phospholipids and total cholesterol — the so-called structural lipids — in the tumour (Sveč erythroleukaemia in rats) display sharp variations during tumour growth.

During intense tumour growth the phospholipids in tumour tissue increase more than five-fold and then drop sharply, whereas the terminal stage of the process exhibits a marked increase in the phospholipid content. The total percentage of cholesterol changes as does phospholipid content. Characteristically the increasing content of structural lipids in tumour tissue is observed against their decrease in the liver of hosts with Sveč erythroleukaemia. The kinetic approach to the study of lipid metabolism during tumour growth revealed also the nature of changes in the content of lipid fractions in the tissues of host organs (Lankin and Neifakh, 1968).

Changes in triglyceride concentrations in host liver were found to be extreme compared with those in other lipid fractions. At the same time the contents of phospholipids, of non-esterified fatty acids and of free cholesterol hardly changed during tumour growth. The content of linoleic acid in mouse liver and blood plasma rose in the early stages of Ehrlich carcinoma and then dropped in the period of fast tumour development, approaching the control level at the terminal stage of tumour growth. The oleic acid content changed in the same way.

The study of changes in the content of individual fatty acids in tumour-bearing animals during the growth of transplanted tumours of a different histogenesis revealed a tendency to a sharp increase in the content of unsaturated acids at the stage of intense tumour growth (Table 53).

TABLE 53   Unsaturated fatty acid content in liver lipids of tumour-bearing animals in relation to normal

Tumour	Fatty acids		
	16:0	18:1	18:2
Ehrlich ascites carcinoma	1.41	3.22	1.38
Ascites form of sarcoma 37	1.63	4.24	1.62
Ascites form of sarcoma 180	2.09	2.33	1.33
Walker carcinosarcoma	1.67	2.94	1.87

Shifts in lipid content during transplanted tumour growth can be caused by several metabolic processes, including peroxidation (Vladimirov and Archakov, 1972). The biogenic inhibitors of free radical reactions, the bio-antioxidants, play an important part in the regulation of peroxidation.

In this connection it would be expedient to discuss the kinetic regularities of the changes in antioxidant activity (AOA) of lipids in tumour growth.

The AOA is a physico-chemical property of the cell lipid fraction related to the capacity to inhibit radical oxidation processes. This capacity is based on the content of bio-antioxidants and synergists in lipids and it can serve as a criterion of the state of cell lipids and this is connected with the structure and function of the biological cell membranes. Such an inter-relationship is confirmed, for instance, by the results of changes in AOA, in phosphoethanol amine content and in the activity of membrane-bound enzymes (glucose-6-phosphatase) presented in Figure 163a.

This is supported by the correlation between AOA changes and the content of non-esterified fatty acids in liver during the development of transplanted leukaemia La (Figure 163b) (Arkhipova et al., 1967).

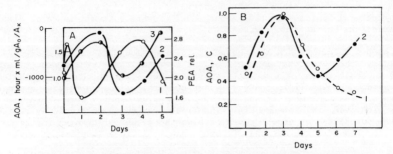

Fig. 163 Composition and AOA of lipids. (a) Changes in
AOA of microsome lipids (1), in phosphatidyl ethanolamine
(2) and in glucose-6-phosphatase activity (3) (Burlakova
et al., 1975); (b) changes in liver lipid AOA (1) and in
unsaturated fatty acid content (2) (Arkhipova *et al.*, 1967).

The change in functional activity of membranes is accompanied by a change in the
antioxidative activity of their lipids. For instance, HeLa cells enter the phase
of DNA synthesis with a sharp drop in the AOA of nuclear lipids (Alesenko and
Burlakova, 1972). It will also be emphasized that the character of AOA changes in
lipids extracted both from tissue homogenate, and from various cell components, is
virtually the same (Alesenko *et al.*, 1973).

The possibility of using lipid AOA as a physico-chemical criterion of the development of various pathological states was discussed in detail in a monograph by
Burlakova *et al.* (1975).

The kinetics of lipid AOA changes with respect to tumour growth was studied for
various forms of carcinogenesis (Burlakova and Molochkina, 1968, 1973), for development of transplanted leukaemia (Burlakova *et al.*, 1966), and for growth of solid
and ascites experimental tumours (Goloshchapov *et al.*, 1973; Burlakova and Palmina,
1967; Burlakova *et al.*, 1966).

Regular lipid AOA changes in tumour tissues and organs of tumour-bearing animals
were observed for all the transplanted tumours studied. The greatest amount of
information was obtained for AOA changes in host liver lipids. Virtually in all
cases AOA arises at the initial stage of tumour growth, reaches a maximum, and then
drops to a level characteristic of healthy animals, or lower.

Inhibition of tumour growth with drugs delays the appearance of the AOA maximum
(Burlakova and Palmina, 1966), whereas an increased inoculum dose induces an earlier
appearance of the AOA maximum (Burlakova and Palmina, 1966; Burlakova *et al.*,
1966).

These regularities of liver lipid AOA changes during tumour growth are supported
by the results in Figure 164.

For transplanted leukaemia La the development of which is accompanied by leukaemic
cell infiltration in host organs, the AOA maximum is observed towards the end of
the induction period, when there is a marked increase in spleen weight, in leucocyte count, and in the haemocytoblast count in bone marrow (Figure 164a). It is
characteristic that liver lipid AOA changes display the same regularity when the
leukaemia development rate is altered by varying the inoculum dose or by administration of an effective antileukaemic drug (of ionol) (Burlakova and Palmina,
1966; Burlakova *et al.*, 1965).

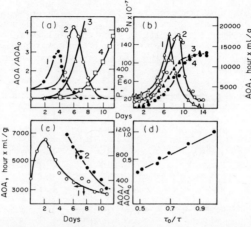

Fig. 164   Changes in liver lipid AOA during experimental
tumour development: (a) leukaemia La: curves for AOA changes
(1 and 2) and the relevant curves for increase in spleen
weight (3 and 4) with different inocula;   (b) Ehrlich ascites
carcinoma: curves for AOA changes (1 and 2) and the relevant
curves for increase in cell number in the ascitic fluid (3
and 4);   (c) hepatoma 22a: changes in tumour lipid AOA (2)
and in host liver (1);   (d) correlation between AOA and
weight-doubling time of hepatoma 22a in the course of tumour
growth.

Ehrlich ascites carcinoma development is accompanied by the same liver lipid AOA
changes (Figure 164b).   The maximum AOA value is attained when the tumour cells
appear in the blood, so the AOA starts dropping from the moment the ascites cells
begin infiltrating the host organs.   A rise of AOA in the period of maximum tumour
development rate (Figure 164c, curve 2) is characteristic for lipids extracted
from ascites cells (Goloshchapov *et al.*, 1973;   Burlakova *et al.*, 1966).

The growth of solid hepatoma 22a is accompanied by extreme changes in the liver
lipid AOA (Figure 164c, curve 1) and by a reduction of the tumour lipid AOA
(Figure 164c, curve 2) (Burlakova and Palmina, 1967).

Calculation of the tumour mass doubling time (with approximation of hepatoma growth
by a power function) yielded a linear dependence (Figure 164d) between tumour lipid
AOA and the doubling time (Burlakova and Palmina, 1967).   Thus the tumour lipid AOA
correlates with changes in proliferative activity, since the AOA changes do not
represent a specific characteristic of tumour growth, but are due to the intensity
of cellular proliferation (Burlakova *et al.*, 1975).

The main conclusions on the regularity of AOA changes in the development of transplanted solid tumours are supported by the results obtained for tumours of different localizations induced by various carcinogens.   Stepwise lipid AOA changes of
the same type were observed for experimental carcinogenesis induced by hepatotropic
carcinogens (Burlakova and Molochkina, 1968), by polycyclic hydrocarbons (Burlakova
and Molochkina, 1973;   Esakova and Tarusov, 1970), or by γ-rays (Burlakova and
Molochkina, 1973).

For instance the administration of o-aminoazotoluene (Burlakova and Molochkina,
1968) first results in a drop in liver lipid AOA activity then in a subsequent

approximately triple rise compared to normal. The phase of AOA drop corresponds
to the stage of low reactivity of liver cells to growth-stimulating treatment. At
the stage of diffuse-focal hyperplasia, when the proliferative activity of cells
rises and the first tumours appear, the liver lipid AOA becomes stronger. Characteristically, when the weight of the induced tumour increases the tumour lipid AOA
drops (Figure 165a).

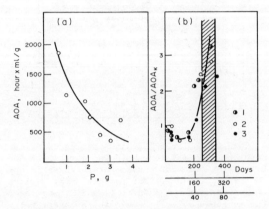

Fig. 165 Changes in lipid AOA for experimental carcinogenesis.
(a) Tumour lipid AOA as a function of induced tumour weight;
(b) normalized curve for liver lipid AOA changes after treatment with o-aminoazotoluene (1), with γ-rays (2) and with
3,4-benzoapyrene (3).

Kinetic curves for changes in the relative AOA value plotted in experiments on
tumour induction by various carcinogenic factors can be generalized by transformation along the time axis to the moment of the appearance of the first tumours
(Figure 165b) (Burlakova et al., 1975). This demonstrates the general nature of
changes in the composition of the cell lipid fraction during the appearance and
growth of tumours.

Regular changes in the lipid AOA of host organs suggested the possibility of using
these results for a rational approach to chemotherapy of tumours. Changes in liver
lipid AOA under the action of various antitumour drugs were studied and their
administration to healthy animals resulted in a substantial and prolonged drop of
liver lipid AOA. The effectiveness of antitumour drugs was found to correlate
with their capacity for decreasing liver lipid AOA.

For instance, a study of the antileukaemic action of various antitumour treatments
(inhibitors of free radical reactions, alkylating drugs, irradiation, hypothermia)
showed that the inhibition coefficient for leukaemia La ($\varkappa*$) was related in a
linear manner to the reciprocal of liver lipid antioxidative activity (Figure 166)
so that

$$\varkappa = 0.53 + 0.64 \cdot 10^3 \ (AOA).$$

The relationship between the changes in these values suggests that antitumour drugs
act on the same system in the body and this involves lipids. The biological
membranes exercise various regulation functions in the cell and seem to represent
such a system.

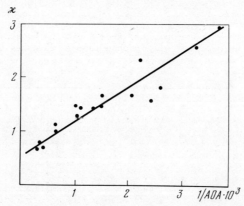

Fig. 166   Relation of antitumour activity coefficient of
drugs to the lipid lipid AOA.

CHAPTER 8

DISTURBANCE OF STRUCTURE AND BIOSYNTHESIS OF INFORMATIONAL MACROMOLECULES IN MALIGNANT GROWTH

Scientific advances during the two last decades have opened up new possibilities for the study of the nature of malignant growth. Study of the molecular mechanisms of malignant growth is a future field for kinetic analysis.

Extensive experimental data support the transport scheme of the gene information:

DNA
$\downarrow\uparrow$
DNA $\rightleftarrows$ RNA $\longrightarrow$ protein

and the elucidation of the structure and function of this process represent basic advances in molecular biology.

Diverse disturbances in the structures which contain the genetic code or in certain links in gene translation or in regulation of these processes seem to be the most probable causes of malignant cell transformation. This stimulated much research in experimental oncology aimed at elucidating the possible disturbances of structures and biosynthesis of informational macromolecules, and biosynthesis regulation during tumour growth.

1. STRUCTURAL CHANGES IN BIOMACROMOLECULES

DEOXYRIBONUCLEIC ACID

The role of DNA as a carrier of the genetic code suggested the need for research aimed at finding the quantitative differences between DNA from normal and tumour tissues. The differences in DNA content have already been discussed in Chapter 7. Many papers give comparative studies of the nucleotide content, physico-chemical properties, nucleotide sequences, and secondary structures of DNA of tumour and normal cells. However, earlier information on physico-chemical and biochemical characteristics of tumour DNA is very contradictory, probably due to differences in experimental conditions, morphological and biochemical heterogeneity of tumours, and inadequate methods of DNA isolation.

Nucleotide Composition

There is no generally accepted concept concerning changes in the DNA nucleotide

261

composition in tumour growth. DNA nucleotide composition does not differ from that in normal tissues. The content of 5-methylcytosine in DNA of leukaemia lymphocytes was found to be five times higher than in lymphocyte DNA of a healthy human, and the content of guanine was two to three times higher and cytosine was 2 to $2\frac{1}{2}$ times higher than normal (Desai et al., 1971). This suggests not only a higher level of DNA methylation, but also an alteration of its nucleotide composition in the leukaemic cell.

In the satellite DNA of tumour and normal liver cells the content of 5-methylcytosine is the same; their buoyant densities are the same too.

The level of DNA methylation in leucocytes of humans with acute and chronic leukaemia was several times higher than that in DNA of normal leucocytes (Silber et al., 1966; Fedorov et al., 1971).

The DNA of animals and humans generally contains one methylated base: 5-methylcytosine. But as a result of incubation of leucocytes with (^{14}C-methyl)methionine, ^{6}M-methyladenine was isolated from DNA hydrolysates along with 5-methylcytosine. 1-Methylguanine, 7-methylguanine, N^2-methylguanine, N^2-dimethylguanine were detected in the DNA of HeLa cells (Culp et al., 1970). 5-Methylcytosine was found to be the only methylated base in HeLa cells (Lawley et al., 1972). A 'chart' was compiled of the position of 5-methylcytosine in DNA of rat Novikoff hepatoma cells which arose in culture. A very small amount of 5-methylcytosine was localized at the 5-terminus of pyrimidine clusters and it was mainly concentrated at the 3'-terminus. Much 5-methylcytosine was also distributed in the inside regions of these clusters (Sneider et al., 1972). Chemical carcinogens such as N-methyl-N-nitrosourea and dimethylnitrosoamine enlarged the spectrum of methylated bases and involved O^6-methylguanine, 7-methylguanine, 3-methylguanine, 1-methyladenine, 3-methyladenine (Maitra and Frei, 1975; Engelse, 1974; Frei and Lawley, 1975).

The anomaous methylation of DNA may result in the malignant transformation of a cell, because depurinization or the formation of non-complementary pairs can cause mutations.

It is impossible at present to establish the relationship between DNA methylation and cell proliferation and differentiation processes.

Primary Structure

The differences between DNA from various strains of mouse myeloma, and differences between tumour and normal DNA were found by the RNA-DNA hybridization method (Greenberg and Uhr, 1967a; Krueger and McCarthy, 1970). For instance, the study of hybridization of RNA from plasmacytoma with DNA from tumour and normal tissues, conducted under conditions making possible binding only with repeated DNA sequences, suggested that the number of repeats in the plasacytoma genome was larger than in the genome of normal spleen. Moreover, the content of satellite DNA in the genomes of various myeloma types was also higher compared to that in the spleen (Greenberg and Uhr, 1967b).

The distribution of pyrimidine nucleotide blocks in DNA after radiation damage, in mouse leukaemia La, and for spontaneous leukaemia of farm animals was studied. Both after radiation and in leukaemia La part of the DNA polypyrimidine blocks disappeared, whereas the relative content of single thymidine nucleotide residues increased. The distribution of polypyrimidine nucleotide blocks of DNA of leucocytes of cows with leukaemia differs statistically from that for normal DNA. With spontaneous leukaemia of cattle and also with erythromyeloblastosis in rats the relative content of certain tri- and di-nucleotide blocks in DNA considerably diminishes. The distribution of nucleotide DNA blocks for leukaemia substantially differs in these animals from the changes which occur on radiation damage and in leukaemia La in mice. This suggests that cell malignancy is connected with various changes in the primary DNA structure (Kritskii *et al.*, 1972a,b, 1973).

DNA reassociation kinetics is used in studying genome changes induced by malignization and differentiation of organs (Britten and Kohne, 1968).

DNA reassociation — the process of helix formation — is observed experimentally as a bimolecular reaction in solution. The limiting stage is formation of the two elements, i.e. the formation of a nucleus involving serveral pairs of bases bound as in the native molecule. This is followed by fast formation of a double helix ('zippering' of the chain). The effect of these stages on the reassociation rates has been discussed theoretically (Wetmur and Davidson, 1968). DNA reassociation is described by a simple equation

$$C/C_0 = 1/(1 + k_2 C_0 t)$$

where C is the concentration of the denatured DNA fragment, C_0 is the initial concentration, k_2 is the reassociation rate constant. Usually k_2 or $C_0\, t_{1/2}$ — the product of initial concentration by the half-life of DNA transformation — are used as a measure of the DNA reassociation rate. Since at $t = t_{1/2}$ $C/C_0 = \frac{1}{2}$, $k_2 = 1/C_0 t_{1/2}$.

If the DNA of various living bodies are fragmented to the same size, the probability of encounter of two complementary fragments (and thus the k_2 value) will increase as the size of the fragments is reduced. The proportionality between $C_0 t_{1/2}$ and the DNA complexity is the basis for kinetic determination of genome size.

Defects of primary structure connected with modifications and with excision of bases hinder the formation of perfect double strand duplexes; this results in a k_2 decrease.

The DNA of mouse liver and of plasmacytoma exhibit very similar reassociation kinetics (Mori *et al.*, 1973). The T_m of reassociated duplexes were the same for the DNA of tumour and liver reassociated to identical $C_0 t$ values.

The DNA reassociation kinetics of rat thymus and ascites hepatoma were also studied. Three basic zones of 'fast', 'intermediate' and 'slow' DNA reassociation will be noted in the kinetic curve. The 'fast-renaturing' fraction represents 10-18%, the 'intermediate' one is 20-25%, and the 'slow' one is 55-60% (Khanson and Zhivotovskii, 1974). The DNA reassociation curves for thymus and tumour of rat virtually coincide in all three zones. However, the authors do not exclude the possibility of various differences between the DNA of normal and neoplastic cells (changes in certain sequences, modifications of bases) undetectable by the method used.

At the same time a comparison of DNA reassociation curves for mouse spleen and plasmacytoma (Timofeeva *et al.*, 1975) revealed certain differences (Figure 167). For instance, the plasmacytoma DNA contains more repeated sequences reassociating within the range $C_0 t = 10^{-2} - 10^2$ and, consequently, less unique sequences. The content of 'fast-reassociating' repeated sequences ($C_0 t < 10^{-2}$) was the same.

Comparison of the reassociation kinetics of DNA from normal and leukaemia leucocytes showed that the rate constant k_2 for acute leukaemia was lower than normal and in chronic leukaemia. This might be due to a greater amount of primary structure defects.

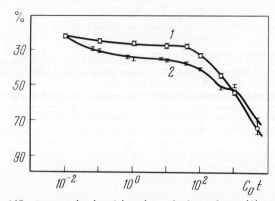

Fig. 167 Reassociation kinetics of the spleen (1) and
plasmacytoma nuclei DNA of mice (Timofeeva et $al.$, 1975).

Secondary Structure

Differences between tumour and normal cell DNA with respect to their physico-
chemical properties have been found recently. It was thought by Fiel et $al.$ (1965)
that DNA isolated from neoplastic cells had a lower molecular weight and a more
rigid configuration than DNA from normal tissues. Moreover, the elastoviscosity
and the intrinsic viscosity of DNA diminish in the process of cell malignization
(Kuzmina and Strazhevskaia, 1970) and there is a change in the DNA melting point.

Comparison of IR spectra of normal and tumour DNA for different relative humidity
levels revealed that the hydration of tumour DNA was weaker at a relative humidity
of 95%, and stronger at lower relative moisture values. Differences were also
found in the parameters characterizing the structures of spin-labelled DNA preparations of DNA from normal liver and hepatoma (Bogdanov and Shmonina, 1975).

An important difference in the behaviour of DNA from normal and tumour cells was
found by studying the conformational transitions in DNA, making use of spin-
labelled ethylene imine (Mil et $al.$, 1973).

A sensitive kinetic formaldehyde (KF) method has been developed recently. It can
fix one defect per 10^4 nucleotide pairs. Local unwound fragments — despiralization
nuclei — appear in the native double-stranded DNA structure under the action of
formaldehyde. The initial rate of formaldehyde-induced DNA despiralization is very
low, but as nuclei accumulate, despiralization occurs mainly at the expense of
these nuclei and thus increases with larger numbers of nuclei. Having attained
the maximum rate, the process starts slowing down due to coalescence of denatured
regions spreading towards each other.

The model proposed for the interaction of native DNA with formaldehyde can also
help with the problem of DNA with secondary structure defects. The following
analytic expression for the kinetic DNA despiralization curve results:

$$\vartheta(t) = \exp\left[-(p\nu + 2\nu c)t - p\nu t^2\right]$$

Here $\vartheta(t)$ is the extent of DNA spiralization, ν is the initial size of the despiralization nucleus, and p and ν are the rates of nucleus initiation and growth, respectively. The concentration of secondary DNA structure defects equal $1/\bar{n}$ by definition, where $\bar{n}$ is the average length of the spiral section between defects (in
nucleotide pairs).

The linear anamorphosis of this curve

$$- \ln \vartheta/t = p\nu + 2\nu c + p\nu t$$

is a straight line crossing the y-axis at point $(p\nu + 2\nu c)$ and its distance from the origin of co-ordinates increases with a larger number of defects, c.

Thus, the KF method permits evaluation of the summary amount of secondary structure defects whatever the nature of chemical damage. It was used to study the stability of the secondary DNA structure in normal and tumour tissues. The amount of denatured DNA loci in the spleen of leukaemic mice and particularly in ascites cells was found to be higher than normal (Figure 168). Secondary DNA structure destabilization may be due to its functional role in cells with elevated mitotic activity, such as tumour cells. Another possible reason for local DNA denaturation may be primary structure damage, such as excess methylation of bases, single-strand cleavages, etc.

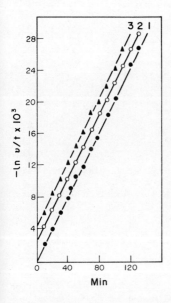

Fig. 168 Linear anamorphoses of the DNA despiralization kinetic curves in the presence of formaldehyde: (1) DNA of intact mouse spleen; (2) DNA of mouse spleen with leukaemia La; (3) DNA of Ehrlich ascites carcinoma.

The presence of secondary structure defects in tumour DNA suggested that the damage caused by physical or chemical factors can be greater in tumour than in normal DNA. Certain experiments were conducted in this connection. DNA specimens were irradiated with X-rays *in vitro* at a dose of 5 krad, and the curves for despiralization in the presence of formaldehyde were analysed. A comparison of these curves with those obtained experimentally in the absence of irradiation showed approximately similar damage of the spleen protein in intact mice and of spleen DNA in mice with leukaemia La, whereas damage to the Ehrlich ascites cells DNA was much greater. This is evidence of a higher radiosensitivity of the ascites cell DNA.

However, the defects in DNA structure do not represent the only source of differences between normal and tumour DNA. For instance, the markedly dissimilar content of pyrimidine blocks of different length in DNA or normal and tumour cells (Kritskii *et al.*, 1972a,b, 1973) is responsible for the different radiosensitivity of these DNA. This was observed by studying *in vitro* radiation-induced DNA damage. A certain correlation between the percentage of radio-damaged bases Z and a parameter such as the extent of grouping β of the most radioresponsive bases — pyrimidines — was observed (Fonarev *et al.*, 1979). This correlation is described by the equation

$$\log [6.4/(Z - C_i) - 1] = 6.49 - 1.23\beta,$$

where C_i is a parameter depending on the mean GC composition of DNA.

The β values for a number of DNA (in terms of its radiosensitivity) were calculated using this equation and the results were in agreement with those obtained by direct chromatographic analysis.

Defects of the secondary DNA structure in tumours can appear in the course of replication (Zhizhina *et al.*, 1975). However, the measurements of defectiveness of the actively synthesizing DNA in regenerating liver showed that the amount of DNA defects is no higher than 1 per 10^4 pairs (1×10^{-4}), which is lower than that in tumour growth ($1.5 - 3.3 \times 10^{-4}$). Moreover, the accumulation of secondary DNA structure defects in the course of Ehrlich ascites carcinoma development occurs within the period corresponding to the slowing down of tumour growth, and by the 8th – 9th day the number of defects becomes 4×10^{-4}. This also supports the conclusion that the contribution of replication to the appearance of secondary DNA structural defects in tumours is insignificant. It might be that the elevated number of DNA defects in tumour cells can be caused by DNA autolysis in the course of mass cell decay at later stages of tumour growth. Chanchalaghvili *et al.* (1975) report microcalorimetric studies of solutions of DNA isolated from normal (liver, spleen, kidney) and tumour (sarcoma M-1, Walker sarcoma and Pliss lymphosarcoma) tissues of white rats. These revealed that the heat absorption characteristics of normal tissue DNA (T_m, ΔT) coincide, whereas those of tissue DNA represent one family differing from normal DNA. The basic heat absorption by tumour DNA within the range 79 – 84°F is shifted towards lower temperatures by 0.7 – 1°F. Weak heat absorption by tumour DNA is observed in the range 73 – 78°F. These effects suggest that the amount of defects in tumour DNA is higher than normal.

The structural defects in spin-labelled DNA isolated from normal and leukaemic cells have been investigated (Mil *et al.*, 1975). The temperature dependence of the label rotational correlation was evaluated by the EPR technique. The temperature of structural transition in spin-labelled leukaemic DNA was found to be lower than normal. This could be due to the increased number of defects and would also be in agreement with the KF results (Table 54).

TABLE 54   Characteristics of a DNA preparation

DNA preparation number	Temperature of structural transition	Amount of defects 10^4
Normal		
K-75	60° ± 0.5	4.1
K-68	57.5° ± 0.5	6.3
Leukaemia		
K-66	49° ± 0.5	12.2
K-64	54° ± 0.5	10.0
K-62	49° ± 0.5	

The effect of radiation on structural transitions in normal and leukaemic DNA cells is different. The temperature of structural transition is substantially

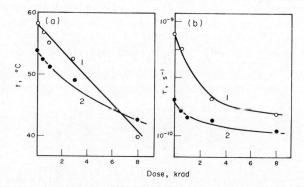

Fig. 169 Structural characteristics of spin-labelled DNA
preparations irradiated with various doses: (a) curves for
change of temperature of structural DNA transition in normal
cells (1) and for leukaemia (2); (b) changes in the
rotational correlation time at 20° in DNA preparations in
normal cells (2) and for leukaemia (2) (Mil et al., 1975).

reduced by radiation and with a big enough dose it approaches the value obtained
for completely denatured DNA (Figure 169a).

The dependence of the structural transition temperature and of the time of the label
rotational correlation (τ_C) on the radiation dose is also markedly different for
DNA of normal and leukaemic cells. With low radiation doses (up to 2 krad) the
structural transition temperature for DNA of leukaemic cells is lower than for the
DNA of normal leucocytes (Figure 169a). The dose dependence of τ_C at 20° also
shows a different radioresponse of leukaemic and normal DNA (Figure 169b).

Though the above results produce evidence for distinct differences between the DNA
in tumour and normal cells, the cause and effect relationship between DNA structural
disturbances and malignant cell transformation cannot be considered as established.

RIBONUCLEIC ACID

Heterogeneous Nuclear and Information RNA

The scanty information reported about the structure of heterogeneous nuclear and
information RNA in tumours has been discussed recently in Busch's book (1974).
This section deals with later research on this problem.

It has been found by the competing hybridization method (Garrett et al., 1973) that
the nuclear RNA in newborn rat liver and in hepatoma 5123C are characterized by the
lack of certain base sequences that are present in nuclear RNA in the liver of
adult animals. Certain differences between the nuclear sequences of RNA in normal
liver and heptoma AH-130 were found by the same method (Ono et al., 1971).

The structure of heterogeneous nuclear RNA from lymphocytes of patients with
chronic lymphatic leukaemic has been studied by Mansson et al. (1975). The number
of poly(A) sites in the nuclei of normal lymphocytes was found to be lower than
that in the lymphocyte nuclei of patients with chronic lymphatic leukaemia.
Presumably the largest molecules of nuclear RNA contain a larger amount of

'recognition sites' for RNA-ase processing.

Double-stranded RNA was found in a number of eukaryotic cells. The functions of these molecules in the metabolism of cell RNA are unknown. However, the ability of very low amounts of double-stranded RNA to inhibit initiation of protein synthesis in acellular systems underlies the hypothesis that these molecules are involved in regulation of RNA translation in eukaryotic cells (Robertson and Matthews, 1973).

It was found that at least in some cell types the double stranded RNA is associated with poly(A)-sequences and possessed metabolic properties characteristic of hetero-geneous nuclear DNA. The presence of a larger amount of poly(A)-containing nuclear RNA in leukaemic cells, compared to normal lymphocytes, has been reported (Torelli and Torelli, 1973). Later on, the same authors conducted more extensive research on double stranded nuclear RNA in leukaemic cells (Torelli et al., 1975).

A new class of nuclear RNA — the low molecular weight nuclear RNA — has been found and characterized recently. Though the functions of most low molecular weight nuclear RNA are unknown, there is evidence of their biological role (Busch, 1974). A difference between the number of fractions of low-molecular weight nuclear RNA in normal rat liver and in Novikoff hepatoma has been reported (Prestayko et al., 1970).

Similar results were obtained by comparing the low molecular weight nuclear RNA of liver and Zaidel hepatoma (Kozlov and Seits, 1975).

Ribosomal RNA

Important differences between the composition and primary structure of RNA from tumour and normal cells, caused by the low content of adenylic and the high content of cytidylic acids in tumour RNA were reported in early papers by Busch (see, for instance, Busch and Smetana, 1970) and by others (for instance, Matsuhisa et al., 1970). Moreover, a higher content of GU and UG nucleotides and a lower content of CG in tumours, compared to normal, were observed in 28 S rRNA of hepatomas (Wikman et al., 1970; Seeber and Busch, 1972).

Competing hybridization (Wikman et al., 1970) of 28 S rRNA from Novikoff hepatoma and from normal liver with nucleolar Novikoff hepatoma DNA revealed that the amount of hybridized 28 S rRNA from normal liver was only 92% of the hybridized 28 S rRNA from Novikoff hepatoma. No such difference was found by the same method for relevant 18 S rRNA. It follows that the 28 S rRNA of normal liver and of Novikoff hepatoma differ in loci containing 300-400 nucleotides, i.e. certain 28 S rRNA sequences of the hepatoma seem to be lacking in the 28 S rRNA of normal liver.

Later analysis of polypurines (Amaldi and Attardi, 1971) and of polypyrimidines (Nazar and Busch, 1972) treated with RNA-ases revealed no differences between the primary structures of normal and tumour tissues. Besides, the 28 S rRNA-^{32}P from HeLa cells competed successfully (at a simultaneous competing hybridization) both with non-labelled 28 S rRNA of HeLa and with RNA of normal human tissues. Also no differences were found in RNA from tumour and normal cells, when the nucleotide composition was evaluated from UV absorption (Busch and Smetana, 1970) and by analysis of nucleotide derivatives (Nazar, 1973).

The data on the resemblance of ribosomal RNA and of their precursors in normal and tumour tissues obtained support in the study of these RNA by the competing hybrid-ization method and by analysis of nucleotides (Sitz et al., 1973).

Thus, both rRNA and their precursors remain unchanged during oncogenesis and, consequently, the data suggesting substantial differences exist between the

nucleotide composition and the distribution of oligonucleotides in the rRNA of
normal and tumour tissues seem to be incorrect: they were obtained using preparations of non-uniformly labelled rRNA.

At the same time the possibility of certain minor differences between rRNA from
normal and tumour tissues cannot be excluded. For instance, it was reported that
the 18 S rRNA from normal mouse tissue contained tetranucleotide and hexanucleotide
that were absent in the RNA of hepatomas (Hashimoto and Muramatsu, 1973).

Transport RNA

A large amount of indirect evidence supporting the suggestion that the tRNA of
tumour cells can differ in structure from that of normal tissues has been obtained
lately. It was found, in particular, that the activity of tRNA-methyltransferase
(Borek and Srinivasan, 1966; Kerr and Borek, 1972; Starr and Sells, 1969) in
extracts from diverse neoplastic tissues including virally transformed cells and
chemically-induced tumours, was several times higher than that in normal tissues
(Borek and Kerr, 1972). A hypothesis was proposed that the increase in methylase
activity results in hypermethylation of tRNA and is related to oncogenesis
(Srinivasan and Borek, 1963, 1964).

A large amount of research on the peculiarities of tRNA methylation in tumour cells
was conducted taking into account the possibility of anomalous methylation of tRNA
in tumour cells. An increased amount of a number of methylated bases was found in
the tRNA of CH3 mouse adenocarcinoma and of the ascites tumour 180, compared to the
tRNA content in mouse liver (Bergquist and Matthews, 1962).

The amount of methylated nucleosides in tRNA from human brain tumours was found to
be higher than that in normal human brain. For instance, an 80-fold increase in
1-methylguanosine was found in the glioblastoma tRNA. A correlation with the
extent of tumour cell deviation from normal was observed, but the increase in
content of methylated bases was not related to the tumour growth rate (Viale, 1971).

However, another study of tRNA from human brain tumour and from normal brain tissues
by the labelling method did not show a considerable increase in the content of
various methylated nucleosides in tumour tRNA (Randerath, 1971; Randerath et al.,
1971). No important differences were found between the general content of modified
bases in the tRNA of normal and tumour brain tissues. These data on the composition
of tumour tRNA bases are consistent with the results obtained by Iwanami and Brown
(1968), Baguley and Staehelin (1968) for tRNA from other malignant sources (leukaemic cells, HeLa and L cells).

The method of chemical labelling of nucleic acid derivatives was used when studying
the composition of tRNA bases in two Morris hepatomas (7777 and 5123D) and in rat
liver (Randerath et al., 1974). The tRNA from Morris hepatomas did not substantially differ from that in rat liver, and no explicit correlation was found between
the extent of tRNA modification and the rate of Morris hepatoma growth. The
differences in the nucleotide composition of tRNA observed earlier could have been
caused by changes in the composition of isoforms in tRNA of hepatomas (Randerath
et al., 1974; Sheid et al., 1971).

It was concluded from studies of tRNA methylation in normal and SV40-transformed
cells that the extent of methylation and the composition of methylated bases in
these cells do not differ, though the tRNA-ase activity in extracts from transformed cells appeared to be higher (Klagsbrun, 1972).

The higher activity of tRNA-methyltransferases in tumours was thought to be
connected with selective methylation of certain tRNA forms. Naturally, essential

differences in the extent of methylation would not be observed for the whole tRNA.

Differences in the extent of base methylation were actually found for tyrosyl- and histidyl-tRNA from normal liver and from Novikoff hepatoma. For instance, the content of 5-methylcytosine and thymine in tyrosyl-tRNA from hepatoma was half that in the liver. 1-Methylguanine was completely absent in liver and was present in a considerable amount in a tyrosyl-tRNA preparation isolated from hepatoma. At the same time the total tRNA preparations from liver and hepatoma virtually did not differ in the extent of base methylation (Nau, 1974; Baliga *et al.*, 1969).

The differences between modifications of tRNA from normal and tumour cells might result in dissimilar spatial structures of tRNA. For instance, it was found that the chromatographic characteristics of labelled phenylalanyl-tRNA, seryl-tRNA and tyrosyl-tRNA from tumour and normal mouse cells were different (Taylor *et al.*, 1967, 1968). Similar results were obtained for normal and leukaemic lymphoblasts of humans (Gallo and Pestka, 1970). Differences were also found between thr tRNA from normal rats and from lysyl-, leucyl-, phenylalanyl- and tyrosyl-tRNA from rats treated with a carcinogen, 3'-methyl-4-dimethylaminoazobenzene (Goldman and Griffin, 1970). Thus, there are qualitative and quantitative differences between the compositions of modified tRNA bases and this seems to be responsible for the dissimilar three-dimensional structure of tRNA molcules in normal and tumour cells.

PROTEINS

Shapot (1975) suggested that no genetically determined protein macromolecules foreign to intact tissue are formed in the cancer cell. However, there are changes in the quantitative ratio and the subcellular localization of certain proteins, especially isoenzymes, in the tumour cell. This disturbs the normal development of certain biochemical processes and the metabolism of tumour tissues.

Electrophoretic comparison of ribosomal proteins from tumour and normal cells showed no substantial differences in the protein composition of the Morris hepatoma 5123 and of normal tissues. At the same time the Yoshida hepatoma demonstrated a considerably increased protein content in ribosomes. Great differences were also observed between proteins of the hepatoma AH-130 ribosomes and those of liver ribosomes, as well as between brain tissue of normal rats and neuroblastoma C-1300 (Chiarugi and Lorenzoni, 1968; Subramanian *et al.*, 1975). The differences in protein content might cause disturbance in translation of genetic information in tumour cells.

There are several comparative studies of chromatin proteins in normal and tumour tissues. The acid proteins of chromatin were found to change in the case of mammary gland cancer (Kadohama and Turkington, 1974) and leukaemia (Desai *et al.*, 1975). The ratio of non-histone to histone proteins in tumour tissue is twice that in normal tissue (Desai *et al.*, 1975; Sawada *et al.*, 1973). The structural and matrix activities of chromatin in a fast-growing Morris hepatoma 5123C and in a slow-growing Morris hepatoma 9618A were very different from those in normal liver (Arnold *et al.*, 1973). The amino acid composition of various histone fractions in tumour and normal tissues (Jungmann *et al.*, 1970) and the electrophoretic mobility of these fractions were also different.

Only the protein groups which might be responsible for disturbance in the regulation of the biosynthesis of informational macromolecules in tumour cells have been discussed above. Yet much information is available also about the functional activity, isomorphism, electrophoretic mobility, antigen properties, etc., of various protein classes and groups in normal and tumour tissues. This information is covered in reviews by Shapot (1975) and McCarty and McCarty (1974).

2. BIOSYNTHESIS OF NUCLEIC ACIDS AND PROTEINS

DNA BIOSYNTHESIS AND ITS REGULATION

This section deals mainly with the replication and regulation mechanisms of DNA synthesis.

DNA Polymerases

Various forms of DNA polymerases with a large spectrum of physico-chemical properties have been found in chromatin, cytoplasm, mitochondria, cytoplasmic membranes
of normal and tumour cells: their functions are repair and replication. The DNA-
polymerases are usually divided into three groups with respect to their localization: the cytoplasmic, the nuclear and the mitochondrial polymerases (Filippovich,
1975). In tumour and normal cells (HeLa cells and normal diploid cells of human
pulmonary tissue) one of the DNA polymerases in the nucleus represents the nuclear
form, and the other resembles the cytoplasmic polymerase (Weissbach *et al.*, 1971).
In rat hepatoma cells the DNA polymerase usually is in its high molecular weight or
cytoplasmic form (Ove *et al.*, 1969) and it differs in its properties from the
enzyme with lower molecular weight present preferentially in nuclei of normal and
regenerating liver. It might be that in cells of normal or regenerating liver the
transition of high molecular weight to low molecular weight DNA polymerase is so
fast that this prevents detection of the high molecular weight enzyme in the
course of purification. At the same time in a hepatoma the DNA polymerase dissociation might be slower, and this could be responsible for the presence of both DNA
polymerase forms in hepatoma cells. Indeed, an additional fraction (mol. weight
70,000 - 80,000) exhibiting polymerase activity appears in the DNA polymerase preparations on prolonged storage (Tanabe and Takahashi, 1973).

Two functional types of enzymes are distinguished: the replicative DNA polymerase
II and the DNA polymerase I to repair DNA (Grishom *et al.*, 1972).

Comparative analysis of DNA polymerases in normal and tumour tissues (thymus and
regenerating rat liver, mouse liver, rat hepatoma, Ehrlich ascites carcinoma cells)
showed the presence of both types of the DNA polymerase in all cells (Baril *et al.*,
1973; Wallace *et al.*, 1971). The amount of replicative DNA polymerase is higher
in actively proliferating tissues, and in the resting cells both forms are found in
equal amounts. Only the DNA polymerase I is found in nuclei of normal rat liver.

Substantial differences were found between the DNA polymerases of normal and tumour
cells. The replicative cell system is known to control the polycondensation of
deoxynucleotides with high precision, using the principle of the complementarity of
bases. The interaction energies of complementary and non-complementary bases
(1-3 kcal/mole) (Loeb *et al.*, 1974) appears to be much lower than would follow from
quantum-mechanical calculations, and this cannot ensure a high precision of base-
pairing. It follows that the DNA polymerase must contribute to the choice of
nucleotides and to the complementarity of bases in DNA biosynthesis.

The DNA polymerases substantially differ in this respect in the precision of
complementary base-pairing. In a model system with polydeoxynucleotides as
matrices the frequency of incorporation of non-complementary nucleotides ('error'
frequency) by the DNA polymerase of leukaemic cells is approximately one 'error'
per 250-800 of incorporated nucleotides (Table 55). In the same system the
'errors' of DNA polymerase from normal lymphocytes stimulated for division were
much less frequent: one 'error' per 2,500 - 91,000 nucleotides (Loeb *et al.*, 1974;
Springgate *et al.*, 1972; Sirover and Loeb, 1974). Thus the number of 'errors' in
the DNA polymerase of leukaemic lymphocytes is ten times higher than that for the
DNA polymerase of normal lymphocytes. The 'errors' in DNA replication are

TABLE 55 Errors in base pairing with DNA-polymerases *in vitro*

Source of the DNA polymerases	Error frequency	Error frequency after treatment with carcinogen (β-propiolactone)	Matrix	References
Normal lymphocytes stimulated with phytohaemagglutinin	1/15000-1/91000	-	Poly(dA-dT)	Loeb *et al.* (1974)
Leukaemia cells	1/250-1/800	-	Poly(dA-dT)	Loeb *et al.* (1974)
Calf thymus	1/12000-1/180000	-	Poly(dA)$_{600}$ x (dT)$_{11}$	Loeb *et al.* (1974)
E. coli, phage T4	1/12000-1/184000	-	Poly(dA-dT)	Loeb *et al.* (1974)
Virus from bird myeloblastosis (reverse transcriptase)	1/579	1/203	Poly(dA)$_{200}$-oligo(dT)$_{18}$	Sirover and Loeb (1974)
Echinus nuclear cells	1/3852	1/2448-1/2626	Poly(dA)$_{200}$-oligo(dT)$_{10}$	Sirover and Loeb (1974)

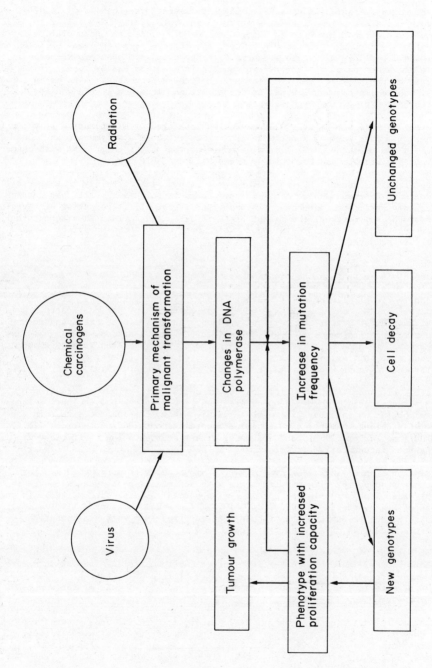

Scheme 6   Accumulation of genetic errors in the course of tumour growth

considered to be the basic cause of malignant alterations (Loeb *et al.*, 1974). Indeed, if the DNA polymerase makes 'errors' in synthesizing DNA, this results in accumulation of proteins with an altered amino acid sequence. Accumulating in cell generations and reaching threshold values, the 'errors' lead to decay or to degeneration and possibly malignancy (Scheme 6). The process of DNA biosynthesis is very often accompanied by 'errors' in genetic information and by repair of these 'errors' by DNA polymerases. The intensity of these processes, balanced in normal cells, can be judged by the kinetics of one strand cleavages of DNA and its depurinization at various temperatures.

Different mechanisms of 'error' accumulation connected with alteration of the ratio of the polymerase to the exonuclease activities in the DNA polymerase as such (Herzfeld and Greengard, 1972) or with modification of the matrix DNA with chemical carcinogens (Sirover and Loeb, 1974) are possible (Table 55).

No specifically 'tumour' DNA polymerases were found with certainty in tumour cells. The forms of DNA-dependent DNA polymerases found in tumours are the same as those in actively proliferating normal tissues. But the quantitative ratios of certain types of DNA polymerases, the extent of their activity, certain physico-chemical properties, and also the precision of their functioning *in vitro* suffer certain changes in tumours.

Structural Aspects of DNA Replication

DNA replication in living cells has not been sufficiently studied. It is not known whether RNA contributes as a primer to initiation of DNA replication in normal and tumour cells. No covalently added ribonucleotides were found in newly synthesized DNA fragments of P-815 cells (Gautschi and Clarkson, 1975), but they were present in HeLa cells (Binkerd and Toliver, 1974). RNA is suggested to contribute to initiation of DNA replication in CHO cells (Taylor *et al.*, 1974), but this was not observed for mouse melanoma cells (Berger, 1974).

The stage of elongation in normal and tumour cells is the time of formation of short polynucleotide fragments which are then linked by the polynucleotide ligase into a continuous daughter line of DNA. It is known, for instance, that in the cells of a Chinese hamster such fragments contain about 1000 nucleotides (10 S) (Schandl and Taylor, 1969), and fragments with a sedimentation coefficient 7 S are synthesized in CHO cells (Taylor *et al.*, 1974).

The distribution of short DNA fragments in tumour cells is more complex. For instance, a number of oligomer fragments with sedimentation constants increasing in the order 4-5 S → 60-100 S → 380 S was observed in mouse sarcoma cells in the course of DNA synthesis (Hyodo *et al.*, 1970). In mouse melanoma cells the newly synthesized DNA is represented by heterogeneous fragments with sedimentation coefficients 30, 40, 50 and 65 S (Berger, 1974).

The process of DNA methylation normally occurs when newly synthesized DNA exists as short pieces. However, in Ehrlich ascites carcinoma cells methylation occurs only after cross-linking of short fragments (9 S) into 30 S fragments. The extent of methylation of the 30 S fragments corresponds to that of the whole DNA cell (Drahovsky and Wacker, 1975).

No fundamental differences between DNA replication in normal and tumour cells have been observed. However, in normal human blood lymphocytes the rate of label incorporation into the short polypyrimidine DNA clusters is higher, compared to clusters of greater length. With chronic lymphatic leukaemia the label incorporation into clusters is the same for any length.

Histone Proteins

The histone proteins contribute directly to the formation of the genetic system in a cell and play an important part in the control of DNA biosynthesis. It was found experimentally that the composition and properties of histones in hepatomas and normal liver are fundamentally different. Arginine-rich histones are predominant in erythroid myelosis cells (Lass, 1973). In a regenerating liver the synthesized histones become bound with the daughter DNA chains in the process of replication.

In accordance with the above, the synthesis of all histone types is connected in time with DNA synthesis, both in normal (Borun *et al.*, 1967) and in malignant (Stein *et al.*, 1975) cells. At various stages of DNA synthesis the histones are modified by methylation, phosphorylation, acetylation, etc. These modifications are of functional importance to the control of DNA replication processes. For instance, the methylation of H4 and H3 histones in Ehrlich ascites carcinoma cells starts immediately after biosynthesis and occurs at different rates. H3 histone methylation is a first order reaction with a rate constant 0.21 hr^{-1} (Figure 170), whereas the dimethylation of histone H4 can be described by a zero order reaction (Thomas *et al.*, 1975).

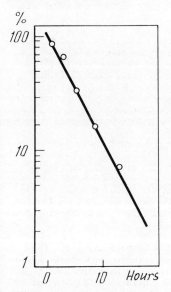

Fig. 170 Kinetics of GC histone methylation in Ehrlich ascites carcinoma cells (Thomas *et al.*, 1975).

Non-Histone Proteins

Non-histone proteins partly or totally prevent histone inhibition of DNA synthesis in the reaction of DNA polymerase (Wang, 1969). Certain nuclear acid proteins are strongly synthesized directly before DNA replication in fibroblasts stimulated for division (Tsuboi and Baserga, 1972). A factor isolated from an Ehrlich ascites carcinoma and capable of stimulating DNA synthesis has been described (Erhan *et al.*, 1970); this may enter the enzymatic system of DNA polymerase, 'recognize' the DNA initiation site, and help in DNA despiralization. Proteins stimulating DNA polymerase activity were isolated also from Novikoff hepatoma (Probst *et al.*, 1975) and from other tissues. These results have mostly been obtained without correct comparative analysis of normal and pathological tissues and this makes their systematization difficult.

Metabolism of DNA Precursors

The activities of certain catabolic and anabolic enzymes of DNA precursors are connected by a direct correlational dependence with the rate of tumour growth. Such a correlation between the key enzymes of nucleic acid metabolism and the hepatoma growth rate was found for thymidylate synthetase and thymidine kinase (Elford *et al*., 1970), DNA polymerase (Ove *et al*., 1969), deoxycytidine monophosphate deaminase (Sneider *et al*., 1969). Hepatoma growth rate was found to be inversely related to catabolism of thymidine (Elford *et al*., 1970), thymine, uracil (Ove *et al*., 1969) and dihydrouracil dehydrogenase activity. Detailed kinetic analysis of the ribonucleotide reductase activity in hepatomas with a different growth rate (Figure 171) suggested that the ribonucleotide reductase reaction limits the rates of DNA synthesis and of cell division (Elford *et al*., 1970).

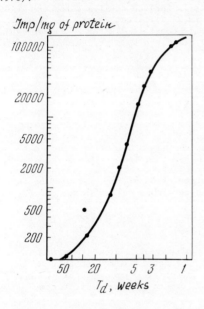

Fig. 171   Relation between the hepatoma doubling time and the specific activity of ribonucleotide reductase (Elford *et al*., 1970).

Isoforms of the metabolism enzymes of DNA precursors not innate to normal tissues were found in tumour cells. Two forms of thymidine kinase with molecular weights 70,000 and 120,000 and Michaelis constants (k_m) differing for ATP (8×10^{-5} and 7×10^{-5} M) and thymidine (3.3×10^{-5} and 3.1×10^{-6} M) were found in all tumours studied (Ehrlich ascites carcinoma, hepatoma AH-130, sarcoma 180, Yoshida sarcoma, Morris hepatoma 7794A and 7793). Only one enzyme form is present in normal tissues (regenerating liver, embryo liver and bone marrow cells) (Okuda *et al*., 1972).

The changes in hepatomas seem to be specific for tumour systems and are not directly related to faster tumour growth, but rather they relate to changes in gene expression in tumours, following from Weber's notions about molecular correlations (Weber and Lea, 1967).

Cyclic Nucleotides

Cyclic nucleotides, such as cyclic 3',5'-AMP (cAMP) and cyclic 3',5'-GMP (cGMP), are regulators of metabolic processes at a cellular level and they contribute directly to processing of genetic information. The amount of these nucleotides in the cell controls the rates and extent of phosphorylation of histones and ribosomal proteins, and also the general level of transcription. Cyclic nucleotides initiate DNA synthesis and cell proliferation and are involved in the action of various metabolism regulators (hormones, prostaglandins, etc.) (Shapot, 1975).

Comparative analysis of normal liver and hepatoma cells revealed no regularities in the cAMP and cGMP contents (Goldberg *et al.*, 1975). The true level of cAMP is dependent not only on the total composition of this nucleotide, but also on the capacity of certain proteins to react with cAMP, and on the antagonist's activities.

The differences between normal and tumour cells can be seen from the intranuclear localization and properties of the enzyme responsible for the metabolism of cyclic nucleotides. For instance, the adenylate cyclase activity in plasma membranes from Yoshida hepatoma cells is ten times lower and less responsive to the stimulating action of adrenalin, glucagon and NaF than it is in the normal liver (Tomasi *et al.*, 1973). The transformation of fibroblasts with the Rous sarcoma virus causes a fast decrease in the intracellular cAMP content. This process correlates with the decreasing adenylate cyclase activity and is connected with changes in the kinetic properties of the enzyme: the K_m value for ATP rises from 0.2 to 1.0 mM. The total activity of the cAMP phosphodiesterase increases with transformation, and the ratio of phosphodiesterases with low to high K_m values suffers a change for cAMP (Pastan *et al.*, 1973).

The following mechanism of malignant transformation is proposed: hormones bind with membrane receptors, transmit the signal to the adenylate cyclase or guanylate cyclase, alter the cAMP and cGMP content and the protein kinase and phosphoprotein kinase activities, resulting in uncontrolled synthesis of DNA, RNA, proteins, etc. (Criss, 1974).

RNA SYNTHESIS AND ITS REGULATION

Important regularities in RNA synthesis and its regulation were first found in tumour cells, and then extended to normal cells without additional experimental grounding. This was possible because the widely accepted assumption that no important differences exist between mechanisms in normal and tumour cells. The deviations observed are of a limited nature and seem to be unspecific for malignant growth.

RNA biosynthesis involves two stages: the first is transcription involving initiation, elongation and termination; the second is the post-transcriptional modification of RNA involving processing (transformation of the high molecular weight RNA precursor to smaller mature forms of various RNA types), methylation of individual RNA nucleotides, and in certain cases covalent binding of the polynucleotides with RNA, etc.

RNA Polymerases

Diverse forms of DNA-dependent RNA polymerases were found both in tumour and in normal cells (Rutter *et al.*, 1972; Jacob, 1973). Various forms of RNA polymerases were studied for the Ehrlich ascites carcinoma (Cereghini and Franze-Fernandez, 1974), neuroblastoma (Maio and Kurnit, 1974), myeloma (Hall and Smuckler, 1974; Heinmann and Roeder, 1974) and leukaemic mouse cells (Babcock and Rich, 1973). The same forms of RNA polymerases were found both in normal and tumour tissues. However, the content of three RNA polymerases in hepatoma H-35 cells was substantially higher than in normal rat liver (Chesterton *et al.*, 1972).

TABLE 56 Activity of nuclear RNA polymerases from tumour and normal cells

Tissue*	Activity of RNA polymerases (units per 1 mg of DNA)				
	Ia	Ib	IIa	IIb	III
Normal	0.31 ± 0.18	0.56 ± 0.19	0.80 ± 0.21	0.89 ± 0.37	0.43 ± 0.18
Kidney (2)	1.29 ± 0.75	0.99 ± 0.34	3.30 ± 0.88	0.35 ± 0.23	0.15 ± 0.06
Liver (2)	0.20 ± 0.12	0.49 ± 0.17	0.91 ± 0.24	0.07 ± 0.03	0.08 ± 0.03
Spleen (2)	0.60 ± 0.49	0.68 ± 0.22	1.67 ± 1.16	0.44 ± 0.34	0.22 ± 0.15
Ehrlich ascites carcinoma (13)	5.93 ± 3.46	1.31 ± 0.82	6.16 ± 4.85	7.59 ± 3.19	1.19 ± 0.50
6C3HED (2)	8.24 ± 4.81	0.92 ± 0.58	5.37 ± 1.84	13.26 ± 5.57	0.45 ± 0.19
TAS (2)	1.85 ± 1.07	0.88 ± 0.55	2.02 ± 0.69	5.48 ± 2.30	0.86 ± 0.36
Average	5.33 ± 2.65	1.04 ± 0.17	4.52 ± 1.79	8.78 ± 3.28	0.83 ± 0.31
Tumours: normal	4.98		6.30		3.77

*Numbers in parentheses refer to the number of measurements

in studying the activities of individual forms of nuclear RNA polymerases in cells of three ascites tumours in mice (Ehrlich carcinoma, lymphosarcoma 6C3HED, adenocarcinoma TAS) (Table 56) it was found that the activity of nuclear RNA polymerases in tumour cells was mich higher than in normal tissues (liver, kidney, spleen) (Blair, 1975). At the same time no specificity with respect to RNA polymerase form was observed for matrix DNA of tumour cells.

It can be concluded that the RNA polymerases in normal and tumour tissues differ not in multiplicity of forms, but only in the quantitative values of their activities.

Heterogeneous Nuclear RNA and mRNA

Extensive reviews deal with the structures and metabolism of heterogeneous nuclear RNA (including nuclear precursors of mRNA, rRNA and tRNA) (Stewart and Letham, 1973; Weinberg, 1973; Brawerman, 1974). However, in spite of the large number of papers, no comparative data on the properties of these RNA in normal tissues and tumours have been reported. This section is concerned with the results obtained for tumour cells.

The experiments on hybridization of fast-labelled RNA from leukaemic cells of mice with homologous DNA revealed three RNA groups differing in the content and half-life of the fast-labelled RNA capable of hybridization. The lifetime of the first group involving 66% of fast-labelled RNA is 10 minutes, that of the second group (33%) is 1 to 1½ hours, that of the third (10%) is 20 hours. Hybridization ability of RNA with longer lifetimes is lower. It has also been found that newly synthesized RNA contains a fast degrading component with a lifetime of 10 to 20 minutes (Meltz and Okada, 1971).

A number of nucleotide sequences of nuclear and microsomal DNA in normal liver of adult and newborn rats and in three hepatomas with minimal deviations were studied by the competing hybridization method. It was found that the nRNA in liver of newborn rats and in hepatoma 5123C were characterized by absence of certain base sequences which are present in the nRNA of normal liver in adult rats (Garrett *et al.*, 1973). At the same time the nRNA of slow-growing Morris hepatoma 9618 did not differ from that of normal liver. A number of base sequences characteristic of RNA in normal liver and hepatoma 5123C are absent from the microsomal RNA in hepatomas 9618 and 7800. This seems to be caused by a different extent of gene switch-off and by a change in the stability of cytoplasmic RNA in various tumours differing in growth-rate and progression.

The kinetics of synthesis and breakdown of pulse-labelled mRNA molecules isolated from the polysomes of exponentially growing HeLa cells was studied by Singer and Penman (1973). Two forms of mRNA were observed: short-lived mRNA with a half-life of 7 hours, representing 33% of the total cell mRNA, and long-lived mRNA with a half-life of 24 hours (stable mRNA) representing 67% of the total cell mRNA. The dissociation of long-lived mRNA was considerably slower than that of the newly synthesized mRNA with a high molecular weight. Spontaneous dissociation of a large amount of newly formed RNA was observed in Ehrlich ascites carcinoma cells (Tigerstrom, 1973).

The poly(A) sequences involved in the mRNA structure (Kates, 1970) were found in polysome mRNA from HeLa cells (Edmonds *et al.*, 1971), ascites cells of mouse sarcoma (Lee *et al.*, 1971) and Morris hepatoma 7800 cells (Tweedie and Pitot, 1974).

Biosynthesis of Ribosomal RNA

Ribosomal RNA synthesis begins with the formation of a 45 S precursor (Percy, 1962; Penman et al., 1966). Then the 45 S-pre-rRNA molecules split to form 18 S and 32 S RNA (Girard et al., 1965). The 18 S rRNA rapidly passes from the nucleolus to the cell cycoplasm in the form of small ribosomal subunits. The 32 S RNA converts in the nucleoli to 28 S RNA and passes to the cytoplasm in the form of 60 S ribosomal particles. Analysis of rRNA from the HeLa cell nucleoli revealed several forms of RNA with sedimentation coefficients 45, 32, 28, 41 S, and a minor component with a sedimentation coefficient 36 S (Weinberg et al., 1967).

The 45 S precursor formed becomes methylated (Greenberg and Penman, 1966).

The following scheme of rRNA processing can be proposed from the above

$$45\ S \longrightarrow 41\ S \underset{(3.1\times10^6)}{\overset{(4.1\times10^6)}{}}$$

$$32\ S\ (2.1\times10^6) \longrightarrow \begin{cases} 28\ S\ (1.7\times10^6) \\ 7\ S\ (5.0\times10^4) \end{cases}$$

$$20\ S\ (0.9\times10^6) \longrightarrow 18\ S\ (6.5\times10^5)$$

The degradation of rRNA precursors seems to be realized by the exonuclease (RNA-ase I) found in the nuclei of Ehrlich ascites carcinoma cells, since the low molecular weight 5'-PO$_4$-oligonucleotides were the major splitting products (Speers and Tigerstrom, 1975). Possibly the processing of rRNA precursors occurs as a limited but specific splitting of molecule-precursors by the endonuclease together with the oxo-RNA-ase II (Perry and Kelly, 1972). An enzyme similar in its properties was found in HeLa cell nuclei (Mirault and Scherver, 1972) and Novikoff hepatoma cells (Harris, 1963).

The synthesis of 45 S and 32 S rRNA and transformation of these to 28 S and 18 S rRNA in normal leucocytes and in leucocytes of patients suffering from forms of acute leukaemia were identical. The only difference was that the 45 S and 32 S RNA accumulated in blast cells were not fully methylated, and the splitting of 45 S RNA occurred at a somewhat slower rate (Torrelli et al., 1970, 1971; Seeber et al., 1974). At the same time the rates of rRNA synthesis and methylation in normal and tumour cells did not essentially differ (Billington and Itzhari, 1974).

Thus there is no essential difference in the rates of synthesis and processing of 45 S RNA precursors.

Biosynthesis of 5 S rRNA

Out of the several RNA types involved in the ribosomal cell composition, the 5 S rRNA differs from the other RNA in that it is synthesized in a mature form (Hatten et al., 1969; Viotti et al., 1973) in the extranucleolic part of the nucleus (Brown and Webex, 1968; Wimber and Steffensen, 1970). The 5 S rRNA is present in large ribosomal subunits together with 28 S RNA in a molar ratio 1:1 (Knight and Darnell, 1967).

In cell nuclei of lymphatic leukaemia in 15178Y mice the newly synthesized 5 S rRNA appears first in the nucleoplasm and then diffuses into the nucleolus (Auger and

Tiollais, 1974). The synthesis kinetics show the time of appearance of 5 S rRNA and 45 S rRNA precursors is the same. The 5 S RNA function is unknown.

The absence of information on 5 S rRNA biosynthesis in homologous normal and tumour tissues makes impossible a comparactive evaluation of these processes. However, taking into account the functional proximity and the relation of 5 S rRNA to the system of 45 S rRNA processing and ribosome assembling, it can be suggested that 5 S rRNA biosynthesis in normal and tumour tissues seems to show no fundamental differences.

Regulation of RNA Biosynthesis

The regulation of transcription in living cells is one of the major differentiation mechanisms. There is no doubt that part of the nuclear proteins (particularly histones), their modifications and non-histone proteins, as well as the low molecular weight nuclear RNA are involved to some extent in the regulation of transcription processes (Ashmarin, 1974). However, there is no specific inform- ation on the regulatory action of these factors both for tumour and normal tissues. However, in certain cases the contribution of protein factors to transcription processes becomes somewhat clearer. For instance, two factors stimulating the activity of partially purified RNA polymerase II were found for Ehrlich ascites tumours. One stimulates RNA synthesis only on DNA matrices from Ehrlich ascites carcinoma cells and rat hepatoma, but does not stimulate it in poly(dAT) or calf thymus DNA.

Further study of this factor showed that it is protein and is inactivated by trypsin or by heating at 60° for 10 minutes. Transcription initiation appeared to be strongly related to ribonuclease H, though suppression of ribonuclease H activity with $MnCl_2$ had no effect on the stimulating activity of this factor.

A protein R with a molecular weight of 38,000, suppressing the RNA polymerase II activity, was isolated from the Ehrlich ascites carcinoma cells. Its inhibiting action manifests at the stage of transcription initiation and has no effect on the RNA polymerase II activity after start of transcription. In the presence of the protein factor of initiation the R protein suppresses preferentially the synthesis of certain RNA forms.

Protein factors stimulating the activity of the DNA-dependent RNA polymerase II *in vitro* were isolated from the Novikoff hepatoma ascites cells (Lee and Dahmus, 1973). These stimulated RNA synthesis only on the native DNA matrix from the Novikoff hepatoma.

The information on other forms of transcription regulation is sparse. However, the data reported indicate a marked drop in the selectivity of mRNA transport from the nucleus to the cytoplasm of tumour cells (Shearer and Smuckler, 1972; Shapot, 1975).

PROTEIN BIOSYNTHESIS AND ITS REGULATION

Level of Protein Biosynthesis

The rate of protein biosynthesis in tumour cells is, as a rule, very different from that in normal cells, though in certain cases it can be almost identical.

In the Morris hepatoma 5123tc the protein biosynthesis intensity was almost three times higher, in its ^{14}C-leucine incorporation, than that in normal living cells (Schreiber *et al.*, 1974).

The synthesis intensity of plasma proteins (albumin, fibrinogen, hepatoglobin, transferrin, β-lipoprotein, β-glucoprotein and α-fetoprotein) in cell culture was highest in tumour tissue, somewhat lower in the normal loci of cancerous liver, and lowest in normal liver tissue (Rioche *et al.*, 1974).

An identical content and rate of albumin synthesis were found for normal liver and for liver of host rats (Ove *et al.*, 1972). The rate of α-globulin synthesis was also the same, but its decay rate was somewhat lower in hepatoma-bearing rats. The albumin synthesis *in vivo* in liver of normal and of hepatoma-bearing rats is approximately the same, whereas in hepatoma microsomes it is eleven times weaker (Ove *et al.*, 1972b).

Ribosomes and Polyribosomes

Ribonucleotide particles occupy the central place in translation of the genetic code. They organize the spacing of matric and adaptor RNA, co-ordinate the functioning of various protein factors of translation, the sequential readout of information in mRNA, and as a result the multiply-repeated peptide bond synthesis results in formation of a complete polypeptide chain. The changes in the protein synthesis level in tumour cells can obviously be due to disturbance of ribosome structures or functions.

The comparactive changes in the composition of ribosomal proteins, in rRNA structur and biosynthesis were discussed in previous sections of this book. Various amounts of free ribosomes and of ribosomes bound with membranes have been found in normal and tumour cells. In normal liver cells the amount of free polyribosomes is 40%. In leukaemic and other tumour cells the amounts of free polyribosomes attains 80-90%. The monoribosomes 80 S in normal mouse liver represent only a small part, in the myeloid leukaemic tumour they constitute about a half, and in Ehrlich ascites tumour and sarcoma 180 they make up almost the whole cell population. At the same time the intensity of protein biosynthesis in such tumour cells is only a little higher than normal (Sacchi *et al.*, 1974).

Normal and tumour cells differ also in the amount of polyribosomes synthesizing albumin: in normal liver it is 9.75%, in Zaidel hepatoma it is 0.74% (Shapot and Berdinskikh, 1975).

The initiating effect of the cytoplasmic fraction of certain normal and tumour tissues on the process of poly(Y) dependent phenylalanine incorporation was studied using the acellular system of liver ribosomes in young rats (Bielka, 1974). It will be seen from the following data that the cytoplasmic fraction of tumours has a great effect on this process.

Source of the cytoplasmic fraction:	Incorporation of phenylalanine (compared to control)
Normal	
Kidney	4.6
Brain	7.8
Liver	10.9
Regenerating liver	17.7
Tumours	
Jensen sarcoma	26.4
Hepatoma Fst	26.5
Zaidel hepatoma	31.4
Walker carcinosarcoma	32.8
Tumour 312	27.2

Thus, the tumour cell ribosomes differ from normal cells in the protein composition and in certain elements of the rRNA structure, in the quantitative ratio of mono- to polyribosomes, as well as in their functional activity.

Translation Mechanism

It has been established by now that protein synthesis in living cells begins with formation of a complex containing a 40 S ribosomal subunit, mRNA, a specific aminoacyl tRNA and a specific initiation factor (Lucas-Lenard and Lipmann, 1971).

The function of the specific aminoacyl tRNA (met-tRNA$_F$) consists in transport and formation of the N-position of the future polypeptide chain. Another met-tRNA (met-tRNA$_M$) transports and incorporates methionine into the internal sections of the synthesizing polypeptide chain. No changes were observed in the met-tRNA$_F$ and met-tRNA$_M$, compared to normal (Drews et al., 1971; Jones and Mach, 1973).

An initiating complex of the 40 S ribosomal subunit, the AUG triplet, the met-tRNA$_F$ and the specific initiating factor was found in virus-transformed cells (Ascione and Vande Woude, 1971), in ascites tumour cells (Smith and Marcker, 1970), and also in hepatoma and normal rat liver (Murty et al., 1974). Consequently, the initiation of protein synthesis occurs in the same way as it does in normal cells. The higher activity of initiating factors is a distinctive feature of this stage (Ascione and Vande Woude, 1971) (Table 57). It will be seen from Figure 172 that the initiation factor obtained from virally infected cells is considerably more active than the other initiation factors.

The results in Table 57 show that the initiation factor of hepatoma in a homologous system increases the binding of phe-tRNA and met-tRNA with the 40 S subunit to a greater extent than does the relevant binding in the homologous system of the host liver (a). The initiation factors from the hepatoma were capable of higher (compared to the liver) stimulation of phe- and met-tRNA-^{14}C binding with the 40 S subunit in the heterologous system (b). On the other hand, the 40S subunits of host hepatoma and liver showed no essential differences in the binding of phe- and met-tRNA.

TABLE 57   phe-tRNA-C^{14} and met-tRNA-C^{14} binding with C 40S subunit
from hepatoma and liver as a function of the protein initiation factor
(Murty et al., 1974)

(A) HOMOLOGOUS SYSTEMS

Source of 40 S-subunit and initiation factor	Incorporation of phe-tRNA, %		Incorporation of met-tRNA, %	
	40 S-subunits	Initation factor	40 S-subunits	Initiation factor
Liver	100	100	100	100
Hepatoma	113 ± 5.6	171 ± 9.4	106 ± 4.7	168 ± 2.2

(B) HETEROLOGOUS SYSTEMS

Source of 40 S-subunit	Source of initiation factor	Incorporation of phe-tRNA-C, imp/min	Incorporation of met-tRNA-C, imp/min
Liver	Hepatoma	215	306
Hepatoma	Liver	152	192

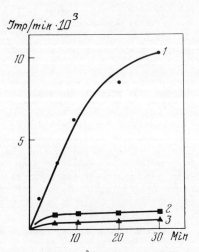

Fig. 172   Incorporation of ³H-aminoacyl-tRNA from guinea
pig liver, induced by various initiation factors: (1)
incorporation with the initiation factor from infected
hamster cells;   (2) incorporation with the initiation
factor from non-infected hamster cells;   (3) incorporation with the initiation factor from guinea pig liver
(Ascione and Vande Woude, 1971).

Thus, the stronger binding of phe- and met-tRNA in the hepatoma acellular system
is due to a higher activity of the hepatoma initiating factor.

Elongation factors also take part in the process of biosynthesis (Lucas-Lenard and
Haenni, 1968).

The function of one of the factors consists in binding aminoacyl-tRNA (in the
presence of GTP) with the ribosomes to form dipeptide.   The other factor is needed
for catalysis of peptidyl-tRNA transport to the 60 S subunit.

Two elongation factors were isolated from normal and tumour cells (T-I and T-II)
(Black and Griffin, 1970).   These factors appeared to be interchangeable with those
in normal rabbit and rat reticulocytes.

It was concluded accordingly that the elongation factors and the whole polysomal
system of protein synthesis are the same for all cells, both in normal mammals and
in those with malignant growths:

Elongation factor*	Imp/min/mg of ribosomal protein
In absence of transport factor	320
T-I from reticulocytes	600
T-II from reticulocytes	492
T-I + T-II from reticulocytes	4160
40-70% $(NH_4)_2SO_4$ from tumours	4640

*The elongation factors were isolated from tumour ascites cells and normal rat
 reticulocytes;   the ribosomes were isolated from normal rat reticulocytes.

Elongation factor*	Imp/min/mg of ribosomal protein
T-I from tumours	2464
T-II from tumours	673
T-I + T-II from tumours	4640
T-I from reticulocytes + T-II from tumours	3350
T-II from reticulocytes + T-I from tumours	8400

The above data give certain comparative characteristics of elongation factors in normal tissues and in tumours. There seems to be no difference between the T-II factor activities, whereas the m T-I activity is much stronger in tumours than in normal cells.

The effect of an elongation inhibitor, cycloheximide (Rajalakshmi et al., 1971), on the reaction of puromycin in an acellular system was found to consist of inhibition of peptidyl puromycin formation in the systems isolated both from normal liver and from host liver (Walker carcinosarcoma (Clark and Goodlad, 1975).

However, it will be seen from Figure 173 that in the presence of cycloheximide peptidyl puromycin formation is retarded to a greater extent in host liver than normal.

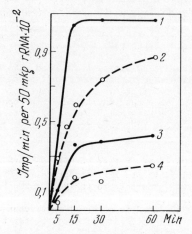

Fig. 173 Effect of cycloheximide on the formation of peptidyl-puromycin-8^{3}H (Clark and Goodlad, 1975): (1) normal; (2) normal + cycloheximide; (3) host; (4) host + cycloheximide.

It was also found that the ribosomes isolated from host muscles were less capable of synthesizing polyphenyl alanine than are the ribosomes from muscle tissue of normal rats. It follows from the data below that the lower polyphenylalanine synthesizing ability of host ribosomes reconstructed from subunits seems to be due to a defective 40 S ribosomal subunit (Clark and Goodlad, 1975).

Incubation conditions	Incorporation, imp/min per 50 μg of ribosomal RNA
N 40 S + N 60 S	2377
Tum 40 S + Tum 60 S	1072
N 40 S + Tum 60 S	2234
Tum 40 S + N 60 S	1292

No comparative data are available on the protein factors of polypeptide chain termination.

Thus, the translation mechanism in tumour cells does not differ, in principle, from normal, and the differences observed are only quantitative.

Isoacceptor tRNA and Regulation of Protein Biosynthesis

The system of activation and transport of amino acids to ribosomes, i.e. the tRNA and aminoacyl-tRNA ligases can also play an important part in regulation of the translation process. Indeed, experimental evidence has recently been obtained by Elska *et al.* (1971) for the hypothesis that the degeneration of the genetic code together with possible alteration of tRNA sets represent the regulation factor of the synthesis rate in the polypeptide chain (Ames and Martin, 1964).

Comparative study of aminoacyl-tRNA in normal and tumour cells revealed differences between the properties of isoacceptor tRNA (Volkers and Taylor, 1971; Gonaco *et al.*, 1973; Yang, 1971; Rennert, 1971; Mushinski, 1974; Ouellette and Taylor, 1973). These differences are due to alteration of the tRNA content and chromatographic behaviour, to appearance or reduction of individual isoforms, and also to changes in the acceptor activity of tRNA. The relevant data available are generalized in Table 58. It will be seen that deviations in aminoacyl-tRNA properties, from those in normal liver, have been established for certain transplanted hepatomas The most essential differences are observed for three tRNA specific of histidine, tyrosine and phenylalanine.

In evaluating the differences in properties of hepatoma and normal liver tRNA it has to be borne in mind that a certain resemblance in chromatographic behaviour and number of isoforms has been observed for hepatomas and embryonic liver (Gonaco *et al.*, 1973; Yang, 1971).

The changes in the isozyme spectrum of aminoacyl-tRNA ligases in tumour tissues, compared to normal, should also be noted (Mittelman, 1971; Gallo and Pestka, 1970).

The data on differences in properties of isoacceptor tRNA forms suggest that the changes in protein biosynthesis rates compared to normal are to a great extent dependent on the consistency of the tRNA isoform spectrum with the 'codon composition' of the tumour cell mRNA.

TABLE 58   Nature of deviations in aminoacyl-RNA properties in hepatomas
(I = content;   II = chromatographic behaviour;   III = appearance of new forms;
IV = isoform reduction;   V = change in acceptor activity)

Aminoacyl-tRNA	Zaidel hepatoma	Morris hepatoma	References
Arginyl-	V	V	Ouellette and Taylor (1973)
Phenylalanyl-	None	III, II, V	Volkers and Taylor (1971); Mushinsky (1974); Ouellette and Taylor (1973)
Propyl-	V	-	
Tyrosyl-	None	II, III, V	Yang (1971); Ouellette and Taylor (1973)
Alanyl-	I	-	
Asparaginyl-	-	II, III	Yang (1971)
Aspartyl-	I	-	
Lysyl-	I	V	Ouellette and Taylor (1973)
Threonyl-	I	-	
Tryptophanyl-	I, V	-	
Glutamyl-	II	-	
Seryl-	II	III, V	Volkers and Taylor (1971); Ouellette and Taylor (1973)
Valyl-	II, V	-	
Histidyl-	-	IV, II, III, V	Volkers and Taylor (1971); Ouellette and Taylor (1973)
Isoleucyl-	-	V	Ouellette and Taylor (1973)
Glycyl-	None	-	
Leucyl	None	-	
Methionyl	None	-	

3. NUCLEIC ACIDS AND MITOCHONDRIAL PROTEINS

The established autonomy of the genetic system and of the systems responsible for
realization of the mitochondrial genetic information justifies a separate discussion
of the properties of the mitochondrial protein synthesizing system of normal and
tumour cells.

Composition, Structure and Replication of Tumour Cell Mitochondrial RNA

The detection in mitochondria of specific DNA (mtDNA) and of the protein synthesizing system elements differing from those in nuclei and cytoplasm suggested that
malignization might involve, along with disturbance of the genetic nuclear structures, also that of mitochondrial genetic structures.

For instance, it has been found that the mitochondria of certain transplanted
tumours contain an eight-to-nine-fold larger amount of DNA than do the mitochondria
of normal tissues. There was also a three-fold larger amount of DNA in hepatoma
mitochondria than in liver mitochondria. It will be noted in this connection that
the process of tissue differentiation is accompanied by a decrease in mtDNA content
(Tanguay and Chaudhary, 1971). A study of the buoyant density of mtDNA from
Zaidel ascites hepatoma, Jensen sarcoma, and Walker carcinosarcoma showed no
essential deviations from the mtDNA properties of homologous normal tissues
(Bottger and Wunderlich, 1973). Electron microscopy of tumour cell mtDNA revealed
a considerable proportion of complex DNA forms, virtually absent from normal cell
mitochondria: these are the macrocyclic catenated dimers and trimers (Figure 174,
II, III).

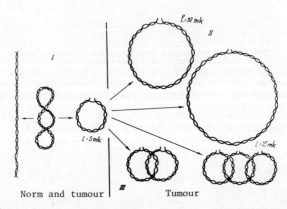

Fig. 174 Mitochondrial DNA in tumour cells: (I) monomers
(supercoiled and open ring molecules) with 5 mk contour
length; (II) circular dimers and trimers with 10 and 15 mk
contour length, respectively; (III) catenated dimers and
trimers.

The monomeric cyclic molecules with a contour length 1 - 4 mk represent an unusual
mtDNA form encountered in tumour cells only.

The macrocyclic dimers found in hepatoma, ascites tumour, leukaemic cells (Smith
and Vinograd, 1973; Clayton *et al.*, 1970) and various tumours in humans (Paoletti
and Riou, 1971) also seem to be characteristic of tumour cells only. The content
of cyclic dimers can change depending on the kind of tumour and its stage of growth.
For instance, their amount in HeLa cells is small (Hudson and Vinograd, 1969), and
in other tumours it attained up to 40% (Clayton *et al.*, 1968).

The catenated forms are characteristic of tumour cells and of embryonic tissues.
A considerable percentage of catenated dimers and oligomers was found in leukaemic
leucocytes (Smith and Vinograd, 1973) and mitochondria of rat ascites hepatoma.
However, there is evidence that the catenated mtDNA forms are encountered with the
same frequency both in tumour and normal cells (Kumar and Fox, 1974).

Supercoiled cyclic mtDNA involving polyribonucleotide fractions were detected in
cells of rat ascites hepatoma (Miyaki *et al.*, 1973) and of HeLa (Wong-Staal *et al.*,
1973).

The buoyant density of the monomer and dimer mtDNA forms were studied in order to
evaluate their correlation. It appeared to be identical and this indicates the
same content of bases. Also no substitution of bases, deletions or additions were
observed within the accuracy of the hybridization method (50 to 100 bases (Clayton
et al., 1970). It is of interest to note the correlation between the content of
complex mtDNA forms and the rate of tissue growth, i.e. the rate of mtDNA biosynthesis. The fast-growing embryonic tissue containing many cyclic dimers is characterized by an elevated rate of mtDNA reduplication (Rabinovitz and Swift, 1970).
The same holds for tumours, since the rate of their mtDNA synthesis is markedly
elevated (Khonson and Ivanova, 1971). It is suggested that the increased content
of mtDNA dimers in tumour cells is due not only to the increased rate of their
mtDNA reduplication, but also results from the recombination of such molecules
under the action of carcinogens (Koike *et al.*, 1975; Vilenchik, 1973).

The mtDNA reduplication process is realized via the DNA-dependent mitochondrial DNA polymerase which differs from the relevant nuclear enzyme, but it coded by the nuclear DNA (Küntzel, 1971). In tumour cells the amount of this enzyme is higher. A factor absent from normal tissues and stimulating mtDNA synthesis was detected in tumours and embryonic cells (Kalf et al., 1971).

The intensity of mtDNA biosynthesis in two hepatomas and host liver depended on the radioactive precursor used. ^{3}H-Thymidine was incorporated into the hepatoma mtDNA eight to thirteen times more intensely than into the host liver. ^{3}H-Cytidine incorporation into the host liver was two to four times more intense than that for the hepatoma mtDNA (Chang et al., 1960).

Mitochondrial RNA of Tumour Cells

All RNA types having analogues in the cytoplasm were isolated from the mitochondria of normal and tumour cells (Aloni and Attardi, 1971; Mitrokhin et al., 1973). A mtRNA fraction complementary to the nuclear DNA was found by means of hybridizing a pulse-labelled in vivo mouse hepatoma with nuclear DNA. Competing hybridization revealed only a partial homology of nucleotide RNA sequences in mitochondria of normal liver and hepatoma hybridized with the nuclear DNA. This is evidence that other RNA types of a nuclear origin appear in the mitochondria of tumour cells. The RNA synthesized in isolated mitochondria of tumours and controls is characterized by complete absence of complementarity to the nuclear DNA.

Proteins and Enzymes of Tumour Cell Mitochondria

The biosynthesis of mitochondrial proteins is realized both in the cytoplasmic and intramitochondrial systems of protein synthesis. Cytochrome b and certain subunits of the cytochrome oxidase and of the oligomycin-responsive ATP-ase synthesize in mitochondria are probably coded by the mtDNA (Schatz and Mason, 1974). All these proteins possess distinct hydrophobic properties and represent an integral part of the functionally active internal membrane of mitochondria.

The proteins of mitochondrial membranes isolated from normal rat liver, host liver and five hepatoma strains (H35, H35-tC$_1$, H35-tC$_2$, 3924A, 9098) were studied by the method of electrophoresis in polyacrylamide gel. The basic protein band observed in the electrophoregram of membrane proteins isolated from normal liver mitochondria either disappeared or markedly diminished for membrane proteins isolated from hepatoma mitochondria. Moreover, the membranes of hepatoma H35 mitochondria exhibited an additional protein component, which was absent in membranes from normal liver (Chang et al., 1971).

The incorporation of ^{14}C-leucine into membrane proteins of the Zaidel hepatoma mitochondria and in normal liver was studied in the cytoplasm under conditions of suppressed protein synthesis with cycloheximide. The label incorporation occurred preferentially into the insoluble fraction of the mitochondrial proteins and was responsive to chloramphenicol. No essential difference was observed in the protein synthesis of mitochondria in normal and tumour cells (Kuzela et al., 1973, 1975).

At the same time possible changes in the primary structure of tumour mtDNA cannot be excluded. These changes might play a distinct part in the incidence and progression of tumours, since proteins with physico-chemical and immunological properties, resembling those of membrane proteins of mitochondria, have been found in the cytoplasm and nuclear membranes.

The enzymatic activity of soluble proteins synthesized outside mitochondria, but involved in the composition of the mitochondrial enzyme systems, is different for

tumour and normal tissues. For instance, the activity of adenylate kinase in
Novikoff solid hepatoma is lower by 30%. and in the Novikoff hepatoma cell culture
it is lower by 60% compared to normal. The activity of NADH-cytochrome-c-reductase
and of aminoxidase is 60% lower than in normal liver; that of succinate dehydrogenase, succinate oxidase and NADH-oxidase is four, five and eight times lower,
respectively, compared to normal liver (White et al., 1974).

Similar data were obtained for hepatomas H35 (Myers and Bosmann, 1974), 9618A,
7800 and 3924A (Pedersen et al., 1970). No deviation from normal in the activities
of cytochrome oxidase and malate dehydrogenase was reported in the papers cited
above.

Thus a thorough study of the protein synthesizing system in mitochondria has
revealed many essential differences in tumour cells. There is a relatively large
number of complex mtDNA forms in the mitochondria of tumours: it is difficult to
say what the contribution of these peculiar forms is to the incidence and progression of tumours, though their relationship to the high rate of mtDNA reduplication is evident. The detection of the RNA fraction of nuclear origin in tumour
cells appears to be important. This fraction might be responsible for the elevated
rate of the mitochondrial protein biosynthesis. Finally, certain peculiarities in
the composition of tumour mitochondrial membrane proteins synthesized under mtDNA
control, their possible contribution to structures of other cell membranes suggest
that along with the disturbances in the regulation mechanism of the nuclear genome,
the disturbance of the mitochondrial genetic system regulation also plays an
important part in tumour growth.

The results discussed in this chapter suggest that the alteration of nucleic acid
and protein structures is not the sole determining factor in the strong disturbances
of metabolism and cell growth parameters of malignant processes. More important in
this respect could be the changes in the synthesis of biopolymers and particularly
in their regulation, i.e. readout, transport and processing of genetic information.
Though all the molecular mechanisms of DNA, RNA and protein synthesis studied so
far are identical for normal and tumour cells, there are marked differences in the
activities, precision of functioning, and ratios of various components in the
complex systems of the biosynthesis of informational macromolecules. The changes
in the protein biosynthesis system and the distinct differences in the isomorphism
of various protein groups and of tRNA deserve attention, since the disturbances of
translation must act on the transcription and replication processes via the system
of feedback in cells.

Changes in the structures of certain types of macromolecules probably underlie
these changes in regulation. Finding these structural disturbances and elucidating
their connection with malignant transformation of cells is an important problem in
the molecular biology of cancer.

Wide use of kinetic methods in such studies will undoubtedly help us to overcome
the difficulties and will make these studies strictly quantitative and objective.

BIBLIOGRAPHY

ABDURASULOV, D.M., NIKOLAEV, A.I. AND GAZIEV, A.I. (1967) The effect of carcinogenic compounds on the content of free radicals in tissues of animals. *Voprosy
Onkologii*, 13, 50-54.

ADACHI, K., YAMASAWA, S., SUSKIND, R.R. and CHRISTIAN, G. (1969) Hexokinase activities in normal hyperplastic and cancerous epidermis of mice. *Nature*, 222, 191-
192.

ADAMS, D.H. AND BOWMAN, B.M. (1963) The chemotherapy of established sarcoma 180
and adenocarcinoma 755 tumors with 6-thioguanine. *Cancer Research*, 23, 883-889.

AGATOVA, A.I. and EMANUEL, N.M. (1966) Deistvie propilgallata na fermenty soder-
zhashchie SH-i S-S-gruppy. *Biokhimiya*, 31, 299-305.

AGATOVA, A.I. and TRESCHCHENKOVA, Iu.A. (1972) Puti izmeneniia aktivnosti laktat-
degridrogenazy v protsesse razvitiia astsitnoi opukholi erlikha. *Voprosy Meditsinkoi Khimmi*, 18, 19-25.

AGATOVA, A.I., VARTANYAN, L.S., GONIKBERG, E.M. and EMANUEL, N.M. (1968) Effect
of polyphenols on enzymes. *Mater vses simp.* pp. 146-154.

AGNEW, D.A. and SKARSGARD, L.D. (1972) Sensitization of anoxic mammalian cells to
radiation by triacetoneamine-n-oxyl. Effect of pre- and postirradiation.
Radiation Research, 51, 97-109.

AISENBERG, A.C. (1961) *The Glycolysis and Respiration of Tumors*. New York:
Academic Press. 224 pp.

AISENBERG, A.C. and MORRIS, H.P. (1961) Energy pathways of hepatoma no. 5123.
Nature, 191, 1314-1315.

ALBERT, R.E., PHILIPS, M.E., BENNETT, P., BURNS, F.J. and HEIMBACH, R.D. (1969)
The morphology and growth characteristics of radiation-induced epithelial skin
tumors in the rat. *Cancer Research*, 29, 658-668.

ALESENKO, A.V., ARCHYPOVA, G.V., BURLAKOVA, E.B., GOBETY, V.N. and TERKHOVA, S.F.
(1973) Abstracts of the Ninth International Congress of Biochemistry at Stockholm.

ALESENKO, A.V. and BURLAKOVA, E.V. (1972) Relation of a change in lipid antioxidative activity with DNA synthesis in the mouse regenerating liver. *Doklady Akademii Nauk SSSR*, 207, 1471-1474.

ALESENKO, A.V., LIPCHINA, L.P. and FRANKFURT, O.S. (1967) Avtoradiografticheskoe issledovanie deistviia rentegonovskogo oblucheniia na kletki astsitnogo limfaticheskogo leikoza myshei. *Tsitologiya*, 9, 217-222.

ALONI, Y. and ATTARDI, G. (1971) Expression of the mitochondria genome in HeLa cells. IV. Titration of mitochondrial genes for 16S, 12S and 4S RNA. *Journal of Molecular Biology*, 55, 271-276.

AMALDI, F. and ATTARDI, G. (1971) A comparison of the primary structures of 28S and 18S RNA from HeLa cells and different human tissues. *Biochemistry*, 10, 1478-1483.

AMES, B.N. and MARTIN, R.G. (1964) Biochemical aspects of genetics: the operon. *Annual Reviews of Biochemistry*, 33, 235-258.

ANON (1958). Metodicheskie ukazaniya po eksperimentalnomu izucheniyu preparatov s predpolagaemoi protivoopukholevoi aktivnostiyu. Vtoroe koordinatisionnoe soveshchanie po khimioterapii raka. Moscow.

ANSFIELD, F.J. (1965) Phase I study of azotomycin. *Cancer Chemotherapy Reports*, 46, 37-40.

ARENDAREVSKII, L.F. (1971) *Onkologiya*. Kiev.

ARKHIPOVA, G.V., BURLAKOVA, E.B. and TERKHOVA, S.F. (1967) Izmenenie kontsentratsii neesterifitsirovannykh zhirnykh kislot v krovi i antiokislitelnoi aktivnosti lipidov pecheni u mysheirazlichnykh liniivnorme, pri luchevoi bolezni i perevivnom leikoze La. *Biofizika*, 12, 560-563.

ARNOLD, E.A., BUKSAS, M.M. and YOUNG, K.E. (1973) A comparative study of some properties of chromatin from two 'minimal deviation' hepatomas. *Cancer Research*, 33, 1169-1176.

ASCIONE, R. and VANDE WOUDE, G.F. (1971) Ribosomal factors effecting the stimulation of cell-free protein synthesis in the presence of foot-and-mouth disease virus RNA. *Biochemical and Biophysical Research Communications*, 45, 14-21.

ASHMARIN, I.P. (1974) *Molekulyarnaya biologiya*. Leningrad: Meditsina.

ASHMORE, J. (1958) Isotope studies of the pathways of glucose-6-phosphate metabolism in the Novikoff hepatoma. *Cancer Research*, 18, 974.

AUGER, M.A. and TIOLLAIS, P. (1974) 5-S RNA: biosynthesis and association to immature ribosomal particles in the nucleus of lymphocytic mouse leukaemia cells L5178Y. *Journal of Biochemistry*, 48, 157-165.

AZHIPA, Ia.I., KAIUSHIN, L.P. and NIKISHKIN, E.I. (1966) Elektronnyi paramagnitnyi rezonans tkanei zhivotnykh pri nekotorykh vidakh tkanevoi giposkii. *Biofizika*, 11, 710-713.

AZHIPA, Ia.I., KAIUSHIN, L.P. and NIKISHKIN, E.I. (1969) Spektry elektronnogo paramagnitnogo rezonansa zhelezosoderzhashchikh kompleksov, voznikaiushchikh v tkaniakh zhivotnykh pri nekotorykh vidakh gipoksii. *Biofizika*, 14, 852-857.

BABCOCK, D.F. and RICH, M.A. (1973) DNA-dependent RNA polymerases from murine spleen cells. *Biochemical Journal*, 133, 797-804.

BABIOR, B.M., KIPNES, R.S. and CURNETTE, J.T. (1973) Biological defense mechanisms. The production by leukocytes of superoxide, a potent bactericidal agent. *Journal of Clinical Investigation*, 52, 741-744.

BAGG, H.J. and JACKSON, J. (1937) *American Journal of Cancer*, 30, 539.

BAGULEY, B.C. and STAEHELIN, M. (1968) Substrate specificity of adenine-specific transfer RNA methylase in normal and leukemic tissues. *European Journal of Biochemistry*, 6, 1-7.

BALDESSARINI, R.J. and GREINER, E. (1973) Inhibition of catechol-o-methyl transferase by catechols and polyphenols. *Biochemical Pharmacology*, 22, 247-256.

BALIGA, B.S., BOREK, E., WEINSTEIN, I.B. and SRINIVASAN, P.R. (1969) Differences in the transfer RNA's of normal liver and Novikoff hepatoma. *Proceedings of the National Academy of Sciences of the USA*, 62, 899-905.

BARIL, E.F., JENKINS, M.D., BROWN, O.E., LASZLO, J. and MORRIS, H.P. (1973) DNA polymerases I and II in regenerating rat liver and Morris hepatomas. *Cancer Research*, 33, 1187-1193.

BARSEL, V.A., MATVEEVA, S.A., DRONOVA, L.M. and KORMAN, D.B. (1976) *Sintez i mekhanizm deistviya fiziologicheskii aktivnykh veshchestv*. Odessa.

BARTLETT, M.S. (1958) *Vvedenie v teoriyu sluchainykh protsessov*.

BASERGA, R. (1963) Mitotic cycle of ascites tumor cells. *Archives of Pathology*, 75, 156-161.

BEAUCHAMP, C. and FRIDOVICH, I. (1970) A mechanism for the production of ethylene from methional. *Journal of Biological Chemistry*, 245, 4641-4646.

BEHAR, D., CZAPSKI, G., RABANI, J., DORFMAN, L.M. and SCHWARZ, H.A. (1970) The acid dissociation constant and decay kinetics of the perhydroxyl radical. *Journal of Physical Chemistry*, 74, 3209-3213.

BEILI, N. (1970) *Matematika v biologii i meditsine*. Moscow: Mir.

BELICH, E.I., EROKHIN, V.N. and EMANUEL, N.M. (1972) Kineticheskie zakonomernosti izmeneniia gematologischeskikh pokazeteleipri razvitii spontannogo leikoza u myshei. *Izvestiia Akademii Nauk SSSR, Seriya Biologicheskaia*, 2, 204-212.

BELOUSOVA, A.K. (1965) *Biokhimicheskie podkhody k khimioterapii opukholei*. Leningrad: Meditsina.

BERENBAUM, N.C. (1969) Dose-response curves for agents that impair cell reproductive integrity. *British Journal of Cancer*, 23, 426-433.

BERGELSON, L.D., DIATLOVITSKAIA, E.V. and KRASOVSKII, E.D. (1967) Sviazyvanie kaliia natriia fosfolipidami normalnykh i opukholevykh tkanei. *Biokhimiia*, 32, 1128-1133.

BERGER, H. (1974) Studies on nascent DNA in mouse myeloma. *Cell*, 2, 23-30.

BERGOLTS, V.M. and RUMYANTSEV, N.V. (1966) *Sravenitelnaya patologiya i etiologiya leikoza cheloveka i zhivotnykh*. Moscow: Meditsina.

BERGQUIST, P.L. and MATTHEWS, R.E.F. (1962) Occurrence and distribution of methylated purines in the ribonucleic acids of subcellular fractions. *Biochemical Journal*, 85, 305-313.

BERLIN, A.A., BOGDANOV, G.N., KONOVALOVA, N.P., LIOGONKII, B.I. and EMANUEL, N.M. (1971) Protivoopukholevaia aktivnost polimerov s sistemoi sopriazhennykh sviazei. *Izvestiia Akademii Nauk SSSR, Seriya Biologicheskaia*, 2, 294-296.

BERTALANFFI, VON L. (1960) Principles and theory of growth. In: *Fundamental Aspects of Normal and Malignant Growth* (Ed. W.W. Nowinskii). New York: Elsevier.

BIELKA, H. (1974) Regulation der translation in eukaryotischen zellen. *Acta Biologica et Medica Germanica*, 32, 175-180.

BILLINGTON, R.W. and ITZHARI, R.F. (1974) Ribosomal RNA synthesis in chronic lymphocytic leukaemia. *British Journal of Cancer*, 318-323.

BINKERD, P. and TOLIVER, A. (1974) RNA linked membrane associated DNA. *Molecular and Cellular Biochemistry*, 5, 177-183.

BLACK, D.D. and GRIFFIN, A.C. (1970) Similarity of the transfer factors in Novikoff ascites tumor and other amino acid-incorporating systems. *Cancer Research*, 30, 1281-1286.

BLAIR, D.G.R. (1975) DNA-dependent RNA polymerases of Ehrlich carcinoma, other murine ascites tumors, and murine normal tissues. *Journal of the National Cancer Institute*, 55, 397-412.

BLOCH-FRANKENTHAL, L., LANGAN, J., MORRIS, H.P. and WEINHOUSE, S. (1965) Fatty acid oxidation and ketogenesis in transplantable liver tumors. *Cancer Research*, 25, 732-736.

BLOKHIN, N., LARIONOV, L., PEREVODCHIKOVA, N., CHEBOTAREVA, L. and MERKULOVA, N. (1958) Clinical experiences with sarcolysin in neoplastic diseases. *Annals of the New York Academy of Sciences*, 68, 1128-1132.

BOGDANOV, G.N., BURLAKOVA, E.B., KONOVALOVA, N.P. and KRUGLYAKOVA, K.E. (1968) *Fenolnye soedineniya i ikh biologicheskie funktsii*. Moscow: Nauka.

BOGDANOV, G.N., KOVTUN, Iu.T. and KONOVALOVA, N.P. (1971) Kineticheskie zakonomernosti raspada DNK v gomogenatakh selezenki v khode razvitiia perevivnogo leukoza La. *Doklady Akademii Nauk SSSR*, 201, 1234-1236.

BOGDANOV, G.N. and SHMONINA, V.M. (1975) Obmen nukleinovykh kislot v normal'noi regeneriruiushchei i neoplasticheskoi tkaniakh pecheni. *Voprosy Onkologii*, 21, 28-32.

BOGDANOV, G.N., SHMONINA, V.M. and EMANUEL, N.M. (1973) Kineticheski zakonomernosti rosta perevivaemykh gepatom s razlichnoi stepen'iu differtsirovki. *Byulleten Eksperimental'noi Biologii I Meditsiny*, 75, 87-89.

BOGDANOV, G.N., VARFOLOMEEV, V.N., PAVLOVA, V.M. and EMANUEL, N.M. (1976) Sviaz' paramagnitnykh svoistv gomologichnykh opykholenykh tkanei so stepen'iu ikh differentsirovki. *Doklady Akademii Nauk SSSR*, 226, 207-209.

BOGDANOV, G.N., VARFOLOMEEV, V.N., PAVLOVSKII, I.V. and EMANUEL, N.M. (1977) Svobodnye radikaly v protesse rosta perevivnoi pigmentonoi melanomy. *Doklady Akademii Nauk SSSR*, 233, 494-497.

BOLSHEV, L.N. and SMIRNOV, N.V. (1965) *Tablitsy matematicheskoi statistiki*. Moscow: Nauka.

BOREK, E. and KERR, S.J. (1972) Atypical transfer RNA's and their origin in neoplastic cells. *Advances in Cancer Research*, 15, 163-190.

BOREK, E. and SRINIVASAN, P.R. (1966) The methylation of nucleic acids. *Annual Review of Biochemistry*, 35, 275-298. .

BORSA, J., WHITMORE, G.F., VALERIOTE, F.A., COLLINS, D. and BRUCE, W.R. (1969) Studies on the persistence of methotrexate, cytosine arabinoside and leucovorin in serum of mice. *Journal of the National Cancer Institute*, 42, 235-242.

BORUKAEVA, M.R., RAIKMAN, L.M., SHABALKIN, V.A. and SAPRIN, A.N. (1969) Vzaimodeistvie kantserogenov s mikrosomal'nymi gemoproteinami. *Doklady Akademii Nauk SSSR*, 189, 651-654.

BORUN, T.W., SCHARFF, M.D. and ROBBINS, E. (1967) Rapidly labeled, polyribosome-associated RNA having the properties of histone messenger. *Proceedings of the National Academy of Sciences of the USA*, 58, 1977-1983.

BOTTGER, M. and WUNDERLICH, V. (1973) Rat liver mitochondrial DNA: unexpected sedimentation behavior and evidence for a molecular heterogeneity. *Acta Biologica et Medica Germanica*, 31, 655-666.

BOX, G.E. and JENKINS, G.M. (1970) *Time Series Analysis, Forecasting and Control*. Holden-Day.

BRAWERMAN, G. (1974) Eukaryotic messenger RNA. *Annual Review of Biochemistry*, 43, 621-642.

BRAY, R.C., PALMER, G. and BEINER, H. (1965) In: *Oxidases and Related Redox Systems*, Vol. 1, p. 359. Proceedings of a Symposium held in Amherst, Mass., July 15-19, 1964 (Eds. T.E. King, H.S. Mason and M. Marrison). New York: Wiley.

BRENK, H.A. VEN DEN, MOORE, V. and SHARPINGTON, C. (1971) Growth of metastases from P-388 sarcoma in the rat following whole body irradiation. *British Journal of Cancer*, 25, 186-207.

BRENNAN, M.J., COLE, T. and SINGLEY, J.A. (1966) A unique hyperfine ESR spectrum in mouse neoplasms analyzed by computer simulation. *Proceedings of the Society for Experimental Biology and Medicine*, 123, 715-718.

BRITTEN, R.I. and KOHNE, D.E. (1968) Repeated sequences in DNA. *Science*, 161, 529-540.

BROWN, D.D. and WEBEX, C.S. (1968) Gene linkage by RNA-DNA hybridization. *Journal of Molecular Biology*, 34, 661-680.

BRUSTAD, T., BUGGE, H., JONES, W.B.Y. and WOLD, E. (1972) Reactions between organic nitroxyl free radicals and radiation-induced transients in the DNA bases. *International Journal of Radiation Biology*, 22, 115-129.

BURLAKOVA, E.B., ALESENKO, A.V., MOLOCHKINA, E.M., PALMINA, N.P. and KHRAPOVA, N.G. (1975) *Bhoantioksidanty v luchevom porazhenii i zlokachestvennom roste*. Moscow: Nauka.

BURLAKOVA, E.B., DUBINSKAIA, N.I., KOPERINA, E.B. and PALMINA, N.P. (1966) Deistvie khlorgidrata 4-oski-3, 5-ditretbutil-alpha-metilbenzilamina na razmnozhenie kletok astsitnogo raka Erlikha. *Biofizika*, 11, 1008-1012.

BURLAKOVA, E.B., DZYUBA, N.M., PALMINA, N.P. and EMANUEL, N.M. (1965) *Doklady Akademii Nauk SSSR*, 163, 1278.

BURLAKOVA, E.B., GAINTSEVA, V.D. and PALMINA, N.P. (1973) Sovmestnoe diestvie rentgenovskogo izlucheniia i ingibitorov radikal'nykh reaktsii na opukhol i organizm zhivotnogo-opukholenositelia. *Doklady Akademii Nauk SSSR*, 213, 1451-1453.

BURLAKOVA, E.B. and MOLOCHKINA, E.M. (1968) Izemenenie antiokislitel'noi aktivnosti lipidov pecheni myshei pri indutsirovanii gepatomy ortoaminoazotoluolom. *Biofizika*, 13, 443-448.

BURLAKOVA, E.B. and MOLOCHKINA, E.M. (1973) Izmenenie antiokislitel'noi aktivnosti lipidov pecheni myshei pri eksperimental'nom kantserogeneze. *Biofizika*, 18, 293-298.

BURLAKOVA, E.B. and MOLOCHKINA, E.M. (1974) Vliianie na protsess kantserogeneza izmenenii antiokislitel'noi aktivnosti lipidov pri deistvii antioksidantov. *Voprosy Onkologii*, 20, 62-66.

BURLAKOVA, E.B. and PALMINA, N.P. (1966) Sinteticheskie ingibitory i prirodyne antioksidanty. *Biofizika*, 11, 258-262.

BURLAKOVA, E.B. and PALMINA, N.P. (1967) Izmenenie antiokislitel'noi aktivnosti lipidov v protsesse razvititiia perevivaemoi gepatomy 22a. *Biofizika*, 12, 1032-1036.

BUSCH, H. (Ed.) (1974) *The Molecular Biology of Cancer*. New York: Academic Press. 638 pp.

BUSCH, H. and SMETANA, K. (1970) *The Nucleolus*. New York: Academic Press. 626 pp.

CAIN, B.F., CALVELEY, S.B., BOREHAM, B.A., WEST, C., PRICE, N.A., WALKER, D.J. and CHURCHOUSE, M.J. (1974) Drug-tumor sensitivity matching procedure diffusion chambers *in vivo*. *Cancer Chemotherapy Reports*, 58, 189-205.

CARTER, S.K., DI MARCO, A. and GHIONE, M. (Eds.) (1972) *Proceedings of the International Symposium on Adriamycin*. New York: Springer-Verlag.

CATES, L.A. (1973) Assay of thiotepa by PMR spectrometry. *Journal of Pharmaceutical Sciences*, 62, 1698-1699.

CEREGHINI, S. and FRANZE-FERNANDEZ, M.T. (1974) Ehrlich ascites cells DNA-dependent RNA polymerases: effect of amino acids and protein synthesis inhibition. *FEBS Letters*, 41, 161-165.

CERIOTTI, G., SPANDRIO, L. and AGRADI, A. (1960) Study of substances of tumor origin with inhibitory action on hepatic catalse *in vivo*. *Tumori*, 46, 486-493.

CHANCHALASHVILI, Z.I., MADZHAGALADZE, G.V., MGELADZE, G.N. and MONASALIDZE, D.R. (1975) *Konformatsionnye izmeneniya biopolimerov v rastvorakh*. Tbilski.

CHANG, L.O., MORRIS, H.P. and LOONEY, W.B. (1968) Comparative incorporation of tritiated thymidine and cytidine into the mitochondrial and nuclear DNA and RNA of two transplantable hepatomas (3924A and H-35t$_Z$) and host livers. *Cancer Research*, 28, 2164-2167.

CHANG, L.O., SCHNAITMAN, C.A. and MORRIS, H.P. (1971) Comparison of the mitochondrial membrane proteins in rat liver and hepatomas. *Cancer Research*, 31, 108-113.

CHERKASOVA, E.V. (1969) Vliianie tsinka na potreblenie kisloroda fagotsitoz i razvitie limfosarkomy plissa. *Voprosy Onkologii*, 15, 81-85.

CHERNOV, V.A. (1964) *Tsitostaticheskie veshchestva v khimioterapii zlokachest-vennykh novoobrazovanii*. Moscow: Meditsina.

CHESTERTON, C.J., HUMPHREY, S.M. and BUTTERWORTH, P.H. (1972) Comparison of the multiple DNA-dependent RNA polymerase forms of whole rat liver and a minimal-deviation rat hepatoma cell line. *Biochemical Journal*, 126, 675-681.

CHIARUGI, V.P. and LORENZONI, C. (1968) Electrophoretic patterns of ribosomal proteins from liver and hepatomas. *Sperimentale*, 118, 475-482.

CHIRIGOS, M.A., COLSKY, J., HUMPHREYS, S.R., GLYNN, J.P. and GOLDIN, A. (1962) Evaluation of surgery and chemotherapy in the treatment of mouse mammary adeno-carcinoma. *Cancer Chemotherapy Reports*, 22, 49-53.

CLARK, C.M. and GOODLAD, G.A.J. (1975) Muscle protein biosynthesis in the tumour-bearing rat. *Biochimica et Biophysica Acta*, 378, 230-240.

CLARKE, D.A., REILLY, H.C. and STOCK, C.C. (1957) A comparative study of 6-diazo-5-oxo-L-serine on sarcoma 180. *Antibiotics and Chemotherapy*, 7, 653-671.

CLAYTON, D.A., DAVIS, R.W. and VINOGRAD, J. (1970) Homology and structural relationships between the dimetric and monometric circular forms of mitochondrial DNA from human leukemic leukocytes. *Journal of Molecular Biology*, 47, 137-153.

CLAYTON, D.A., SMITH, C.A., JORDAN, J.M., TEPLITZ, M. and VINOGRAD, J. (1968) Occurrence of complex mitochondrial DNA in normal tissues. *Nature*, 220, 976-979.

COMFORT, A. (1965) *The Process of Ageing*. London: Weidenfeld and Nicolson.

COMIS, R.L., BRODER, L.E. and CARTER, S.K. (1972) 1-(2-chloroethyl)-3-(4-methyl-cyclohexyl)-1-nitrosourea (Me CCNU) NSC 95441. Clinical brochure of the Division of Cancer Treatment of the National Cancer Institute.

COMMONER, B. and TERNBERG, J.L. (1961) Free radicals in surviving tissues. *Proceedings of the National Academy of Sciences of the USA*, 47, 1374-1384.

COMMONER, B., TOWNSEND, J. and PAKE, G.E. (1954) Free radicals in biological materials. *Nature*, 174, 689-693.

CORBETT, T.H., GRISWOLD, D.P., MAYO, J.G., LASTER, W.R. and CHABEL, F.M. (1975) Cyclophosphamide-adriamycin combination chemotherapy of transplantable murine tumors. *Cancer Research*, 35, 1568-1573.

COSTA, A. (1932) Untersuchungen uber die zur Übertragung experimentallen Tumoren der Hühner und Saugetiere durch Gehirnbrei von an Tumoren erkrankten Tieren. *Zeitschrift fur Krebsforschung*, 36, 399-408.

CRISS, W.E. (1974) Second messenger system in neoplasia. *Oncology*, 30, 43-80.

CROW, J.F. and KIMURA, M. (1970) *An Introduction to Population Genetics Theory*. New York: Harper and Row. 591 pp.

CULP, L.A., DORE, E. and BROWN, G.M. (1970) Methylated bases in DNA of animal origin. *Archives of Biochemistry and Biophysics*, 136, 73-79.

DEDRICK, R.L., ZAHARKO, D.S., BENDER, R.A., BLEYER, W.A. and LUTZ, R.J. (1975) Pharmacokinetic considerations on resistance to anticancer drugs. *Cancer Chemo-therapy Reports*, 59, 795-805.

DENISOV, E.T. (1971) *Konstanty skorosti gomoliticheskikh zhidkofaznykh reaktsii.* Moscow: Nauka.

DENNOSUKE, J., SANAE, T., JUNYA, S. and MASANORI, O. (1961) *Bulletin of the Cancer Institute of the Okayama University Medical School,* 1, 106.

DESAI, L.S., WULFF, U.C. and FOLEY, G.E. (1971) Human leukemia cells. *Experimental Cell Research,* 65, 260-263.

DESAI, L.S., WULFF, U.C. and FOLEY, G.E. (1975) Properties of chromosomal proteins of human leukemic cells. *Biochimie,* 57, 315-323.

DEWYS, W.D. (1972) Studies correlating the growth rate of a tumor and its metastases and providing evidence for tumor-related systemic growth. *Cancer Research,* 32, 374-379.

D'IACHKOVSKAIA, R.F. (1973) Unpublished thesis. Moscow.

D'IACHKOVSKAIA, R.F. and KONOVALOVA, N.P. (1973) Kinetika rosta kartsionomy 755 v zavisimosti ot vozrasta inokuluma i pola zhivotnykh. *Izvestiya Akademii Nauk SSSR, Seriya Biologicheskaia,* 1, 147-149.

D'IACHKOVSKAIA, R.F., PARKHOMENKO, I.I., VASILEVA, L.S., SURKOVA, N.I., SHUPPE, N.G., KONOVALOVA, N.P., BOGDANOV, G.N. and EMANUEL, N.M. (1969) Protivoopukholevaia aktivnost'preparatov riada fenoksazinovykh krasitelei. *Farmakologiya i Toksikologiya,* 32, 84-87.

DINGMAN, C.W. and SPORN, M.B. (1965) Actinomycin D and hydrocortisone: intracellular binding in rat liver. *Science,* 149, 1251-1254.

DISVETOVA, V.V., GENIEVA, E.N., EVSEENKO, L.S., RATKEVICH, G.I. and BOGOSLOVSKAYA, E.P. (1968a) Lechenie luchevykh porazhenii kozhi dibunolom. *Meditsinskaia radiologiia,* 13, 43-46.

DISVETOVA, V.V., GENIEVA, E.N., EVSEENKO, L.S., RATKEVICH, G.I. and BOGOSLOVSKAYA, E.P. (1968b) Primenenie antioksidantov pri troficheskikh porazheniiakh kozhi. *Klinicheskaia Meditsina,* 46, 126-130.

DIXON, R.L. and ADAMSON, R.G. (1965) Antitumor activity and pharmacologic disposition of cytosine arabinoside. *Cancer Chemotherapy Reports,* 48, 11-16.

DODD, N.J. and GIRON-CONLAND, J.M. (1975) Electron spin resonance study of changes during the development of a mouse myeloid leukaemia. *British Journal of Cancer,* 32, 451-455.

DOST, F.H. (1968) *Grundlagen der Pharmakokinetik.* Stuttgart.

DRAHOVSKY, D. and WACKER, A. (1975) *Naturwissenschaft,* 62, 189-190.

DREWS, J., HOGENAUER, G., UNGER, F. and WEIN, R. (1971) Incorporation of methionine from met-tRNA-Met-F into internal positions of polypeptides by mouse liver polysomes. *Biochemical and Biophysical Research Communications,* 43, 905-912.

DRISCOLL, D.H., DETTMER, C.M., WALLACE, J.D. and NEAVES, A. (1967) Variation of ESR signal amplitude with duration of tumor growth. *Currents in Modern Biology,* 1, 275-278.

DRONOVA, L.M. (1968) Unpublished thesis. Moscow.

DRONOVA, L.M., BELICH, E.I., EROKHIN, V.N. and EMANUEL, N.M. (1966) *Izvestiya Akademii Nauk SSSR, Seriya Biologischeskaia*, 5, 743.

DRONOVA, L.M., BELICH, E.I., TIURINA, E.P., EROKHIN, V.N. and KRENTSEL, B.A. (1966) Sravenie protivoopukholevoi aktivnosti etoksena i ego polimerov na kineticheskoi modeli leikoza. *Izvestiia Akademii Nauk SSSR, Seriya Biologicheskaia*, 6, 896–900.

DYATLOVITSKAYA, E.V. (1970) Unpublished thesis. Moscow.

EDMONDS, M., VAUGHAN, M.H. and NAKAZATO, H. (1971) Polyadenylic acid sequences in the heterogeneous nuclear RNA and rapidly labeled polyribosomal RNA of HeLa cells: possible evidence for a precursor relationship. *Proceedings of the National Academy of Sciences of the USA*, 68, 1336–1340.

EDWARDS, A.J., SUMNER, M.R. and ROWLAND, G.F. (1971) Changes in lymphoreticular tissues during growth of a murine adenocarcinoma. *Journal of the National Cancer Institute*, 47, 301–311.

EFIMOV, M.L. and BERNSHTEIN, V.A. (1968) Napriazhenie kislorida v astsiticheskoi zhidkosti v raznye sroki posle perevivki opukholi Erlikha. *Voprosy Onkologii*, 14, 95–97.

EHRLICH, P.Z. (1907) *Krebsforsch*, 5, 132.

EIGHTEN, J.G. and MARUYAMA, Y. (1968) Site difference for solid tumor growth. *Growth*, 32, 211–219.

EIGEN, M. (1973) *Samoorganizatsiya materii i evolyutsiya biologichsekikh makromolekul*. Moscow: Mir.

ELFORD, H.L., FREESE, M., PASSAMANI, E. and MORRIS, H.P. (1970) Ribonucleotide reductase and cell proliferation. *Journal of Biological Chemistry*, 245, 5228–5233.

ELSKA, A.V., MATSUKA, G.K., MATIASH, U.M., NASARENKO, J.J. and SEMENOVA, N.A. (1971) t-RNA and aminoacyl-tRNA synthetases during differentiation and various functional states of the mammary gland. *Biochemica et Biophysica Acta*, 247, 430–440.

ELTSINA, N.V. (1965) Unpublished thesis. Moscow.

EMANUEL, N.M. (1965) Perspektivy kineticheskogo izuchenia biokhimicheskikh protsessov v ratsional'noi khimioterapii raka. *Vestnik Akademii Meditsinskikh Nauk SSSR*, 20, 86–94.

EMANUEL, N.M. (1973) Kinetics and the free-radical mechanisms of tumor growth. *Annals of the New York Academy of Sciences*, 222, 1010–1030.

EMANUEL, N.M. (1974a) Kinetika i svobodnoradikal'nye mekhanizmy opukholevogo rosta. *Izvestiia Akademii Nauk SSSR, Seriya Biologicheskaia*, 6, 773–784.

EMANUEL, N.M. (1974b) Obshchaia zakonomernost' izmereniia soderzhaniia svobodnykh radikalov pri zlokachestvennom roste. *Doklady Akademii Nauk SSSR*, 217, 245–248.

EMANUEL, N.M. (1976) Free radicals and the action of inhibitors of radical processes under pathological states and ageing in living organisms and in man. *Quarterly Review of Biophysics*, 9, 283–308.

EMANUEL, N.M., DEDERER, L.I., KUKUSHKINA, G.V. and GORBACHEVA, L.B. (1976) Tormozhenie sinteza RNK propilgallatom v RNK-polimeraznoi sisteme. *Izvestiia Akademii Nauk SSSR, Seriya Biologicheskaia*, 4, 517–519.

EMANUEL, N.M., DENISOV, E.T. and MAIZUS, Z.K. (1965) *Tsepnye reaktsii okisleniya uglevodorodov z zhidkoi faze*. Moscow: Nauka.

EMANUEL, N.M., DRONOVA, L.M., EROKHIN, V.N. and BELICH, E.I. (1970) Vliianie nekotorykh protivoopukholevykh veshchestv na razvivshiisia eritromieloz Shvesta u krys. *Izvestiya Akademii Nauk SSSR, Seriya Biologicheskaia*, 1, 87-92.

EMANUEL, N.M., DRONOVA, L.M., GAGARINA, A.B. and KONOVALOVA, N.P. (1964) *Doklady Akademii Nauk SSSR*, 155, 220.

EMANUEL, N.M. and EVSEENKO, L.S. (1970) *Quantitative Basis of Clinical Oncology*. Moscow: Medizina.

EMANUEL, N.M., GORBACHEVA, L.B. and KUKUSHKINA, G.V. (1964) Suppression of plant biosynthesis in Ehrlich ascites cancer cells by chemical compounds of different classes. *Biochemical Pharmacology*, 13, 241-247.

EMANUEL, N.M., GUMANOV, L.L., KONOVALOVA, N.P., BOGDANOV, G.N., VASILEVA, L.S. and PLUGINA, L.A. (1968) Protivoleikemicheskoe deistvie 1,2-bis-diazoatsetiletana v eksperimente. *Doklady Akademii Nauk SSSR*, 183, 724-726.

EMANUEL, N.M., KISELEVA, E.G., D'IACHKOVSKAIA, R.F., KONOVALOVA, N.P. and VOLKOVA, L.M. (1975) Kineticheskii analiz rosta perevivnykh opukholei i ikh metastazov. *Voprosy Onkologii*, 21, 90-96.

EMANUEL, N.M., KONOVALOVA, N.P. and DRONOVA, L.M. (1962) *Doklady Akademii Nauk SSSR*, 143, 737.

EMANUEL, N.M., SHULAIKOVSKAIA, T.S. and KONDRATEVA, V.A. (1973) Izmenenie soderzhaniia svobodnykh radikalov v tkaniakh organizma pri toksicheskom deistvii khimicheskikh soedinenii. *Doklady Akademii Nauk SSSR*, 209, 1213-1214.

EMANUEL, N.M., VERMEL, E.M., KRUGLYAK, S.A., DRONOVA, L.M., OSTROVSKAIA, L.A. and BELICH, E.M. (1966) *Supermutageny*. Moscow: Nauka.

EMANUEL, N.M., VERMEL, E.M., OSTROVSKAIA, L.A. and KUKHARENKO, Yu.A. (1970) Kineticheskoe izuchenie protivoopukholevoi aktivnosti n-nitrozoalkilmochevin v eksperimente. *Voprosy Onkologii*, 16, 46-54.

EMMERSON, P.T. (1967) Enhancement of the sensitivity of anoxic *Escherichia coli* B-r to X-rays by triacetoneamine-N-oxyl. *Radiation Research*, 30, 841-849.

ENGELSE, L. DEN (1974) The formation of methylated bases in DNA by dimethylnitrosamine and its relation to differences in the formation of tumours in the livers of GR and C3HF mice. *Chemico-Biological Interactions*, 8, 329-338.

ERHAN, S., REISHER, S., FRANKO, E.A., KAMATH, S.A. and RUTMAN, R.J. (1970) Evidence for 'the wedge', initiator of DNA replication. *Nature*, 225, 340-342.

EROKHIN, V.N. (1968) Unpublished thesis. Moscow.

ERUKHIMOV, L.S. (1966) Lechenie opukhole mochevogo puzyria gossipolom i ionolom v sochetanii s khirurgicheskim vmeshatelstvom. *Voprosy Onkologii*, 12, 29-34.

ESAKOVA, T.D. and TARUSOV, B.N. (1970) *Fiziko-khimicheskie mekhanismy zlokachestvennogo rosta*. Moscow: Nauka.

EVSEENKO, L.S., MAKSIMOV, V.M., NIKOLAITSEVA, O.V. and SHIYATAYA, O.K. (1971) Nekotorye aspeckty primeniia kineticheskogo metoda v kolichestvennoi onkologii.

Izvestiia Akademii Nauk SSSR, Seriya Biologicheskaia, 5, 704-709.

FEDOROV, N.A., BOROVKOVA, T.V. and KIMERAL, R.E. (1971) *Patogenez, lechenie i epidemiologiya leikozov*. Moscow: Riga.

FELISTOVICH, G.I. (1964) Vliianie timina na techenie spontannogo leikoza u myshei Afb. *Voprosy Onkologii*, 10, 82-84.

FELL, P.J. and STEVENS, M.T. (1975) Pharmacokinetics — uses and abuses. *European Journal of Clinical Pharmacology*, 241-248.

FELLER, V. (1967) *Vvedenie v teoriyu veroyatnostei i eye prilozheniya*. Moscow: Mir.

FERDINANDUS, J.A., MORRIS, H.P. and WEBER, G. (1971) Behaviour of opposing pathways of thymidine utilization in differentiating, regenerating and neoplastic liver. *Cancer Research*, 31, 550-556.

FERRER, J.F. and MIHICH, E. (1967) Dependence of the regression of Sarcoma 180 in vitamin B_6-deficient mice upon the immunological competence of the host. *Cancer Research*, 27, 451-461.

FERRER, J.F. and MIHICH, E. (1968) Prevention of therapeutically induced regression of Sarcoma 180 by immunologic enhancement. *Cancer Research*, 28, 245-250.

FIEL, R.J., BARDOS, T.J., CHMIELEWICZ, Z.F. and AMBRUS, J.L. (1965) Biochemical parameters of neoplasia. II. Some macromolecular properties of DNA from normal and neoplastic human tissue. *Cancer Research*, 25, 1244-1253.

FILIPPOVICH, I.V. (1975) DNK-zavisimye DNK-polimerazy kletok eukariotov. *Uspekhi Sovremennoi Biologii*, 80, 147-165.

FLEISCHMANN, W., PRICE, H.G. and FLEISCHMANN, S.K. (1968) Pathways of excretion of colchicine in the golden hamster. *Pharmacology*, 1, 48-52.

FONAREV, A.B., SHUGALII, A.V., TIKHONRAVOV, A.L., KHANSON, K.P. and TODOROV, I.N. (1979) Osobennosti kinetiki reasstsiatsii bystrykh povtarov termolabil'nykh fraktsii DNK gepatomyzaidela. *Molekuliarnaia Biologiia*, 13, 30-37.

FRANKFURT, O.S. (1975) *Kletochnyi tsikl v opukholiakh*. Moscow: Meditsina.

FREI, J.V. and LAWLEY, P.D. (1975) Methylation of DNA in various organs of C57Bl mice by a carcinogenic dose of N-methyl-N-nitrosourea and stability of some methylation products up to 18 hours. *Chemico-Biological Interactions*, 10, 413-427.

FRIDOVICH, I. (1974) Superoxide dismutases. *Advances in Enzymology*, 41, 35-97.

FRIDOVICH, I. (1977) In: *Free Radicals in Biology* (Ed. W.A. Pryor). New York: Academic Press.

FRIEDELL, G.H., SHERMAN, J.D. and SOMMERS, S.C. (1961) Growth curves of human cancer transplants during experimental chemotherapy. *Cancer*, 14, 1117-1121.

FRINDEL, E., MALAISE, E.P., ALPEN, E. and TUBIANA, M. (1967) Kinetics of cell proliferation of an experimental tumor. *Cancer Research*, 27, 1122-1131.

FURTH, J. (1935) Transmission of myeloid leukemia of mice. *Journal of Experimental Medicine*, 61, 423-446.

FURTH, J. and KAHN, M.C. (1937) Transmission of leukemia of mice with single cells. *American Journal of Cancer*, 31, 276-282.

FURTH, J., SEIBOLD, H.R. and RATHBONE, R.R. (1933) Experimental studies on lymphomatosis of mice. *American Journal of Cancer*, 19, 521-604.

GALE, G.R. (1964) Effect of hydroxyurea on the incorporation of thymidine into Ehrlich ascites tumor cells. *Biochemical Pharmacology*, 13, 1377-1382.

GALLO, R.C. and PESTKA, S. (1970) Transfer RNA species in normal and leukemic human lymphoblasts. *Journal of Molecular Biology*, 52, 195-213.

GARRETT, C.T., MOORE, R.E., KATZ, C. and PITOT, H.C. (1973) Competitive DNA-RNA hybridization of nuclear and microsomal RNA in normal, neoplastic and neonatal liver tissue. *Cancer Research*, 33, 2469-2475.

GARSOU, J. (1956) Effets biologiques des radicauz libres semi-quinoniques. *Revue Belge de Pathologie et de Medecine Experimentale*, 25, 477-487.

GAUTSCHI, J.R. and CLARKSON, J.M. (1975) Discontinuous DNA replication in mouse P-815 cells. *European Journal of Biochemistry*, 50, 403-412.

GELSHTEIN, V.I. (1966) Unpublished thesis. Moscow.

GERSTENBERG, E. (1965) Due wachstumsgeschwindigkeit maligner tumoren. *Radiobiologia, Radiotherapia*, 6, 325-331.

GIASUDDIN, A.S.M., CAYGILL, C.P.J., DIPLOCK, A.T. and JEFFERY, E.H. (1975) The dependence on vitamin E and selenium of drug demethylation in rat liver microsomal fractions. *Biochemical Journal*, 146, 339-350.

GIRARD, M., LATHAM, H., PENMAN, S. and DARNELL, J.E. (1965) Entrance of newly formed messenger RNA and ribosomes into HeLa cell cytoplasm. *Journal of Molecular Biology*, 11, 187-201.

GOLDBERG, M.L., BURKE, G.C. and MORRIS, H.P. (1975) Cyclic AMP and cyclic GMP content and binding in malignancy. *Biochemical and Biophysical Research Communications*, 62, 320-327.

GOLDBERG, L.E., FILIPPOSIANTS, S.T. and STEPANOVA, E.S. (1973) K voprosu o kumuliativnykh svoistvakh protivoopukholevogo antibiotika. *Antibiotiki*, 18, 701-706.

GOLDBERG, G., KLEIN, E. and KLEIN, G. (1950) The nucleic acid content of mouse ascites tumor cells. *Experimental Cell Research*, 1, 543-570.

GOLDIN, A., VENDITTI, J.M., MEAD, J.A.R. and GLYNN, J.P. (1964) Antileukemic activity of hydroxyurea and other urea derivatives. *Cancer Chemotherapy Reports*, 40, 57-74.

GOLDMAN, M. and GRIFFIN, A.C. (1970) Transfer RNA patterns in livers of rats fed diets containing 3'-methyl-4-dimethylaminoazobenzene. *Cancer Research*, 30, 1677-1680.

GOLOSHCHAPOV, A.N., ALESENKO, A.V., BOGDANOV, G.N. and BURLAKOVA, E.B. (1973) Fizio-khimicheskie kharakteristiki lipidov i belkov pri razvitii perevivaemykh opukholei. *Biofizika*, 18, 1047-1051.

GOLOSHCHAPOV, A.N. and BURLAKOVA, E.B. (1973) Deistvie sinteticheskogo ingibitora radikal'nykh reaktsii na protsessy privitoi sopolimerizatsii v lipidakh i belkakh organov zhivotnykh. *Biofizika*, 18, 177-183.

GOMPERTZ, B. (1825) On the nature of the function expressive of the law of human mortality, and on a new mode of determining the value of life contingencies. *Philosophical Transactions of the Royal Society of London*, 115, 513-585.

GONACO, F., PIRRO, G. and SILVETTI, S. (1973) Foetal liver tRNA^{phe} in rat hepatoma. *Nature, New Biology*, 242, 236-237.

GONCHAROVA, S.A., KONOVALOVA, N.P., LIPCHINA, L.P. and FRANKFURT, O.S. (1973) Kletochonyi tsich perevivaemoi leikemii L 1210. *Voprosy Onkologii*, 19, 60-65.

GONCHAROVA, S.A., KONOVALOVA, N.P. and SHEVTSOVA, V.N. (1976) Vliianie diazana na mitoticheskii tsikl kletok leikemii L1210. *Voprosy Onkologii*, 22, 68-72.

GONIKBERG, E.M. (1968) Unpublished thesis.

GORBACHEVA, L.B. and KUKUSHKINA, G.V. (1970) Some aspects of the mechanism of action of 1-propyl-1-nitrosourea. *Biochemical Pharmacology*, 19, 1561-1568.

GORBACHEVA, L.B., KUKUSHKINA, G.V. and PETROV, O.E. (1968) *Fenolnye soedineniya i ikh biologicheskie funktsii*. Moscow: Nauka.

GORDY, W. (1958) In: *Symposium on Information Theory in Biology*, Gatlinburg, Tenn., October 29-31, 1956 (ed. H.P. Yockey). New York: Pergamon Press. 418 pp.

GORKOV, V.A. (1971) Unpublished thesis. Moscow.

GORKOV, V.A. (1976) *Matematicheskaya teoriya biologicheskikh protsessov*. Kalingrad.

GORKOV, V.A. (1977) Otsenka parametrov asimptoticheskikh krivykh rosta opukholei. *Voprosy Onkologii*, 23, 51-54.

GORKOV, V.A., DISVETOVA, V.V., EVSEENKO, L.S. and MATVEEVA, S.A. (1970) O biologicheskoi aktivnosti butiloksitoluola. *Voprosy Pitaniya*, 29, 65-72.

GORKOV, V.A., MATVEEVA, S.A., NORIKOV, Iu.D. and EVSEENKO, L.S. (1969) Kinetika postupleniia i vyvedeniia 2,6-di-tret. *Izvestiia Akademii Nauk SSSR, Seriya Biologicheskaia*, 6, 843-851.

GORKOV, V.A. and OSTROVSKAIA, L.A. (1977) Sviaz vremeni zhizni zhivotnykh — opukholnositelei s kinetikoi razvitiia zlokachestvennogo protsessa pri perevivnom leikoza La u myshei. *Izvestiia Akademii Nauk SSSR, Seriya Biologicheskaia*, 3, 444-447.

GORKOV, V.A. and VASILEVA, L.S. (1973) Kineticheskii analiz rosta limfosarkomy Plissa. *Voprosy Onkologii*, 19, 91-93.

GOTLIB, V.Ia., PELEVINA, I.I., AFANASEV, G.G. and LIPCHINA, L.P. (1970) Izmenenie letal'nogo effekta oblucheniia pri pomoshchi khimicheskikh soedinenii v usloviiakh kul'tivirovaniia kletok vne organizma. *Doklady Akademii Nauk SSSR*, 192, 1367-1370.

GREENBERG, H. and PENMAN, S. (1966) Methylation and processing of ribosomal RNA in HeLa cells. *Journal of Molecular Biology*, 21, 527-535.

GREENBERG, L.J. and UHR, J.W. (1967a) DNA-RNA hybridization studies of myeloma tumors in mice. *Proceedings of the National Academy of Sciences of the USA*, 58, 1878-1882.

GREENBERG, L.J. and UHR, J.W. (1967b) Myeloma tumor satellite DNA: a role in ribosomal RNA synthesis. *Biochemical and Biophysical Research Communications*, 27, 523-528.

GREENSTEIN, J.P. (1954) *Biochemistry of Cancer*, 2nd edn. New York: Academic Press. 658 pp.

GRENANDER, U. (1961) Sluchainye protsessy i statisticheskie vyvody. Moscow.

GRISHAM, J.W., KAUFMAN, D.G. and STENSTROM, M.L. (1972) 3H-d TTP incorporating activities in isolated rat liver nuclei. *Biochemical and Biophysical Research Communications*, 49, 420-427.

CROPPER, L. and SHIMKIN, M.B. (1967) Combination therapy of 3-methylcholanthrene-induced mammary carcinoma in rats: effect of chemotherapy, ovariectomy and food restriction. *Cancer Research*, 27, 26-32.

GUERIN, M. and GUERIN, P. (1934) Epithelioma de l'uterus du rat, lymphotrope et transplantable. *Bulletin de l'Association Francaise pour l'Etude du Cancer*, 23, 632-646.

GUMANOV, L.L., KONOVALOVA, S.D. and NORENKO, N.P. (1966) *Supermutageny*. Moscow: Nauka.

HAGGMARK, A. (1962) Studies on resistance against 5-fluorouracil thymidylate synthetase from drug resistant tumor lines. *Cancer Research*, 22, 568-572.

HALL, S.H. and SMUCKLER, E.A. (1974) Murine myeloma DNA-dependent RNA polymerase. *Biochemistry*, 13, 3795-3805.

HARDING, H.E. and PASSEY, R.D.J. (1930) *Pathol. Bacteriol.*, 33, 417.

HARDING, H.R., ROSEN, F. and NICHOL, C.A. (1964) Depression of alanine transaminase activity in the liver of rats bearing Walker carcinoma 256. *Cancer Research*, 24, 1318-1323.

HARRIS, H. (1963) Breakdown of RNA in the cell nucleus. *Proceedings of the Royal Society of London*, B158, 79-87.

HARRIS, J.W., SHON, B. and MENESES, J. (1973) Relationship between growth and radiosensitivity in the P388 murine leukemia. *Cancer Research*, 33, 1780-1784.

HARRIS, T.E. (1963) *The Theory of Branching Processes*. New Jersey: Prentice Hall. 231 pp.

HARTMAN, S.C. (1962) Glutamine-phosphoribosyl pyrophosphate amidotransferase. *Federation Proceedings*, 21, 244.

HASHIMOTO, S. and MURAMATSU, M. (1973) Differences in nucleotide sequences of ribosomal RNA between the liver and a hepatoma of C3H/He mice. *European Journal of Biochemistry*, 33, 446-458.

HATLEN, L.E., AMALDI, F. and ATTARDI, G. (1969) Oligonucleotide pattern after pancreatic ribonuclease digestion at the 3' and 5' termini of 5S RNA from HeLa cells. *Biochemistry*, 8, 4989-5005.

HEIDELBERGER, C., GRIESBACH, L., MONTAG, B.J., MOOREN, D., CRUZ, O., SCHNITZER, R.J. and GRUNBERG, E. (1958) Studies on fluorinated pyrimidines. II. Effects on transplanted tumors. *Cancer Research*, 18, 305.

HEIKKILA, R.E. and COHEN, G. (1973) 6-Hydroxydopamine: evidence for superoxide radical as an oxidative intermediate. *Science*, <u>181</u>, 456-457.

HERZFELD, A. and GREENGARD, O. (1972) The dedifferentiated pattern of enzymes in livers of tumor-bearing rats. *Cancer Research*, <u>32</u>, 1826-1832.

HEWITT, H.B. and BLAKE, E.R. (1968) The growth of transplanted murine tumours in pre-irradiated sites. *British Journal of Cancer*, <u>22</u>, 808-824.

HILL, B.T. (1972) Studies on the transport and cellular distribution of chlorambucil in the Yoshida ascites carcinoma. *Biochemical Pharmacology*, <u>21</u>, 495-502.

HOUGLUM, J.E., MORRIS, H.P. and ABUL-HAJJ, Y.J. (1974) Steroid Δ^4-reductase activity in hepatomas of different growth rates. *Cancer Research*, <u>34</u>, 938-941.

HUDSON, B. and VINOGRAD, J. (1969) Sedimentation velocity properties of complex mitochondrial DNA. *Nature*, <u>221</u>, 332-337.

HUMPHREY, E.W. (1963) Tumor growth in potassium-deficient mice. *Cancer Research*, <u>23</u>, 1121-1124.

HYODO, M., KOYAMA, H. and ONO, T. (1970) Intermediate fragments of the newly replicated DNA in mammalian cells. *Biochemical and Biophysical Research Communications*, <u>38</u>, 513-519.

ILINA, K.P. and MERKLE, K. (1973) Chislennost' populiatsii i raschet vremeni generatsii kletok astsitnoi kartsinomy Erlika. *Voprosy Onkologii*, <u>19</u>, 70-74.

INGREM, D. (1972) *Elektronnyi paramagnitnyi rezonans v biologii*. Moscow: Mir.

INSTITORIS, L., DZURILLAY, E., SEBESTYEN, J.H., JENEY, A. and PETHES, C. (1971) Untersuchungen über den Zusammenhang von biologischen Wirkungsunterschieden und Vertailungsparametern bei 1,6-Dibromhexiten. *Zeitschrift fur Krebsforschung*, <u>75</u>, 133-145.

ITO, K. and McKEAN, H.P. (1965) *Diffusion Processes and their Sample Paths*. Berlin: Springer-Verlag. 321 pp.

IWANAMI, Y. and BROWN, G.M. (1968) Methylated bases of transfer RNA from HeLa and L cells. *Archives of Biochemistry and Biophysics*, <u>124</u>, 472-482.

IYER, V.N. and SZYBALSKI, W. (1958) The mechanism of chemical mutagenesis. *Proceedings of the National Academy of Sciences of the USA*, <u>44</u>, 446-456.

JACOB, S.T. (1973) Mammalian RNA polymerase. *Progress in Nucleic Acid Research and Molecular Biology*, <u>13</u>, 93-126.

JEFFREE, G.M. (1958) Hydrogen peroxide and cancer. *Nature*, <u>182</u>, 892.

JOHNSON, R.E., HARDY, W.G. and ZELEN, M. (1966) Chemotherapeutic effects on mammalian tumor cells. *Journal of the Cancer Institute*, <u>36</u>, 15-20.

JOHNSON, R.E., ZELEN, M. and KEMP, N.H. (1965) Chemotherapeutic effects on mammalian tumor cells. *Journal of the National Cancer Institute*, <u>34</u>, 277-290.

JONES, G. and MACH, B. (1973) The function of MET-tRNA_F in the initiation of protein synthesis in mouse myeloma tumors. *Biochimica et Biophysica Acta*, <u>312</u>, 399-402.

JUNGMANN, R.A., SCHWEPPE, J.S. and LESTINA, F.A. (1970) Studies on adrenal histones. *Journal of Biological Chemistry*, 245, 4321-4326.

KADOHAMA, N. and TURKINGTON, R. (1974) In: *Hormones and Cancer* (Ed. K.W. McKerns). New York: Academic Press. 394 pp.

KALF, G.F., D'AGOSTINO, M.A. and HUNTER, G.R. (1971) DNA biosynthesis by isolated mitochondria stimulation by cytoplasmic factors from neoplastic and regenerating tissues. *Cancer Research*, 31, 2054-2058.

KARLIN, S. (1971) *Osnovy teorii sluchainykh protsessov*. Moscow: Mir.

KASS, L. (1973) Erythroid histones in chronic erythemic myelosis. *Proceedings of the Society for Experimental Biology and Medicine*, 144, 887-891.

KASSIRSKII, I.A. (1964) *Vvedenie v klinicheskuyu gematologiyu*. Moscow: Meditsina.

KASSIRSKII, I.A., EMANUEL, N.M., KLOCHKO, E.V., KOVALENKO, O.A., PINZUR, V.I., KRUGYLAKOVA, K.E. and CHIBRIKIN, V.M. (1967) Izmenenie soderzhaniia svobodnykh radikalov v leikotsitakh pri leikozakh. *Problemy Gematologii i Perelivaniia Krovi*, 12, 11-15.

KATES, J. (1970) Transcription of the Vaccinia virus genome and the occurrence of polyriboadenylic acid sequences in messenger RNA. *Symposia on Quantitative Biology*, 35, 743-752.

KERR, S.J. and BOREK, E. (1972) The tRNA methyltransferases. *Advances in Enzymology*, 36, 1-27.

KERSTEN, H. (1962) Action of mitomycin C on nucleic acid metabolism in tumor and bacterial cells. *Biochemica et Biophysica Acta*, 55, 558.

KESSEL, D., BOTTERILL, V. and WODINSKY, I. (1968) Uptake and retention of daunomycin by mouse leukemic cells as factors in drug resistance. *Cancer Research*, 28, 936-941.

KHALD, A. (1856) *Matematicheskaya statistika s tekhnicheskimi prilozheniyami*, Moscow.

KHANSON, K.P. AND IVANOVA, L.V. (1971) Mitokhondrial'naia dezoksiribonukelinovaia kislota zhivotnykh. *Uspekhi Sovremennoi Biologii*, 72, 3-23.

KHANSON, K.P. and ZHIVOTOVSKII, B.D. (1974) Kinetika reassotsiatsii DNK timusa i astsitnoi gepatomy krysy. *Byulleten Eksperimental'noi Biologii i Meditsiny*, 78, 92-94.

KHENNAN, E. (1964) *Analiz vremennykh ryadov*. Moscow: Nauka.

KHENNAN, E. (1974) *Mnogomernye vremennye ryady*. Moscow: Mir.

KHOLMS, B. (1956) *Ioniziruyushchie izlucheniya i kletochnyi metabolizm*. Moscow: Mir.

KHRISTIANOVICH, D.S., DRONOVA, L.M., VARFOLOMEEV, V.N., BOGDANOV, G.N. and EMANUEL, N.M. (1977) Izmeneniia soderzhaniia svobodnykh radikalov v pecheni kak pokazatel' razvitiia eksperimental'nykh leikozov. *Doklady Akademii Nauk SSSR*, 236, 1011-1014.

KISELEVA, E.G. (1971) Unpublished thesis. Moscow.

KISELEVA, E.G., BOGDANOV, G.N., KONOVALOVA, N.P. and EMANUEL, N.M. (1969) *Izvestiia Akademii Nauk SSSR, Seriya Biologicheskaia*, 1, 149.

KISELEVA, E.G., BOGDANOV, G.N., KONOVALOVA, N.P. and EMANUEL, N.P. (1970) Tipy kineticheskikh krivykh rosta sarkomy 45 pri vozdeistvii alkiliruiushchikh soedinenii. *Izvestiia Akademii Nauk SSSR, Seriya Biologicheskaia*, 4, 530-534.

KIT, S. and GROSS, A.L. (1959) Quantitative relationships between DNA content and glycolysis of histones of diploid and tetraploid cells. *Biochemica et Biophysica Acta*, 36, 185.

KLAGSBRUN, M. (1972) The contrast between the methylation of transfer RNA *in vivo* and *in vitro* by normal and SV40 transformed 3T3 cells. *Journal of Biological Chemistry*, 247, 7443-7451.

KLEIN, G. and REVESZ, L.J. (1953) *Journal of the National Cancer Institute*, 14, 229.

KLEPIKOV, N.P. and SOKOLOV, S.N. (1964) *Analiz i planirovanie eksperimentov metodom maksimuma pravdopodobiya*. Moscow: Nauka.

KLINE, I., GANG, M., TYRER, D.D., MANTEL, N., VENDITTI, J.M. and GOLDIN, A. (1968) Duration of drug levels in mice as indicated by residual antileukemic efficiency. *Chemotherapy*, 13, 28-41.

KNIGHT, E. and DARNELL, J.E. (1967) Distribution of 5S RNA in HeLa cells. *Journal of Molecular Biology*, 28, 491-502.

KNOEPP, L.F., LETSON, W.M., DANNA, S.J. and MOORE, Y.W. (1964) Effects of perfusion with thiotepa on carcinoma Vx2 in hind legs of rabbits. *Cancer Chemotherapy Reports*, 41, 1-5.

KNOX, W.E., JAMDAR, S.C. and DAVIS, P.A. (1970) Hexokinase differentiation and growth rates of transplanted rat tumors. *Cancer Research*, 30, 2240-2244.

KOENIGSFELD, H. and PRAUSNITZ, G. (1914) *G. Zbl. Bakteriol.*, 74, 70.

KOGARKO, I.N., KOGARKO, B.S. and EVSEENKO, L.S. (1970) Tsitokhimicheskoe issledovanie nukleinovykh kislot limfoidnoi tkani pri khronicheskom limfaticheskom leikoze cheloveka. *Izvestiia Akademii Nauk SSSR, Seriya Biologicheskaia*, 3, 348-355.

KOIKE, K., KOBAYASHI, M., FUJISAWA, T. and TANAKA, S. (1975) Abnormal synthesis of mitochondrial DNA in the presence of N-methyl-N'-nitro-N-nitrosoguanidine *in vitro*. *Biochemica et Biophysica Acta*, 402, 351-362.

KONOPLEV, V.P. (1960) *Modeli i metody eksperimentalnoi onkologii*. Moscow.

KONOVALOVA, N.P. (1975) Unpublished thesis. Moscow.

KONOVALOVA, N.P., BOGDANOV, G.N., MILLER, V.B., NEIMAN, M.M., ROZANTSEV, E.G. and EMANUEL, N.M. (1964) Protivoopukholevaia aktivnost' stabil'nykh svobodnykh radikalov. *Doklady Akademii Nauk SSSR*, 157, 707-709.

KONOVALOVA, N.P., BOGDANOV, G.N., VASILEVA, L.S., DRONOVA, L.M., MATVEEVA, A.A. and EMANUEL, N.M. (1966) Stroenie i antileikemicheskoe deistvie v riadu zameshchennykh fenolov. *Doklady Akademii Nauk SSSR*, 168, 1419-1421.

KONOVALOVA, N.P., D'IACHKOVSKAIA, R.F. and KISELEVA, E.G. (1973) Toksichnost' i protivoopukholevaia aktinost' novogo analoga tioTEFa. *Voprosy Onkology*, 19, 58-63.

KONOVALOVA, N.P., D'IACHKOVSKAIA, R.F., NAIDICH, V.V. and EMANUEL, N.M. (1976)

Tropnost' i farmako-kineticheskoe povedenie paramgnitnogo analoga tiofosfamida. *Izvestiia Akademii Nauk SSSR, Seriya Biologicheskaia*, 5, 751-754.

KONOVALOVA, N.P., D'IACHKOVSKAIA, R.F., VASILEVA, L.S. and BOGDANOV, G.N. (1968) *Sovremennye sostoyanie khimioterapii zlokachestvennykh opukholei*. Moscow: Riga.

KORENMAN, I.M. (1967) *Analiticheskaya khimiya malykh kontsentratsii*. Moscow: Khimiya.

KOZLOV, A.P. (1973) Svobodnye radikaly i ikh rol v normalnykh i patologicheskikh protsessakh. *Izd. Mgu.*

KOZLOV, A.P. and SEITS, I.F. (1975) Sravnitel'noe izuchenie nizkomolekuliarnykh iadernykh RNK krysy i gepatomy zaidela. *Voprosy Onkologii*, 21, 68-71.

KOZLOV, L.V., GINODMAN, L.M. and OREKHOVICH, V.N. (1967) Inaktivatsiia pepsina alifaticheskimi diazokarbonil'nymi soedineniiami. *Biokhimiia*, 32, 1011-1019.

KRAMER, G. (1948) *Metody matematicheskoi statistiki*. Moscow.

KRASHILINA, A.Ya. (1960) *Modeli i metody eskperimentalnoi onkologii*. Moscow: Medgiz.

KRITSKII, G.A., ALEKSANDROV, S.V., BATISHEV, A.I. and LITAVRIN, V.A. (1973) *Radiobiologiya*, 13, 323.

KRITSKII, G.A., ALEKSANDROV, S.V., KOROMYSLOV, G.F. and GRITSENKO, M.N. (1972b) Anomal'nost raspredeleniia primidinovykh nukleotidnykh blokov DNK pri leikozakh i luchevom porzhenii. *Doklady Akademii Nauk SSSR*, 206, 230-232.

KRITSKII, G.A., BATISHEV, A.I., ALEKSANDROV, S.V., FEDOROV, N.A. and ABRAMOV, R.E. (1972a) Sravnitel'naia kharakteristika nukleotidnykh blokov DNK pri luchevom porazhenii i leikoze. *Doklady Akademii Nauk SSSR*, 203, 233-236.

KRUEGER, R.G. and McCARTHY, B.J. (1970) Hybridization studies with nucleic acids from murine plasma cell tumors. *Biochemical and Biophysical Research Communications*, 41, 944-951.

KRUGLIAKOVA, K.E., NIKOLAEVA, N.V., ZAKHAROVA, N.A. and EMANUEL, N.M. (1964) Radiatsionnyi raspad DNK kak eksperimental'naia model'dlia otsenko effektivnosti radiozashchitnykh veshchestv. *Doklady Akademii Nauk SSSR*, 157, 979-981.

KUKUSHKINA, G.V., GORBACHEVA, L.B. and EMANUEL, N.M. (1966) Tormozhenie biosinteza belka i nukleinovykh kislot fenol'nymi soedineniiami v optakh in vivo. *Voprosy Meditsinkoi Khimii*, 12, 452-455.

KUKUSHKINA, G.V., SOKOLOVA, I.S., OSTROVSKAIA, L.A. and GORBACHEVA, L.B. (1972) Vliianie nitrozome tilmocheviny (NMM) na kineticku rosta i biosintez belka v kletkakh leikemii L1210. *Izvestiia Akademii Nauk SSSR, Seriya Biologicheskaia*, 5, 731-736.

KUMAR, P.M. and FOX, B.W. (1974) An electron microscope study of mitochondrial DNA in spontaneous human tumours and chemically induced animal tumours. *British Journal of Cancer*, 29, 447-461.

KUNTZEL, H. (1971) In: *Current Topics in Microbiology*, p. 94.

KUZELA, S., KOLAROV, J. and KREMPASKY, V. (1973) Electrophoretic properties of the product of protein synthesis in mitochondria of rat liver and Zajdela hepatoma.

Neoplasma, 20, 623-630.

KUZELA, S., KREMPASKY, V., KOLAROV, J. and UJHAZY, V. (1975) Formation, size, and solubility in chloroform/methanol of products of protein synthesis in isolated mitochondria of rat liver and Zajdela hepatoma. *European Journal of Biochemistry*, 58, 483-491.

KUZMINA, S.V. and STRAZHEVSKAIA, N.B. (1970) Sravnitel'naia kharakteristika fiziko-khimicheskikh svoistv DNK normal'nykh i malignizirovannykh myshinykh fibroblastov v kul'ture tkani. *Biofizika*, 15, 1133-1136.

LAIRD, A. (1964) *British Journal of Cancer*, 28, 3.

LANKIN, V.Z. and GUREVICH, S.M. (1976) Ingibirovanie pereokisleniia lipidov i detoksikatsiia lipoperekiasei zashchitnymi fermentativnymi sistemami pri eksperimental'nom zlokachestvennom roste. *Doklady Akademii Nauk SSSR*, 226, 705-708.

LANKIN, V.Z. and NEIFAKH, E.A. (1968) Vysshie zhirnye kisloty v protsesse zlokachestvennogo rosta. *Izvestiia Akademii Nauk SSSR, Seriya Biologicheskaia*, 2, 263-268.

LARIONOV, L.F. (1962) *Khimioterapiya zlokachestvennykj opukholei*. Moscow: Meditsina.

LASTER, W.R., MAYO, J.G., SIMPSON-HERREN, L., GRISWOLD, D.P., LLOYD, H.H., SCHABEL, F.M. and SKIPPER, H.E. (1969) Success and failure in the treatment of solid tumors. *Cancer Chemotherapy Reports*, 53, 169-188.

LAW, L.W., DUNN, T.B., BOYLE, P.Y. and MILLER, J.H. (1949) *Journal of the National Cancer Institute*, 10, 179.

LAWLEY, P.D. (1968) Methylation of DNA by N-methyl-N-nitrosourethane and N-methyl-N-nitroso-N'-nitroguanidine. *Nature*, 218, 580-581.

LAWLEY, P.D., CRATHORN, A.R., SHAH, S.A. and SMITH, B.A. (1972) Biomethylation of DNA in cultured human tumor cells (HeLa). *Biochemical Journal*, 128, 133-138.

LAZAREV, N.V. and MIULLER, N.R. (1970) O rezistentnosti zlokachestvennykh opukholei k khimoterapevticheskim vozdeistviiam. *Voprosy Onkologii*, 16, 40-44.

LEA, M.A., MORRIS, H.P. and WEBBER, G. (1966) Comparative biochemistry of hepatomas. VI. Thymidine incorporation into DNA as a measure of hepatoma growth rate. *Cancer Research*, 26, 465-469.

LEE, S. and DAHMUS, M.E. (1973) Stimulation of eukaryotic DNA-dependent RNA polymerase by protein factors. *Proceedings of the National Academy of Sciences of the USA*, 70, 1383-1387.

LEE, S., MENDECKI, J. and BRAWERMAN, G. (1971) A polynucleotide segment rich in adenylic acid in the rapidly-labeled polyribosomal RNA component of mouse sarcoma 180 ascites cells. *Proceedings of the National Academy of Sciences of the USA*, 68, 1331-1335.

LERMAN, M.I., ABAKUMOVA, O.Yu., KUCENCO, N.G., GORBACHEVA, L.B., KUKUSHKINA, G.V. and SEREBRYANYI, A.M. (1974) Different degradation rates of alkylated RNA protein and lipids in normal and tumor cells. *Cancer Research*, 34, 1536-1541.

LEVENBERG, B., MELNIC, I. and BUCHANAN, J.M. (1957) Biosynthesis of the purines. *Journal of Biological Chemistry*, 225, 163.

LEVIN, W., LU, A.Y.H., JACOBSON, M., KUNTZMAN, R., POYER, J.L. and McCAY, P.B. (1973) Lipid peroxidation and the degradation of cytochrome P-450 heme. *Archives of Biochemistry and Biophysics*, 158, 842-852.

LINDER, M., MUNRO, H. and MORRIS, H.P. (1970) Rat ferritin isoproteins and their response to iron administration in a series of hepatic tumors and in normal and regenerating liver. *Cancer Research*, 30, 2231-2239.

LIPPMAN, M.M., LASTER, W.R., ABBOTT, B.J., VENDITTI, J. and BARATTA, M. (1975) Antitumor activity of macromomycin B (NSC 170105) against murine leukemias, melanoma and lung carcinoma. *Cancer Research*, 35, 939-945.

LO, K.W., MILLER, E.E., MORRIS, H.P. and TSOU, K.C. (1973) Chemotherapy of Morris hepatoma 3924A: correlation of size and weight of tumor and preliminary data with 5-fluoro-2-deoxyuridine. *Cancer Chemotherapy Reports*, 57, 245-249.

LOEB, L.A., SPRINGGATE, C.F. and BATTULA, N. (1974) Errors in DNA replication as a basis of malignant changes. *Cancer Research*, 34, 2311-2321.

LOONEY, W.B., MAYO, A.A., ALLEN, P.M., MORROW, J. and MORRIS, H.P. (1973) A mathematical evaluation of tumour growth curves in rapid, intermediate and slow growing rat hepatomata. *British Journal of Cancer*, 27, 341-344.

LOVELES, A. and HAMPTON, C.L. (1969) Inactivation and mutation of coliphage T2 by N-methyl and N-ethyl-N-nitrosourea. *Mutation Research*, 7, 1-12.

LUCAS-LENARD, J. and HAENNI, A.L. (1968) Requirement of guanosine-5'-triphosphate for ribosomal binding of aminoacyl-sRNA. *Proceedings of the National Academy of Sciences of the USA*, 59, 554-560.

LUCAS-LENARD, J. and LIPMAN, F. (1971) Protein biosynthesis. *Annual Reviews of Biochemistry*, 40, 409-448.

McCARTY, K.S. and McCARTY, K.S. (1974) Protein modification metabolic controls, and their significance in transformation in eukaryotic cells. *Journal of the National Cancer Institute*, 53, 1509-1514.

McCord, J.M. and Fridovich, I. (1969) Superoxide dismutase. *Journal of Biological Chemistry*, 244, 6049-6055.

McCREDIE, J.A., INCH, W.R., KRUUV, J. and WATSON, T.A. (1965) *Growth*, 29, 331.

MacDOWELL, E.C., TAYLOR, M.J. and POTTER, J.S. (1934) Immunization of mice naturally susceptible to a transplantable leukemia. *Proceedings of the Society for Experimental Biology and Medicine*, 32, 84-86.

MAILER, C., SWARTZ, H.M., KONIECZNY, M., AMBEGAONKAR, S. and MOORE, V.L. (1974) Identity of the paramagnetic element found in increased concentrations in plasma of cancer patients and its relationship to other pathological processes. *Cancer Research*, 34, 637-642.

MAIO, J.J. and KURNIT, D.M. (1974) Transcription of mammalian satellite DNA's by homologous DNA-dependent RNA polymerases. *Biochimica et Biophysica Acta*, 349, 305-319.

MAITRA, S.C. and FREI, J.V. (1975) Organ-specific effects of DNA methylation by alkylating agents in the inbred Swiss mouse. *Chemico-Biological Interactions*, 10, 285-293.

MAKSUMOVA, Z.A., AFANASEV, G.G., GOTLIB, V.Y. and PELEVINA, I.I. (1972b) *Radiotsitologiya-72; operativno-informatsionnye materialy*. Leningrad.

MAKSUMOVA, Z.A., AFANASEV, G.G. and PELEVINA, I.I. (1972a) Izmeneie radiochuvstvitel'nosti kletok HeLa pridlitel'nom kul'tivirovanii. *Radiobiologiia*, 12, 541-548.

MALENVO, E. (1975) *Statisticheskie metody ekonometrii*, Vol. 1. Moscow: Statistika.

MALENVO, E. (1976) *Statisticheskie metody ekonometrii*, Vol. 2. Moscow: Statistika.

MALLARD, J.R. and KENT, M. (1964) Differences observed between electron spin resonance signals from surviving tumour tissues and from their corresponding normal tissues. *Nature*, 204, 1192.

MANAILOV, S.E. (1971) *Biokhimicheskie osnovy zlokachestvennogo rosta*. Leningrad: Meditsina.

MANSSON, P.E., HOLMQUIST, L., DEUTSCH, A. and NORDEN, A. (1975) Heterogeneous nuclear RNA from lymphocytes of chronic lymphocytic leukaemia: adenylate-rich and double-stranded regions. *Scandinavian Journal of Haematology*, 14, 42-56.

MARKLUND, S. and MARKLUND, G. (1974) Involvement of the superoxide anion radical in the autoxidation of pyrogallol and a convenient assay for superoxide dismutase. *European Journal of Biochemistry*, 47, 469-474.

MARTIN, G.S., VENUTA, S., WEBER, M. and RUBIN, H. (1971) Temperature-dependent alterations in sugar transport in cells infected by a temperature sensitive mutant of Rous Sarcoma virus. *Proceedings of the National Academy of Sciences of the USA*, 68, 2739-2741.

MASSEY, V. and GHISLA, S. (1974) Role of charge-transfer interactions in flavoprotein catalysis. *Annals of the New York Academy of Sciences*, 227, 446-465.

MATIENKO, N.A. (1970) Unpublished thesis. Novosibirsk.

MATIENKO, N.A., MARTYNOVA, R.P. and SALGANIK, R.I. (1967) Vliianie dezoksiribonukleazy na techenie spontannogo limfoleikoza u myshei vysokoleikoznoi linii AKR. *Doklady Akademii Nauk SSSR*, 172, 1457-1459.

MATSUHISA, T., HIGASHI, K., GOTOH, S. and SAKAMOTO, Y. (1970) Changes in the nucleotide compositions of nucleolar 45S RNA of azo dye-induced hepatoma. *Cancer Research*, 30, 162-166.

MEINELL, D.Z.H. and MEINELL, E. (1967) *Eksperimentalnaya mikrobiologiya*. Moscow: Mir.

MELETT, L.B. and WOODS, L.A. (1960) Fluorometric estimation of mechlorethamine (Mustargen) and its biological disposition in the dog. *Cancer Research*, 20, 518-532.

MELTZ, M. and OKADA, S. (1971) Characterization of the rapidly labeled hybridizable RNA synthesized in L5178Y mouse leukemic cells. *Biophysical Journal*, 11, 582-594.

MERKER, P.C. and HURLEY, J. (1962) A study of human epidermoid carcinoma growing in cortisone-conditioned Swiss mice. *Cancer Research*, 22, 646-650.

MIL, E.M., BOBOVICH, S.I., AZIZOV, Iu.M., KRINITSKAIA, L.A., ZHILTSOVA, V.M., ZHIZHINA, G.P. and KRUGLIAKOVA, K.E. (1975) Strukturnye perekhody v DNK, vydelennoi iz normal'nykh i opukholevykh kletok. *Biofizika*, 20, 757-761.

MIL, E.M., KOZLOVA, L.E. and SAPRIN, A.N. (1971) Sravnitel'noe izuchenie spektrov electronnogo paramagnitnogo rezonansa opukholevykh tkanei i nitrozil'nykh kompleksov gemoproteinov. *Izvestiia Akademii Nauk SSSR, Seriya Biologicheskaia*, 6, 901-906.

MIL, E.M., ZAVRIEV, S.K., GRIGORIAN, G.L. and KRUGLIAKOVA, K.E. (1973) Izuchenie strukturnykh perekhodov spin-mechenoi DN. *Doklady Akademii Nauk SSSR*, 209, 217-220.

MINENKOVA, E.A., EROKHIN, V.N., KRUGLYAK, S.A., VERMEL, E.M. and EMANUEL, N.M. (1967) *Izvestiia Akademii Nauk SSSR, Seriya Biologicheskaia*, 4, 517.

MINENKOVA, E.A., KRUGLYAK, S.A., VERMEL, E.M. and EMANUEL, N.M. (1968) *Izvestiia Akademii Nauk SSSR, Seriya Biologicheskaia*, 4, 475.

MIRAULT, M.-E. and SCHERRER, K. (1972) In vitro processing of HeLa cell peribosomes by a nucleolar endoribonuclease. *FEBS Letters*, 20, 233.

MISHENEVA, V.S. and GORIUKHINA, T.A. (1973) Aktivnost gliutationreduktazy v razlichnykh opukholiakh cheloveka i zhivotnykh. *Voprosy Onkologii*, 19, 58-63.

MISRA, H.P. and FRIDOVICH, I. (1972) The role of superoxide anion in the autoxidation of epinephrine and a simple assay for superoxide dismutase. *Journal of Biological Chemistry*, 247, 3170-3175.

MITROKHIN, Yu.I., GALKIN, A.P., BARDASH, L.A. and TODOROV, I.N. (1973) *Ukr. Biochim. Zhurn.*, 45, 294.

MITROPOLSKII, A.K. (1971) *Tekhnika statisticheskikh vychislenii*. Moscow: Nauka.

MITTELMAN, A. (1971) Patterns of isoaccepting phenylalanine transfer RNA in human leukemia and lymphoma. *Cancer Research*, 31, 647-650.

MIYAKI, M., KOIDE, K. and ONO, T. (1973) RNase and alkali sensitivity of closed circular mitochondrial DNA of rat ascites hepatoma cells. *Biochemical and Biophysical Research Communications*, 50, 252-258.

MIZUNO, N.S., HOF, H. and COLLIN, M. (1968) RNA fractions in normal rat liver and Morris 5123D hepatoma. *Biochimica et Biophysica Acta*, 166, 656.

MONTGOMERY, J.A. and STRUCK, R.F. (1973) The relationship of the metabolism of anticancer agents to their activity. *Progress in Drug Research*, 17, 320-409.

MORAN, P.A.P. (1962) *The Statistical Processes of Evolutionary Theory*. Oxford: Clarendon Press. 200 pp.

MORI, K., WINZERITH, M. and MANDEL, P. (1973) Reassociation of normal mouse DNA and mouse plasmocytoma DNA. *FEBS Letters*, 35, 7-10.

MORRIS, H.P. (1965) Studies on the development, biochemistry and biology of experimental hepatomas. *Advances in Cancer Research*, 9, 227-302.

MORRIS, H.P., DYER, H.M., WAGNER, B.P. and RECHCIGL, M. (1964) Some aspects of the development, biology and biochemistry of rat hepatomas of different growth rate. *Advances in Enzyme Regulation*, 2, 321-334.

MOSIENKO, V.S. and PIVNIUK, V.M. (1968) Raspredelenie tiotefa i tsiklofosfana v organizme krys. *Voprosy Onkologii*, 14, 73-76.

MURTY, C.N., VERNEY, E. and SIDRANSKY, H. (1974) Studies of initiation factors in protein synthesis of host liver and transplantable hepatoma. *Cancer Research*, 34, 410-418.

MUSHINSKI, J.F. (1974) Hepatoma-foetal Phe-tRNA also present in normal rat liver. *Nature*, 248, 332-334.

MYERS, M.W. and BOSMAN, H.B. (1974) Mitochondrial protein content and enzyme activity of Reuber hepatoma H-35. *Cancer Research*, 34, 1989-1994.

NAKAHARA, W. (1925) Resistance to spontaneous mouse cancer induced by injections of oleic acid. *Journal of Experimental Medicine*, 41, 347.

NALIMOV, V.V. (1971) *Teoriya eksperimenta.* Moscow: Nauka.

NAU, F. (1974) Differences in *in vivo* methylation patterns of tyrosine and histidine transfer RNA's from rat liver and Novikoff hepatoma. *Biochemistry*, 13, 1105-1109.

NAZAR, R.N. (1973) Evidence for non-uniform labeling in comparisons of ^{32}P-labeled RNAs from rat liver and the Novikoff hepatoma. *Federation Proceedings*, 32, 853.

NAZAR, R.N. and BUSCH, H. (1972) A comparison of polypyrimidine fragments in 28S ribosomal RNA from rat liver and the Novikoff hepatoma. *Cancer Research*, 32, 2322-2331.

NEBERT, D.W. and MASON, H.S. (1963) An electron spin resonance study of neoplasms. *Cancer Research*, 23, 833-840.

NEIFAKH, E.A. (1976) Toksichnost'lipidov 12 organov zhivotnykhopukholenositelei. *Doklady Akademii Nauk SSSR*, 230, 1470-1473.

NEIFAKH, E.A. and KAGAN, V.E. (1969) Obnaruzhenie perekislei'lipidov v organakh normal'nykh zhivot'nykh in vivo. *Biokhimiia*, 34, 511-517.

NEIMAN, M.B., ROZANTSEV, E.G. and MAMEDOVA, Yu.G. (1962) Free radical reactions involving no unpaired electrons. *Nature*, 196, 472-474.

NIKODEJEVIC, B., SENOH, S., DALY, J.W. and CREVELING, C.R. (1970) Catechol-o-methyltransferase. *Journal of Pharmacology and Experimental Therapeutics*, 174, 83-93.

NIKOL'SKAIA, T.A., EROKHIN, V.N. and EMANUEL, N.M. (1975) Kineticheskie zakonomernosti razvitiia novogo shtamma leukoza mysehi. *Doklady Akademii Nauk SSSR*, 221, 967-969.

NIKOL'SKAIA, T.A. and LIPCHINA, L.P. (1968) Virusnye chastitsy v kletkakh linii LL. *Doklady Akademii Nauk SSSR*, 182, 1223-1225.

NIKOL'SKAIA, T.A., LIPCHINA, L.P., POROCHENKO, G.G. and AKSYUTINA, M.S. (1969) Novaia liniia kletok limfaticheskogo leikoza. *Tsitologiia*, 11, 486-492.

NOTARI, R.E. (1971) *Biopharmaceutics and Pharmacokinetics: An Introduction.* New York: M. Dekker. 319 pp.

ODINTSOVA, S.P. and KRUGLIAKOVA, K.E. (1976) O dvoistvennom kharaktere deistviia propilgallata pri obluchenii DNK. *Doklady Akademii Nauk SSSR*, 226, 456-459.

OKUDA, H., ARIMA, T., HASHIMOTO, T. and FUJII, S. (1972) Multiple forms of deoxythymidine kinase in various tissues. *Cancer Research*, 32, 791-794.

ONISHI, T., HEMINGTON, J., LANOVE, K.F., MORRIS, H. and WILLIAMSON, J. (1973) Electron paramagnetic resonance studies of iron-sulfur centers in mitochondria prepared from three Morris hepatomas with different growth rates. *Biochemical and Biophysical Research Communications*, 55, 372-381.

ONO, T., KAWAMURA, M., HYODO, M. and WAKABAYASHI, K. (1971) Difference of RNA population between normal liver and hepatoma AH-130. *Gann*, 62, 31-40.

ORME-JOHNSON, N.R., HANSEN, R.E. and BEINERT, H. (1974a) Electron paramagnetic resonance-detectable electron acceptors in beef heart mitochondria. I. *Journal of Biological Chemistry*, 249, 1922-1927.

ORME-JOHNSON, N.R., HANSEN, R.E. and BEINERT, H. (1974b) Electron paramagnetic resonance-detectable electron acceptors in beef heart mitochondria. II. *Journal of Biological Chemistry*, 249, 1928-1939.

OSTROVSKAIA, L.A. (1968) Unpublished thesis. Moscow.

OSTROVSKAIA, L.A., DRONOVA, L.M., VERMEL, E.M., KRUGLYAK, S.A. and EMANUEL, N.M. (1964) *Materialy konferentsii po voprosam lekarstvennoi terapii v onkologicheskoi klinike.* Leningrad: Meditsina.

OSTROVSKAIA, L.A. and EMANUEL, N.M. (1976) *Materialy Sov-Amer simpoziuma po protivoopukholevym antibiotikam.* Moscow.

OSTROVSKAIA, L.A. and FRANKFURT, O.S. (1977) Vliianie n-nitrozo-N-metilmocheviny na kletochnuiu kinetiku v opukholiakh. *Voprosy Onkologii*, 23, 88-93.

OSTROVSKAIA, L.A., KRUGLIAK, S.A. and VERMEL, E.M. (1968) *Spetsifichnost khimicheskogo mutageneza.* Moscow: Nauka.

OSTROVSKAIA, L.A., SEREBRIANYI, A.M. and RAPOPORT, I.A. (1977) Sravnitel'noe izuchenie proticoopukholevoi effektivnosti riada nitrozoalkilmochevin. *Izvestiia Akademii Nauk SSSR, Seriya Biologicheskaia*, 2, 264-272.

OSTROVSKAIA, L.A. and VERMEL, E.M. (1975) Kinetika rosta perevivemykh opukholei molochnykh zhelez myshei. *Voprosy Onkologii*, 21, 77-88.

OUELLETTE, A.J. and TAYLOR, M.W. (1973) Elevated levels of acceptor activity of hepatoma transfer RNA. *Biochemistry*, 12, 3542-3546.

OVE, P., BROWN, O.E. and LASZLO, J. (1969) Separation of DNA polymerase from rat liver and hepatomas. *Cancer Research*, 29, 1562-1567.

OVE, P., COETZEE, M.L. and CHEN, J. (1972a) Synthesis and degradation of serum proteins in normal and hepatoma-bearing rats. *Journal of Cell Biology: Abstracts of 12th Annual Meeting Am. Soc. for Cell Biology*, 55, 197.

OVE, P., COETZEE, M.L., CHEN, J. and MORRIS, H.P. (1972b) Differences in synthesis and degradation of serum proteins in normal and hepatoma-bearing animals. *Cancer Research*, 32, 2510-2518.

OVE, P., LASZLO, J., JENKINS, M.D. and MORRIS, H.P. (1969) Increased DNA polymerase activity in a series of rat hepatomas. *Cancer Research*, 29, 1557-1561.

OWEN, D.B. (1962) *Handbook of Statistical Tables.* Reading, Mass: Addison-Wesley. 580 pp.

PAOLETTI, C. and RIOU, G. (1971) In: *Progress in Molecular and Subcellular Biology*. Berlin: Springer-Verlag.

PARKANSKII, M.I. and KONOVALOVA, N.P. (1973) Kineticheskaia kharakteristica rosta eksperimentalnykh opukholei posle khirurgicheskogo vozdeistviia. *Izvestiia Akademii Nauk SSSR, Seriya Biologicheskaia*, 4, 593-597.

PARKANSKII, M.I., KONOVALOVA, N.P. and EMANUEL, N.M. (1973) Kinetika regressi i retsidiva kartsinosarkomy Uokera pri deistvii alkiliruiushchikh soedinenii. *Izvestiia Akademii Nauk SSSR, Seriya Biologicheskaia*, 1, 144-146.

PASTAN, J., WILLINGHAM, M., CARCHAN, R. and ANDERSON, W.B. (1973) In: *Role of Cyclic Nucleotides in Carcinogenesis* (Ed. J. Schultz and H.G. Gratzner). New York: Academic Press. 373 pp.

PAVLOVA, N.I. and LIVENSON, A.R. (1965) Spektry elektonnogo paramagnitnogo resonansa (EPR) krovi cheloveka v norme i pri leukozakh. *Biofizika*, 10, 169-171.

PECHURKIN, N.S. and TERSKOV, I.A. (1975) *Analiz kinetiki rosta i evolyutsii mikrobnykh populyatsii*. Novosibirsk: Nauka.

PEDERSEN, P.L., GREENAWALT, J.W., CHAN, T.L. and MORRIS, H.P. (1970) A comparison of some ultrastructural and biochemical properties of mitochondria from Morris hepatomas 9618A, 7800 and 3924A. *Cancer Research*, 30, 2620-2626.

PELEVINA, I.I. (1973) Unpublished thesis. Moscow.

PELEVINA, I.I., AFANASEV, G.G., LIPCHINA, L.P., ANDREEV, V.M. and EMANUEL, N.M. (1966) *Izvestiia Akademii Nauk SSSR, Seriya Biologicheskaia*, 6, 841.

PELEVINA, I.I., AFANASEV, G.G., LIPCHINA, L.P. and EMANUEL, N.M. (1968) Kinetika rosta solidioi limfosarkomy NKLy pri vozdei'stvii razlichnykh pod ioniziruiushchego izlucheniia. *Izvestiia Akademii Nauk SSSR, Seriya Biologicheskaia*, 1, 99-108.

PENMAN, S., SMITH, I. and HOLTZMAN, E. (1966) Ribosomal RNA synthesis and processing in a particulate site in the HeLa cell nucleus. *Science*, 154, 786-789.

PERRY, R.P. (1962) The cellular sites of synthesis of ribosomal and 4S RNA. *Proceedings of the National Academy of Sciences of the USA*, 48, 2179-2186.

PERRY, R.P. and KELLY, D.E. (1972) Production of ribosomal RNA from high molecular weight precursors. *Journal of Molecular Biology*, 70, 265-279.

PETERS, R.A. and BUFFA, P. (1949) The *in vivo* formation of citrate induced by fluoroacetate and its significance. *Journal of Physiology*, 110, 488.

PETYAEV, M.M. (1972) *Biofizicheskie pokhody k diagnostike zlokachestvennykh opukholei*. Moscow: Meditsina.

PHILLIPS, M.E. (1966) Studies on the kinetics of transplantation immunity. *Cancer Research*, 26, 40-47.

PHILIPS, F.S., STERNBERG, S.S., SCHWARTZ, H.S., CRONIN, A.P., SODERGREN, J.E. and VIDAL, P.M. (1967) Hydroxyurea. I. Acute cell death in proliferating tissues in rats. *Cancer Research*, 27, 61-74.

PIETRO, S.di and GIACOMELLI, V. (1954) Problemi teorici e clinici della chemioterapia dei tumori con sostanze antimitotiche. *Minerva medica*, 1, 373-379.

PLACKETT, R.L. (1960) *Principles of Regression Analysis*. Oxford: Clarendon Press. 173 pp.

PLUGINA, L.A., ORLOVA, Zh.I. and GUMANOV, L.L. (1972) O mekhanizme deistviia diazoketonov. *Doklady Akademii Nauk SSSR*, 204, 1489-1491.

PLUGINA, L.A., SHUPPE, N.G., ORLOVA, Zh.I., VOLKOVA, L.M. and GUMANOV, L.L. (1969) Vliianie diazketonov na sintez makromolekul v bakterial'nykh i zhivotnykh kletkakh. *Doklady Akademii Nauk SSSR*, 188, 934-936.

PLUGINA, L.A., SHUPPE, N.G., ORLOVA, Zh.I., VOLKOVA, L.M. and GUMANOV, L.L. (1971) O mekhanizme biologicheskogo deistviia diazoketonov. *Biokhimiia*, 36, 304-310.

POLIAKOV, V.M., LANKIN, V.Z. and GUREVICH, S.M. (1976) Okislenie ksenobiotikov pri khimicheskom kantserogeneze i eksperimental'nom zlokachestvennom roste. *Doklady Akademii Nauk SSSR*, 226, 471-473.

PRESTAYKO, A.W., TONATO, M. and BUSCH, H. (1970) Low molecular weight RNA associated with 28S nucleolar RNA. *Journal of Molecular Biology*, 47, 505-515.

PRIGOZHINA, E.L. and VENDROV, E.L. (1971) O neobkhodimosti tsitogeneticheskogo kontrolia opukholevykh shtammov. *Voprosy Onkologii*, 17, 83-85.

PROBST, G.S., STALKER, D.M., MOSBAUGH, D.W. and MEYER, R.R. (1975) Stimulation of DNA polymerase by factors isolated from Novikoff hepatoma. *Proceedings of the National Academy of Sciences of the USA*, 72, 1171-1174.

PROKHOROV, Yu.V. and ROZANOV, Yu.A. (1973) *Teoriya veroyatnostei*. Moscow: Nauka.

PRYOR, W.A. (Ed.) (1976) *Free Radicals in Biology*. New York: Academic Press.

PUCK, T.T., MARCUS, P.I. and CIECIURA, S.J. (1956) Clonal growth of mammalian cells *in vitro*. *Journal of Experimental Medicine*, 103, 273-284.

QUEENER, S.F., MORRIS, H.P. and WEBER, G. (1971) Dihydrouracil dehydrogenase activity in normal, differentiating, and regenerating liver and in hepatomas. *Cancer Research*, 31, 1004-1009.

RABINOWITZ, M. and SWIFT, H. (1970) Mitochondrial nucleic acids and their relation to the biogenesis of mitochondria. *Physiological Reviews*, 50, 376-427.

RAIKHLIN, N.T. and SMIRNOVA, E.A. (1967) Gistokhimicheskoe obnaruzhenie. Nekotorykh fermentov energeticheskogo obmena v opukholiakh s razlichnoi skorost'iu rosta. *Voprosy Onkologii*, 13, 93-98.

RAJALAKSHMI, S., LIANG, H., SARMA, D.S.R. and KSILEVSKI, R. (1971) Cycloheximide, an inhibitor of peptide chain termination or release in liver *in vivo* and *in vitro*. *Biochemical and Biophysical Research Communications*, 42, 259-265.

RANDERATH, E., CHIA, L.S.Y., MORRIS, H.P. and RANDERATH, K. (1974) Transfer RNA base composition studies in Morris hepatomas and rat liver. *Cancer Research*, 34, 643-653.

RANDERATH, K. (1971) Applications of a tritium derivative method to human brain and brain tumor transfer RNA analysis. *Cancer Research*, 31, 658-661.

RANDERATH, K., MacKINNON, S.K. and RANDERATH, E. (1971) An investigation of the minor base composition of transfer RNA in normal human brain and malignant brain tumors. *FEBS Letters*, 15, 81.

RECHCIGL, M., PRICE, V.E. and MORRIS, H.P. (1962) Studies on the cachexia of tumor-bearing animals. II. Catalase activity in the tissues of hepatoma-bearing animals. *Cancer Research*, 22, 874-880.

REICH, E. (1963) Biochemistry of actinomycins. *Cancer Research*, 23, 1428-1441.

REICHARD, P., SKOLD, O., KLEIN, G., REVESZ, L. and MAGNUSSON, P. (1962) Studies on resistance against 5-fluorouracil. I. Enzymes of the uracil pathway during development of resistance. *Cancer Research*, 22, 235-243.

RENNERT, O.M. (1971) Transfer RNA's of embryonic tissue. *Cancer Research*, 31, 637-638.

RICHTER, M.N. and MACDOWELL, E.C. (1933) Studies on leukemia in mice. *Journal of Experimental Medicine*, 57, 1.

RIEGELMAN, S., LOO, J.C.K. and ROWLAND, M. (1968) Shortcomings in pharmacokinetic analysis by conceiving the body to exhibit properties of a single compartment. *Journal of Pharmaceutical Sciences*, 57, 117-123.

RIOCHE, M., QUELIN, S. and MESSEYEFF, R. (1974) Synthèse de proteines plasmatiques par les hepatocytes humains cancereux et normaux en culture. *Pathologie Biologie*, 22, 867-876,

ROBERTSON, H.D. and MATHEWS, M.B. (1973) Double-stranded RNA as an inhibitor of protein synthesis and as a substrate for a nuclease in extracts of Krebs II ascites cells. *Proceedings of the National Academy of Sciences of the USA*, 70, 225-229.

ROMANOVSKII, I.V., AGATOVA, A.I. and NOVIKOVA, E.N. (1973) Kinetika izmenenii sul'fgidril'nykh i disul'fidnykh grupp i belka v protsesse razvitiia astsitnoi opukholi Erlikha. *Voprosy Onkologii*, 19, 60-64.

ROMANOVSKII, Yu.M., STEPANOVA, N.V. and CHERNAVSKII, D.S. (1975) *Matematichesko modelirovanie v biofizike.* Moscow: Nauka.

ROSENKRANZ, H.S., ROSENKRANZ, S. and SCHMIDT, R.M. (1969) Effects of nitroso-methylurea and nitrosomethylurethan on the physical chemical properties of DNA. *Biochemica et Biophysica Acta*, 195, 262.

ROSS, U. (1964) *Biologicheskie alkiliruyushchie veshchestva.* Moscow: Meditsina.

ROZANTSEV, E.G. (1970) *Svobodnye iminiksilnye radikaly.* Moscow: Khimiya.

RUTMAN, R.J., CANTAROW, A. and PASCHKIS, K.E. (1954) Studies in 2-acetylamino-fluorene carcinogenesis. I. The intracellular distribution of nucleic acids and protein in rat liver. *Cancer Research*, 14, 111.

RUTMAN, R.J., CHUN, E.H. and LEWIS, F.S. (1968) Permeability difference as a source of resistance to alkylating agents in Ehrlich tumor cells. *Biochemical and Biophysical Research Communications*, 32, 650-657.

RUTTER, W.T., MORRIS, P.W., GROLDBERG, M., PAULE, M. and MORRIS, R.W. (1972) In: *The Biochemistry of Gene Expression in Higher Organisms* (Eds. J.K. Pollack and J.W. Lee). Boston: Reidel.

RUUGE, E.K., KERIMOV, T.M. and PANEMANGLOR, A.V. (1976) O vliianii liofilizatsii na svobodnoradikal'nye sostoianiia kletok zhivotnykh. *Biofizika*, 21, 124-128.

RUUGE, E.K. and KORNIENKO, I.A. (1969) O spektrakh EPR zamorozhennykh tkanei zhivotnykh. *Biofizika*, 14, 752-754.

SACCHI, A., DELPINO, A., GRECO, C. and REFFINI, U. (1974) Analisti strutturale e funzionalita in vitro dei ribosomi 80S isolati da cellule tumorale del topo. *Tumori*, 60, 1-16.

SALYAMOV, L.S. (1974) *Rak i disfunktsiya kletki*. Leningrad: Nauka.

SANDS, R.H. and DUNHAM. W.R. (1974) Spectroscopic studies on two-iron ferredoxins. *Quarterly Reviews of Biophysics*, 7, 443-504.

SAPRIN, A.N., KHOLMUKHAMEDOVA, N.M., AGEENKO, A.I. and EMANUEL, N.M. (1971) Tezisy simpoziuma svobodnoradikalnye sostoyaniya i ikh rol pri luchevom porazhenii i zlokachestvennom roste. Moscow.

SAPRIN, A.N., MINENKOVA, E.A., NAGLER, N.G., KRUGLYAK, S.A., KRUGLIAKOVA, K.E. and EMANUEL, N.M. (1967) Kinetika izmeneniia soderzhaniia svobodnykh radikalov pri razvitii kartsinosarkomy. *Biofizika*, 12, 1099-1103.

SAPRIN, A.N., SHABALKIN, V.A., KOZLOVA, L.E., KRUGLYAKOVA, K.E. and EMANUEL, N.M. (1968) Obnaruzhenie i issledovaie novogo tipa signalov EPR. *Doklady Akademii Nauk SSSR*, 181, 1520-1523.

SAWADA, H., GILMORE, V.H. and SAUNDERS, G.F. (1973) Transcription from chromatins of human lymphocytic leukemia cells and normal lymphocytes. *Cancer Research*, 33, 428-434.

SCHABEL, F.M., JOHNSTON, T.P., McCABEL, G.S., MONTGOMERY, J.A., LASTER, W.R. and SKIPPER, H.E. (1963) Experimental evaluation of potential anticancer agents. VIII. Effects of certain nitrosoureas on intracerebral L1210 leukemia. *Cancer Research*, 23, 725-733.

SCHANDL, E.K. and TAYLOR, J.H. (1969) Early events in the replication and integration of DNA into mammalian chromosomes. *Biochemical and Biophysical Research Communications*, 34, 291-300.

SCHATZ, G. and MASON, T.L. (1974) The biosynthesis of mitochondrial proteins. *Annual Review of Biochemistry*, 43, 51-87.

SCHMID, F.A., CAPPUCCINO, J.G., MERKER, P.C., TARNOWSKI, G.S. and STOCK, C.C. (1966) Chemotherapy studies in an animal tumor spectrum. I. Biologic characteristics of the tumors. *Cancer Research Supplement*, 26, 173-180.

SCHRECK, R. (1935) *American Journal of Cancer*, 24, 807.

SCHREIBER, M., SCHREIBER, G. and KARTENBECK, J. (1974) Protein and ribonucleic acid metabolism in single-cell suspensions from Morris hepatoma 5123tc and from normal rat liver. *Cancer Research*, 34, 2143-2150.

SEEBER, S. and BUSCH, H. (1972) Differences in the primary structure of nucleolar and ribosomal high molecular weight RNA of the Novikoff hepatoma and rat liver, and possible therapeutic implications. *Zeitschrift for Krebsforschung*, 78, 265-281.

SEEBER, S., KADING, J., BRUCKSCH, K.P. and SCHMIDT, C.G. (1974) Defective rRNA synthesis in human leukaemic blast cells? *Nature*, 248, 673-675.

SEKIGUCHI, M. and TAKAGI, Y. (1959). Synthesis of DNA by phage-infected *Escherichia coli* in the presence of mitomycin C. *Nature*, 183, 1134-1135.

SEKIGUCHI, M. and TAKAGI, Y. (1960) Effect of mitomycin C on synthesis of bacterial and viral DNA. *Biochemica et Biophysica Acta*, 41, 434.

SEMENOVA, L.P., NIKOLSKAIA, T.A. and EMANUEL, N.M. (1965) Podavlenie propilgallatom okislitelnogo fosforilirovaniia i dykhaniia v mitokhondriiakh pecheni i solidnoi gepatomy myshei. *Doklady Akademii Nauk SSSR*, 163, 774-776.

SEREBRIANYI, A.M. and MNATSAKANIAN, R.M. (1972) Issledovanie molekuliarnogo mekhanizma mutagennogo deistviia nitrozoalkilnochevin. *Doklady Akademii Nauk SSSR*, 199, 657-660.

SEREBRIANYI, A.M., SMOTRIAEVA, M.A. and KRUGLIAKOVA, K.E. (1969a) Metilirovanie DNK N-nitrozo-N-metilmochevinoi. *Izvestiia Akademii Nauk SSSR, Seriya Biologicheskaia*, 4, 607-608.

SEREBRIANYI, A.M., SMOTRIAEVA, M.A., KRUGLIAKOVA, K.E. and KOSTYANOVSKII, R.G. (1969b) Karbamoilirovanie DNK N-nitrozo-N-metilmochevinoi. *Doklady Akademii Nauk SSSR*, 185, 847-849.

SHANIN, A.P. (1959) *Pigmentnye opukholi*. Moscow: Medgiz.

SHAPOT, V.S. (1972) Some biochemical aspects of the relationship between the tumour and the host. *Advances in Cancer Research*, 15, 253-286.

SHAPOT, V.S. (1973) Biologicheskie kharakteristiki progressii opukholei. *Voprosy Onkologii*, 19, 89-92.

SHAPOT, V.S. (1975) *Biokhimicheskie aspeckty opukholevogo rosta*. Moscow: Meditsina.

SHAPOT, V.S. and BERDINSKIKH, N.K. (1975) O mekhanisme gipoal' buminemii pri eksperimental'nykh opukholiiakh. *Voprosy Onkologii*, 21, 57-62.

SHARMA, R.M., SHARMA, C., ANDREW, A.J., MORRIS, H.P. and WEINHOUSE, S. (1965) Glucose-ATP phosphotransferases during hepatocarcinogenesis. *Cancer Research*, 25, 193-200.

SHEARER, R.W. and SMUCKLER, E.A. (1972) Altered regulation of the transport of RNA from nucleus to cytoplasm in rat hepatoma cells. *Cancer Research*, 32, 339-342.

SHEID, B., WILSON, S.M. and MORRIS, H.P. (1971) Transfer RNA methylase activity in normal rat liver and some Morris hepatomas. *Cancer Research*, 31, 774-777.

SHELTON, E. and RICE, M. (1958) *Journal of the National Cancer Institute*, 21, 1.

SHONK, C.E., MORRIS, H.P. and BOXER, G.E. (1965) Patterns of glycolytic enzymes in rat liver and hepatoma. *Cancer Research*, 25, 671-676.

SHORTLEY, G. and WILKINS, J.R. (1965) Independent-action and birth-death models in experimental microbiology. *Bacteriological Reviews*, 29, 102-141.

SIDORIK, E.P. (1969) Unpublished thesis. Kiev.

SILBER, R., BERMAN, E., GOLDSTEIN, B., STEIN, H., FARNHAM, G. and BERTINO, J.R. (1966) Methylation of nucleic acids in normal and leukemic leukocytes. *Biochimica et Biophysica Acta*, 123, 638.

SINGER, R.H. and PENMAN, S. (1973) Messenger RNA in HeLa cells: kinetics of formation and decay. *Journal of Molecular Biology*, 78, 321-334.

SIROVER, M.A. and LOEB, L.A. (1974) Erroneous base-pairing induced by a chemical carcinogen during DNA synthesis. *Nature*, 252, 414-416.

SITZ, T.O., NAZAR, R.N., SPOHN, W.H. and BUSCH, H. (1973) Similarity of ribosomal and ribosomal precursor RNA's from rat liver and the Novikoff ascites hepatoma. *Cancer Research*, 33, 3312-3318.

SKIPPER, H.E., SCHABEL, F.M. and WILCOX, W.S. (1964) Experimental evaluation of potential anticancer agents. *Cancer Chemotherapy Reports*, 35, 1-111.

SMITH, A.E. and MARCKER, K.A. (1970) Cytoplasmic methionine transfer RNAs from eukaryotes. *Nature*, 226, 607-610.

SMITH, C.A. and VINOGRAD, J. (1973) Complex mitochondrial DNA in human tumors. *Cancer Research*, 33, 1065-1070.

SMOTRYAEVA, M.A., SEREBRYANYI, A.M. and KRUGLIAKOVA, K.E. (1972) *Khimicheskii mutagenez i sozdanie selektsionnogo materiala*. Moscow: Nauka.

SNEIDER, T.W. (1972) Methylation of mammalian DNA. *Journal of Biological Chemistry*, 247, 2872-2875.

SNEIDER, T.W., POTTER, V.R. and MORRIS, H.P. (1969) Enzymes of thymidine triphosphate synthesis in selected Morris hepatomas. *Cancer Research*, 29, 40-54.

SPEERS, E.A. and TIGERSTROM, R.G. von (1975) Degradation of RNA in nuclei from Ehrlich ascites cells. *Canadian Journal of Biochemistry*, 53, 79-90.

SPRINGGATE, C.F., SEAL, G. and LOEB, L.A. (1972) Infidelity of DNA synthesis in human leukemia. *Journal of Cell Biology, Abstracts of 12th Annual Meeting of Amer. Soc. for Cell Biology*, 55, 248a.

SPIRIN, A.S. and GAVRILOVA, L.P. (1971) *Ribosoma*. Moscow: Nauka.

SRINIVASAN, P.R. and BOREK, E. (1963) The species variation of RNA methylase. *Proceedings of the National Academy of Sciences of the USA*, 49, 529-533.

SRINIVASAN, P.R. and BOREK, E. (1964) Enzymatic alteration of nucleic acid structure. *Science*, 145, 548-553.

STARR, J.L. and SELLS, B.H. (1969) Methylated ribonucleic acids. *Physiological Reviews*, 49, 623-669.

STEEL, G.G. and LAMERTON, L.F. (1966) The growth rate of human tumours. *British Journal of Cancer*, 20, 74-86.

STEIN, J.L., THRALL, C.L., PARK, W.D., MANS, R.J. and STEIN, G.S. (1975) Hybridization analysis of histone messenger RNA: association with polyribosomes during cell cycle. *Science*, 189, 557-558.

STEWART, P.R. and LETHAM, D.S. (Eds.) (1973) *The Ribonucleic Acids*. New York: Springer. 268 pp.

STRELER, B. (1964) *Vremay, kletki i starenie*. Moscow: Mir.

STUKOV, A.P. (1966) Sochetannoe deistvie eleuterokokka i sarkolizina na limfosarkomu lio-1 u myshei. *Voprosy Onkologii*, 12, 57-60.

SUBRAMANIAN, A.R., GILBERT, J.M. and KUMAR, A. (1975) Comparison of ribosomal proteins from neoplastic and non-neoplastic cells. *Biochemica et Biophysica Acta*, <u>383</u>, 93-96.

SUGIURA, K. (1959) Studies on a tumor spectrum. VIII. The effect of mitomycin C on the growth of a variety of mouse, rat and hamster tumors. *Cancer Research*, <u>19</u>, 438.

SUGIURA, K. (1962) Studies in a spectrum of mouse, rat and hamster tumors. *Cancer Research Supplement*, <u>22</u>, 93-135.

SUGIURA, K. and STOCK, C.C. (1955) Studies in a tumor spectrum. III. The effect of phosphoramides on the growth of a variety of mouse and rat tumors. *Cancer Research*, <u>15</u>, 38.

SUMMERS, W.C. (1966) Dynamics of tumor growth: a mathematical model. *Growth*, <u>30</u>, 333-338.

SVEC, F., HLAVAY, E. and THURZO, P., (1957) *Acta Haematologica*, <u>17</u>, 34.

SWARTZ, H.M. (1972) Electron spin resonance studies of carcinogenesis. *Advances in Cancer Research*, <u>15</u>, 227-252.

SWARTZ, H.M., MAILER, C., AMBEGAONKAR, S., ANTHOLINE, W.E., McNELLIS, D.R. and SCHNELLER, S.J. (1973) Paramagnetic changes during development of a transplanted AKR/J leukemia in mice as measured by electron spin resonance. *Cancer Research*, <u>33</u>, 2588-2595.

SWEENEY, M.J., ASHMORE, J., MORRIS, H.P. and WEBER, G. (1963) Comparative bio-chemistry of hepatomas. IV. Isotope studies of glucose and fructose metabolism in liver tumors of different growth rates. *Cancer Research*, <u>23</u>, 995-1002.

SYRKIN, A.B. (1965) *Biologiya zlokachestvennogo rosta*. Moscow: Meditsina.

TAGI-ZADE, S.B. and SHAPOT, V.S. (1970) Stimuliatsiia vkliucheniia S35-metionina v belki eksperimental'nykh opukholei pri povyshennom snabzhenni organizma kisloro-dom i gliukozoi. *Voprosy Meditsinkoi Khimmi*, <u>16</u>, 142-147.

TANABE, K. and TAKAHASHI, T. (1973) Conversion of DNA polymerase extracted from rat ascites hepatoma cells. *Biochemical and Biophysical Research Communications*, <u>53</u>, 295-301.

TANGUAY, R. and CHAUDHARY, K.D. (1971) Studies on mitochondria. *Canadian Journal of Biochemistry*, <u>49</u>, 357-367.

TANNOCK, I.F. and STEEL, G.G. (1970) Tumor growth and cell kinetics in chronically hypoxic animals. *Journal of the National Cancer Institute*, <u>45</u>, 123-133.

TAPER, H.S., WOOLLEY, G.W., TELLER, M.N. and LARDIS, M.P. (1966) A new transplant-able mouse liver tumor of spontaneous origin. *Cancer Research*, <u>26</u>, 143-148.

TARNOWSKI, G.S. and STOCK, C.C. (1957) Effects of combinations of azaserine and of 6-diazo-5-oxo-L-norleucine with purine analogs and other antimetabolites on the growth of two mouse mammary carcinomas. *Cancer Research*, <u>17</u>, 1033.

TAYLOR, J.H., WU, M. and ERICKSON, L.C. (1974) Functional subunits of chromosomal DNA from higher eukaryotes. *Cold Spring Harbor Symposia on Quantitative Biology*, <u>38</u>, 225-231.

TAYLOR, M.W., BUCK, C.A., GRANGER, G.A. and HOLLAND, J.J. (1968) Chromatographic alterations in transfer RNA's accompanying speciation, differentiation and tumor formation. *Journal of Molecular Biology*, <u>33</u>, 809-828.

TAYLOR, M.W., GRANGER, G.A., BUCK, C.A. and HOLLAND, J.J. (1967) Similarities and differences among specific tRNA's in mammalian tissues. *Proceedings of the National Academy of Sciences of the USA*, <u>57</u>, 1712-1719.

THOMAS, G., LANGE, H.W. and HEMPEL, K. (1975) Kinetics of histone methylation *in vivo* and its relation to the cell cycle in Ehrlich ascites tumor cells. *European Journal of Biochemistry*, <u>51</u>, 609-615.

TIGERSTROM, G. von (1973) *Canadian Journal of Biochemistry*, <u>51</u>, 495.

TIMOFEEVA, M.Ia., EISNER, G.I. and KUPRIIANOVA, N.S. (1975) Sravnitel'noe issledovanie povtoriaiushchikksia nukleotidnykh posledovatel'nosv v DNK differentsirovannykh tkanei i pri malignizatsii. *Molekuliarnaia Biologiia*, <u>9</u>, 126-133.

TOBEY, R.A. (1972) Effects of cytosine arabinoside, daunomycin, mithramycin, azacytidine, adriamycin and camptothecin on mammalian cell cycle traverse. *Cancer Research*, <u>32</u>, 2720-2725.

TOLNAI, S. and MORGAN, J.F. (1962) Studies on the *in vitro* antitumor activity of fatty acids. *Canadian Journal of Biochemistry*, <u>40</u>, 869-875.

TOMASI, V., RETHY, A. and TREVISANI, A. (1973) In: *Role of Cyclic Nucleotides in Carcinogenesis* (eds. J. Schultz and H.G. Gratzner). New York: Academic Press.

TORELLI, U.L. and TORELLI, G.M. (1973) Poly(A)-containing molecules in heterogeneous nuclear RNA of normal PHA-stimulated lymphocytes and acute leukaemia blast cells. *Nature, New Biology*, <u>244</u>, 134-136.

TORELLI, U.L., TORELLI, G.M., ANDREOLI, A. and MAURI, C. (1970) Partial failure of methylation and cleavage of 45S RNA in the blast cells of acute leukaemia. *Nature*, <u>226</u>, 1063-1165.

TORELLI, U.L., TORELLI, G.M., ANDREOLI, A. and MAURI, C. (1971) Impaired ribosomal precursor RNA in blast cells of acute leukemia. *Acta Haematologica*, <u>45</u>, 201-208.

TORELLI, U.L., TORELLI, G.M. and CADOSSI, R. (1975) Double stranded RNA in human leukemic blast cells. *European Journal of Cancer*, <u>11</u>, 117-121.

TRUBY, F.K. and GOLDZIEHER, J.W. (1958) Electron spin resonance investigations of rat liver and rat hepatoma. *Nature*, <u>182</u>, 1371-1372.

TSEITLIN, P.I., KRUGLIAKOVA, D.E. and ZOZ, N.N. (1975) Fizikokhimicheskie izmeneniia v DNK i DNP pod deistviem N-nitrozo-N-metilmocheviny. *Doklady Akademii Nauk SSR*, <u>222</u>, 232-235.

TSOU, K.C., MORRIS, H.P., LO, K.W. and MUSCATO, J.J. (1974) 5'-nucleotide phosphodiesterase activity in rat hepatoma. *Cancer Research*, <u>34</u>, 1295-1298.

TSUBOI, A. and BASERGA, R. (1972) Synthesis of nuclear acidic proteins in density-inhibited fibroblasts stimulated to proliferate. *Journal of Cellular Physiology*, <u>80</u>, 107-118.

TUGARINOV, O.A. (1971) Unpublished thesis. Moscow.

TWEEDIE, J.W. and PITOT, H.C. (1974) Polyadenylate-containing RNA of polyribosomes isolated from rat liver and Morris hepatoma 7800. *Cancer Research*, 34, 109-114.

URBAKH, V.Yu. (1964) *Biometricheskie metody*. Moscow: Nauka.

VARFALOMEEV, V.M., BOGDANOV, G.N., D'IAKOVA, V.V., PAVLOVA, V.M. and EMANUEL, N.M. (1976) Paramagnitnye svoistva tkanei pecheni i perevivaemykh gepatom. *Biofizika*, 21, 881-886.

VASILEVA, L.S., BOGDANOV, G.N. and KONOVALOVA, N.P. (1974) Kinetika rosta melanomy B-16. *Izvestiia Akademii Nauk SSSR, Seriya Biologicheskaia*, 2, 299-300.

VASILEVA, L.S., BOGDANOV, G.N., KONOVALOVA, N.P. and EMANUEL, N.M. (1969) Kinetika rosta perevivnoi pigmentnoi melanomy. *Izvestiia Akademii Nauk SSSR, Seriya Biologicheskaia*, 6, 926-929.

VASILEVA, L.S., GUMANOV, L.L., D'IACHKOVSKAIA, R.F., KONOVALOVA, N.P., SURKOVA, N.I. and EMANUEL, N.M. (1973) Vliianie bifunktsional'nogo proizvodnogo nitrozoalkil-mocheviny na rost nekotorykh eksperimental'nykh opukholei. *Izvestiia Akademii Nauk SSSR, Seriya Biologicheskaia*, 5, 737-739.

VATANEBE, T. (1967) *Okayama Igakkai Zasshi*, 79, 211.

VEDRICH, M., GREENE, M.O. and GREENBERG, J. (1961) Cloudman mouse melanoma S-91 as a potential screening tool in cancer chemotherapy. *Cancer Research Supplement*, 21, 359-376.

VENTTSEL, A.D. (1975) *Kurs teorii sluchainykh protsessov*. Moscow: Nauka.

VERMEL, E.M., KORMAN, N.P., MILONOV, B.V., EVSEENKO, L.S. and ORLOVA, R.S. (1970) Klinicheskoe izuchenie N-nitrozometilmocheviny. *Voprosy Onkologii*, 16, 31-37.

VESELY, J., RIMAN, J. and SEIFERT, J. (1960) A quantitative and qualitative study of postirradiation myelogenic leukaemia in C57 black mice. *Neoplasma*, 7, 172-186.

VIALE, G.L. (1971) Transfer RNA and transfer RNA methylase in human brain tumors. *Cancer Research*, 31, 605-608.

VILENCHIK, M.M. (1973) Izmeneie tsitoplazmaticheskoi DNK pri malignizatsii kletki. *Uspekhi Sovremennoi Biologii*, 75, 388-405.

VIOTTI, A., SOAVE, C., SALA, E., NUCCA, R. and GALANTE, E. (1973) 5-S RNA: Metabolic stability of the 5' terminal phosphates. *Biochimica et Biophysica Acta*, 324, 72-77.

VITHAYATHIL, A.J., TERNBERG, J.L. and COMMONER, B. (1965) Changes in electron spin resonance signals of rat liver during chemical carcinogenesis. *Nature*, 207, 1246-1249.

VLADIMIROV, Yu.A. and ARCHAKOV, A.I. (1972) *Perekisnoe okislenie lipidov v biologicheskikh membranakh*. Moscow: Nauka.

VOLKERS, S.A.S. and TAYLOR, M.W. (1971) Chromatographic comparison of the transfer RNAs of rat livers and Morris hepatomas. *Biochemistry*, 10, 488-497.

VORONINA, S.S., GRIGORIAN, G.L. and PELEVINA, I.I. (1972) Izmenenie effektivnosti oblucheniia svobodnymi iminoksil'nymi radikalami. *Izvestiia Akademii Nauk SSSR, Seriya Biologicheskaia*, 5, 723-730.

VULLI, D. (1954) *Uchenie ob antimetabolitakh*. Moscow: Mir.

WAGNER, J.G. (1971) *Biopharmaceutics and Relevant Pharmacokinetics*. Illinois: Drug Intelligence Publications. 375 pp.

WALLACE, J.D., DRISCOLL, D.H. and KALOMIRIS, C.G. (1970) A study of free radicals occurring in tumorous female breast tissue and their implication to detection. *Cancer*, 25, 1087-1090.

WALLACE, P.G., HEWISH, D.R., VENNING, M.M. and BURGOYNE, L.A. (1971) Multiple forms of mammalian DNA polymerase. *Biochemical Journal*, 125, 47-54.

WANG, T.Y. (1969) Diametric effects of histones and the non-histone proteins on DNA replication *in vitro*. *Experimental Cell Research*, 57, 467-469.

WATT, K.E.F. (1968) *Ecology and Resource Management: A Quantitative Approach*. New York: McGraw Hill. 450 pp.

WATTENBERG, L. (1972) Inhibition of carcinogenic and toxic effects of polycyclic hydrocarbons by phenolic antioxidants and ethoxyquin. *Journal of the National Cancer Institute*, 48, 1425-1430.

WATTENBERG, L. (1973) Inhibition of chemical carcinogen-induced pulmonary neoplasia by butylated hydroxyanisole. *Journal of the National Cancer Institute*, 50, 1541-1544.

WEBER, G. (1961) Behavior of liver enzymes in hepatocarcinogenesis. *Advances in Cancer Research*, 6, 403-494.

WEBER, G. (1974) Molecular correction concept. In: *The Molecular Biology of Cancer* (Ed. H. Busch. New York: Academic Press. 638 pp.

WEBER, G., BANERJEE, G. and MORRIS, H.P. (1961) Comparative biochemistry of hepatomas. I. Carbohydrate enzymes in Morris hepatoma 5123. *Cancer Research*, 21, 933-937.

WEBER, G., HENRY, M.C., WAGLE, S.R. and WAGLE, D.S. (1964) Correlation of enzymes activities and metabolic pathways with growth rate of hepatomas. *Advances in Enzyme Regulation*, 2, 335-346.

WEBER, G. and LEA, M.A. (1966) The molecular correlation concept of neoplasia. *Advances in Enzyme Regulation*, 4, 115-148.

WEBER, G. and LEA, M.A. (1967) In: *Methods in Cancer Research* (Ed. H. Busch). New York: Academic Press.

WEBER, G. and MORRIS, H.P. (1963) Comparative biochemistry of hepatomas. III. Carbohydrate enzymes in liver tumors of different growth rates. *Cancer Research*, 23, 987-994.

WEBER, G., MORRIS, H.P., LOVE, W.C. and ASHMORE, J. (1961) Comparative biochemistry of hepatomas. *Cancer Research*, 21, 1406-1411.

WEINBERG, R.A. (1973) Nuclear RNA metabolism. *Annual Reviews of Biochemistry*, 42, 329-354.

WEINBERG, R.A., LOENING, U., WILLEMS, M. and PENMAN, S. (1967) Acrylamide gel electrophoresis of HeLa cell nucleolar RNA. *Proceedings of the National Academy of Sciences of the USA*, 58, 1088-1095.

WEINMANN, R. and ROEDER, R.G. (1974) Role of DNA-dependent RNA polymerase III in the transcription of the tRNA and 5S RNA genes. *Proceedings of the National Academy of Sciences of the USA*, 71, 1790-1794.

WEISS, G.H. and ZELEN, M. (1963) A stochastic model for the interpretation of clinical trials. *Proceedings of the National Academy of Sciences of the USA*, 50, 988-994.

WEISSBACH, A., SCHLABACH, A., FRIDLENDER, B. and BOLDEN, A. (1971) DNA polymerase from human cells. *Nature, New Biology*, 231, 167-170.

WENNER, C.E., HACKNEY, J.H. and MOLITERNO, F. (1958) The hexose monophosphate shunt in glucose catabolism in ascites tumor cells. *Cancer Research*, 18, 1105.

WETMUR, J.G. and DAVIDSON, N. (1968) Kinetics of renaturation of DNA. *Journal of Molecular Biology*, 31, 349-370.

WHEELER, G.P. and ALEXANDER, J.A. (1974) Duration of inhibition of synthesis of DNA in tumors and host tissues after single doses of nitrosoureas. *Cancer Research*, 34, 1957-1964.

WHEELER, G.P. and BOWDON, B.J. (1965) Some effects of 1,3-bis (2-chloroethyl)-1-nitrosourea upon the synthesis of protein and nucleic acids *in vivo* and *in vitro*. *Cancer Research*, 25, 1770-1778.

WHEELER, G.P., BOWDON, B.J., GRIMSLEY, J.A. and LLOYD, H.H. (1974) Interrelationships of some chemical, physicochemical and biological activities of several 1-(2-haloethyl)-1-nitrosoureas. *Cancer Research*, 34, 194-200.

WHITE, M.T., ARYA, D.V. and TEWARI, K.K. (1974) Biochemical properties of neoplastic cell mitochondria. *Journal of the National Cancer Institute*, 53, 553-559.

WIKMAN, J., QUAGLIAROTTI, G., HOWARD, E., CHOI, Y.C. and BUSCH, H. (1970) A comparison of ^{32}P distribution in oligonucleotides of ribosomal 28S RNA from normal liver and Novikoff hepatoma ascites cells. *Cancer Research*, 30, 2749-2759.

WILCOX, W.S., GRISWOLD, D.P., LASTER, W., SCHABEL, F.M. and SKIPPER, H.E. (1965) Experimental evaluation of potential anticancer agents. *Cancer Chemotherapy Reports*, 47, 27-39.

WILKS, S.S. (1962) *Mathematical Statistics*. New York: Wiley.

WILLIAMSON, M.H. (1975) *Analysis of Biological Population*. Crane-Russak Co.

WILLS, E.D. (1969) Lipid peroxide formation in microsomes. *Biochemical Journal*, 113, 333-341.

WILSON, D.F. and MERZ, R. (1969) Inhibition of mitochondrial respiration by uncouplers of oxidative phosphorylation. *Archives of Biochemistry and Biophysics*, 129, 79-85.

WIMBER, D.E. and STEFFENSEN, D.M. (1970) Localization of 5S RNA genes on Drosophila chromosomes by RNA-DNA hybridization. *Science*, 170, 639-641.

WINDHEUSER, J.J., SUTTER, J.L. and AUEN, E. (1972) 5-fluorouracil and derivatives in cancer chemotherapy: determination of 5-fluorouracil in blood. *Journal of Pharmaceutical Sciences*, 61, 301-303.

WONG-STAAL, F., MENDELSOHN, J. and GOULIAN, M. (1973) Ribonucleotides in closed circular mitochondrial DNA from HeLa cells. *Biochemical and Biophysical Research*

Communications, 53, 140-148.

WOOD, P.M. (1974) The redox potential of the system oxygen-superoxide. *FEBS Letters*, 44, 22-24.

WOODS, M.W. and VLAHAKIS, G. (1973) Anaerobic glycolysis in spontaneous and transplanted liver tumors of mice. *Journal of the National Cancer Institute*, 50, 1497-1511.

WOOLUM, J.C. and COMMONER, B. (1970) Isolation and identification of a paramagnetic complex from the livers of carcinogen-treated rats. *Biochimica et Biophysica Acta*, 201, 131-140.

WU, C. and HOMBERGER, H.A. (1969) Responsiveness of enzymes in liver to growth of Novikoff hepatoma. *British Journal of Cancer*, 23, 204-209.

WU, R. and RACKER, E. (1959) Regulatory mechanisms in carbohydrate metabolism. *Journal of Biological Chemistry*, 234, 1036.

WUNDERLICH, V., SCHUTT, M., BOTTGER, M. and GRAFFI, A. (1970) Preferential alkylation of mitochondrial DNA by N-methyl-N-nitrosourea. *Biochemical Journal*, 118, 99-109.

YANG, W. (1971) Isoaccepting transfer RNA's in mammalian differentiated cells and tumor tissues. *Cancer Research*, 31, 639-643.

YOKOYAMA, H.O., WILSON, M.E., TSUBOI, K.K. and STOWELL, R.E. (1953) Regeneration of mouse liver after partial hepatectomy. *Cancer Research*, 13, 80-85.

YUDENFREND, S. (1965) *Fluorestsentnyi analiz v biologii i meditsine*. Moscow: Mir.

YUHAS, J.M. and PAZMINO, N.H. (1974) Inhibition of subcutaneously growing line 1 carcinomas due to metastatic spread. *Cancer Research*, 34, 2005-2010.

YUHAS, J.M., PAZMINO, N.H. and WAGNER, E. (1975) Development of concomitant immunity in mice bearing the weakly immunogenic line 1 lung carcinoma. *Cancer Research*, 35, 237-241.

ZAHARKO, D.S. (1972) Pharmacokinetics. *Cancer Chemotherapy Reports*, 3, 21-28.

ZHIZHINA, G.P., BOBOVICH, S.I., ALESENKO, A.V., PETROV, O.E. and KRUGLIAKOVA, K.E. (1975) K voprosu o vozmozhnykh prichinakh izmeneiia vtorichnoi struktury DNK v protsesse opukholevogo rosta. *Doklady Akademii Nauk SSSR*, 222, 973-975.

INDEX